APPLETON & LANGE'S REVIEW OF

PSYCHIATRY

FIFTH EDITION

William M. Easson, M.D.
Professor, Department of Psychiatry
Louisiana State University School of Medicine
New Orleans

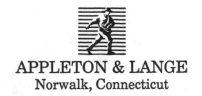

APPLETON & LANGE
Norwalk, Connecticut

ISBN: 0-8385-0247-4

Copyright © 1994 by Appleton & Lange
Paramount Publishing Business and Professional Group
Copyright © 1974, 1978, 1983 by Arco Publishing, Inc.
Copyright © 1989 by Appleton & Lange.

95 96 97 98 / 10 9 8 7 6 5 4 3 2

Prentice Hall International (UK) Limited, *London*
Prentice Hall of Australia Pty. Limited, *Sydney*
Prentice Hall Canada, Inc., *Toronto*
Prentice Hall Hispanoamericana, S.A., *Mexico*
Prentice Hall of India Private Limited, *New Delhi*
Prentice Hall of Japan, Inc., *Tokyo*
Simon & Schuster Asia Pte. Ltd., *Singapore*
Editora Prentice Hall do Brasil Ltda., *Rio de Janeiro*
Prentice Hall, *Englewood Cliffs, New Jersey*

Library of Congress Card Number: 93-074167

Acquisitions Editor: Jamie Mount

PRINTED IN THE UNITED STATES OF AMERICA

Contents

Preface

The candidate in a national examination needs to recognize certain facts about these examinations and prepare accordingly.

Because these examinations are given nationally (and often internationally), the subject matter of each question and answer must be agreed on and accepted nationally. The examinee will not be asked questions that are based on regional interests or reflect individual clinical opinions. Since new medical information and treatments take several years to become nationally accepted, it is unlikely that new clinical or research knowledge or recently developed treatments will appear as the subject for a question for at least 1 to 2 years after general acceptance. The questions in the examinations thus tend to be conservative in outlook and approach.

It may seem unnecessary to emphasize, but the candidate should appreciate that questions can only be asked where there is solid data about a subject. Some very important clinical topics appear in the examinations rarely or not at all because there is no definite data. Questions about the cause of many psychiatric syndromes are missing, usually because the cause is not known or is debatable. For example, death and dying are most important clinical problems but are rarely the focus of questions because there is so little definite data available. If a subject is controversial or sensitive in some way, it is unlikely to be an examination question. Abortion is a very important clinical problem but the candidate will most likely not encounter a question on the psychiatry exam about this controversial clinical situation.

The candidate should recognize that there are only a finite number of topics that can be asked about in each clinical examination. In psychiatry, there are probably not more than 200 separate possible examination subjects. The examination candidate will note that, in this book and in the examinations, questions are frequently repeated, but with a different emphasis each time.

In any board examination, there are only a limited number of questions, new and old, that can be asked. In the psychiatry examinations, 75–85% of the questions posed in any examination are old questions; only 15–25% are new questions. The candidate who knows the old examination questions thoroughly should have no trouble passing the examination, but in the process of learning and understanding the old questions will have thoroughly learned psychiatry.

This edition marks the passing of an era in psychiatry. Questions about psychoanalytic theory and treatment are not posed as frequently. Questions about social and community psychiatry are much less common. Questions dealing with the history and development of psychiatric diagnosis and treatment are few and far between. Now the examinations deal with DSM-IIIR and soon to be DSM-IV diagnoses as if these were definite diseases rather than the syndromes they are. The questions focus on pharmacological treatments of syndromes with as much fervor as the psychodynamic treatments were espoused, and with as little scientific basis. This too will change with continued research into the causes and treatment of mental illness, and the changes will be reflected in future examinations and future editions of this book.

Since the first edition of this book twenty years ago, when she proofread everything written, my wife has supported and tolerated the writing of each edition. We have shared and learned much together and I am eternally grateful.

William M. Easson, MD
New Orleans, August 1993

Introduction

This book has been designed to help you review psychiatry for your clerkship course, the United States Medical Licensing Examination (USMLE) Step 2 and Step 3, and residency-in-training examinations. Here, in one package, is a comprehensive review resource with over 900 "Exam-type" multiple-choice questions with referenced, paragraph-length discussions of each answer. In addition, the last 120 questions have been set aside as a Practice Test for self-assessment purposes. The entire book has been designed to help you assess your areas of relative strength and weakness.

ORGANIZATION OF THIS BOOK

This book is divided into 12 chapters. Eight chapters provide a review of the major areas of psychiatry. There is one chapter of matching-type questions, one of one-best-answer questions, and one of case history questions. The last chapter is a Practice Test, which integrates all of these areas into one simulated examination.

This introduction provides information on question types, question-taking strategies, various ways you can use this book, and specific information on the USMLE Step 2.

The United States Medical Licensing Examination, Step 2

The USMLE Step 2 is a 2-day examination consisting of approximately 800 questions testing your knowledge in the clinical sciences. It contains three different types of questions (or "items," in testing parlance) organized within three dimensions: 1) System; 2) Process; and 3) Organizational Level. Although each dimension is weighted, the projected percentage for each is subject to change from exam to exam. The application materials illustrate the percentage breakout and offer a detailed content outline to aid you in your review.

In general, on the examination, the breakdown of question types is approximately 70% "one best answer–single item" questions, 20% "one best answer–matching sets," and 10% "extended–matching set" questions. In some cases, a group of two or three questions may be related to a situational theme. In addition, some questions have illustrative material (graphs, x-rays, tables) that require understanding and interpretation on your part. Moreover, each question may be categorized at one of three levels of difficulty depending on the level of skill needed to answer it: rote memory, a clear understanding of the problem, or both understanding and judgment. Since the USMLE seems to prefer questions requiring judgment and critical thinking, we have attempted to emphasize these questions. Finally, some of the questions are stated in the negative. In such instances, we have printed the negative word in capital letters (eg, "All of the following are correct EXCEPT"; "Which of the following choices is NOT correct?" and "Which of the following is LEAST correct?").

Question Format

One Best Answer–Single Item Question. The majority of the questions are posed in the A-type, or "one best answer–single item" format. This is the most popular question format in most exams. It generally consists of a brief statement, followed by five options of which only ONE is entirely correct. The options on the USMLE are lettered A,B,C,D, and E. Although the format for this question type is straightforward, these questions can be difficult because some of the distractors may be partially right. The instructions you will see for this type of question will generally appear as below:

DIRECTIONS: Each of the numbered items or incomplete statements in this section is followed by answers or by completions of the statement. Select the ONE lettered answer or completion that is BEST in each case.

The following is an example of this question type:

1. Electroconvulsive therapy is often very effective in

   (A) opioid abuse
   (B) ulcerative colitis
   (C) conversion disorder
   (D) schizophrenia, catatonic type
   (E) phobic disorder

In the question above, the best answer is (D) catatonic schizophrenia, especially the excited type, as it often responds well to a course of electroconvulsive therapy. Apathetic or stuporous catatonia may show symptomatic improvement, but relapse is common. Convulsive therapy would not be indicated for ulcerative colitis, conversion of phobic disorders, or opioid abusers.

**STRATEGIES FOR ANSWERING
ONE BEST ANSWER–SINGLE ITEM QUESTIONS**

1. Remember that only one choice can be the correct answer.
2. Read the question carefully to be sure that you understand what is being asked. Pay attention to key words like "most" or "least."
3. Quickly read each choice for familiarity. (This important step is often not done by test takers.)
4. Go back and consider each choice individually.
5. If a choice is partially correct, tentatively consider it to be incorrect. (This step will help you lessen your choices and increase your odds of choosing the correct answer.)
6. Consider the remaining choices and select the one you think is the answer. At this point, you may want to quickly scan the stem to be sure you understand the question and your answer.
7. Fill in the appropriate circle on the answer sheet.
8. If you do not know the answer, make an educated guess. Your score is based on the number of correct answers, not the number you get incorrect. **Do not leave any blanks.**
9. The actual examination is timed for an average of 50 seconds per question. It is important to be thorough to understand the questions, but it is equally important for you to keep moving.

One Best Answer–Matching Sets. This format presents lettered options followed by several items related to a common topic. The directions you will generally see for this type of question are as follows:

DIRECTIONS (Questions 2 through 6): Each set of matching questions in this section consists of a list of 4 to 26 lettered options followed by several numbered items. For each item, select the ONE best lettered option that is most closely associated with it. Each lettered heading may be selected once, more than once, or not at all.

(A) haloperidol
(B) methylphenidate
(C) dimercaprol
(D) methadone
(E) imipramine

For each disorder, select the correct treatment.

2. Attention deficit hyperactivity disorder

3. Functional enuresis, enuresis

4. Tourette's disorder

5. Chronic mercury poisoning

6. Heroin addiction

Note that unlike the single-item questions, the choices in the matching sets *precede* the actual questions. However, as with the single-item questions, only one choice can be correct for a given question.

**STRATEGIES FOR ANSWERING
ONE BEST ANSWER–MATCHING SETS QUESTIONS**

1. Remember that the lettered choices are followed by the numbered questions.
2. As with single-item questions, only one answer will be correct for each item.
3. Quickly read each choice for familiarity.
4. Read the question carefully to be sure that you understand what is being asked. Pay attention to key words like "most" or "least."
5. Go back and consider each choice individually.
6. If a choice is partially correct for a particular item, tentatively consider it to be incorrect. (This step will help you eliminate choices and increase your odds of choosing the correct answer.)
7. Consider the remaining choices and select the one you think is the answer.
8. Fill in the appropriate circle on the answer sheet.
9. If you do not know the answer, make an educated guess. Your score is based on the number of correct answers, not the number you get incorrect. **Do not leave any blanks.**
10. Again, the actual examination allows an average of 50 seconds per question.

Extended One Best Answer–Extended Matching Sets Questions. The USMLE step 2 uses a new type of matching question that is similar to the one above, but can contain up to 26 lettered options followed by several items. The directions you will see for this type of question will generally read the same as the ones listed for the best answer–matching sets since this is another version of the same question. An example of this type of question is:

(A) sarcoidosis
(B) tuberculosis
(C) histoplasmosis
(D) coccidiomycosis
(E) amyloidosis
(F) bacterial pneumonia
(G) mesothelioma
(H) carcinoma
(I) fibrosing alveolitis
(J) silicosis

7. A right lower lobectomy specimen contains a solitary 1.2-cm diameter solid nodule. The center of the nodule is fibrous. The periphery has granulomatous inflammation. With special stains, multi-

ple 2 to 5 μm budding yeasts are evident within the nodule. Acid-fast stains are negative.

8. A left upper lobectomy specimen is received containing a 4.6-cm nodule with central cystic degeneration. Microscopically, the nodule is composed of anaplastic squamous cells. Similar abnormal cells are seen in a concomitant biopsy of a hilar lymph node.

9. After a long history of multiple myeloma, a 67-year-old male is noted to have abundant acellular eosinophilic deposits around the pulmonary microvasculature at autopsy. A Congo red special stain demonstrates apple green birefringence.

10. A large pleural-based lesion is found on chest x-ray of an asbestos worker. Electron microscopy of the biopsy shows abundant long microvilli.

Note that, like other matching sets, the lettered options are listed first.

STRATEGIES FOR ANSWERING EXTENDED ONE BEST ANSWER–EXTENDED MATCHING SETS QUESTIONS

1. Read the lettered options through first.
2. Work with one item at a time.
3. Read the item through, then go back to the options and consider each choice individually.
4. As with the other question types, if the choice is partially correct, tentatively consider it to be incorrect.
5. Consider the remaining choices and select the answer.
6. Fill in the appropriate circle on the answer sheet.
7. Remember to make a selection for each item.
8. Again, the test allows for 50 seconds per item.

Answers, Explanations, and References

In each of the sections of this book, the question sections are followed by a section containing the answers, explanations, and references for the questions. This section (1) tells you the answer to each question; (2) gives you an explanation/review of why the answer is correct, background information on the subject matter, and why the other answers are incorrect; and (3) tells you where you can find more in-depth information on the subject matter in other books and/or journals. We encourage you to use this section as a basis for further study and understanding.

If you choose the correct answer to a question, you can then read the explanation (1) for reinforcement and (2) to add to your knowledge about the subject matter (remember that the explanations usually tell not only why the answer is correct, but also why the other choices are incorrect). **If you choose the wrong answer** to a question, you can read the explanation for a learning/reviewing discussion of the material in the question. Furthermore, you can look up the references cited (eg, "Last, pp 478–484"), look up the full source in the bibliography

at the beginning of the chapter (eg, "Last JM, Wallace RB, Barrett-Connor E. *Maxcy-Rosenau-Last Public Health and Preventive Medicine.* 13th ed. Norwalk, Conn: Appleton & Lange; 1992."), and refer to the pages cited for a more in-depth discussion.

HOW TO USE THIS BOOK

There are two logical ways to get the most value from this book. We will call them Plan A and Plan B.

In **Plan A,** you go straight to the Practice Test and complete it according to the instructions given on page 158. After taking the practice test, you check your answers and then tick off the ones you got wrong on the subspecialty list on page 179. The *number* of questions you got wrong will be a good indicator of your initial knowledge state, and the *types* of questions you got wrong will help point you in the right direction for further preparation and review. At this point, you can use the first 11 chapters of the book, with the lists and discussions, to help you improve your areas of relative weakness.

In **Plan B,** you go through the book chapters in succession from Chapter 1 to Chapter 11. Once you have completed this process, you can take the practice test, check your answers as described above, and see how well prepared you are at this point. If you still have a major weakness, it should be apparent in time for you to take remedial action.

In Plan A, by taking the practice test first, you get quick feedback regarding your initial areas of strength and weakness. You may find that you know all of the material very well, indicating that perhaps only a cursory review is necessary. This, of course, would be good to know early on in your exam preparation. On the other hand, you may find that you have many areas of weakness. In this case, you could then focus on these areas in your review—not just with this book, but also with textbooks of psychiatry.

It is, however, unlikely that you will not do some studying prior to taking the USMLE Step 2 (especially since you have this book). Therefore, it may be more realistic to take the practice test *after* you have reviewed (as in Plan B). This, of course, will probably give you a more realistic test-type situation since very few of us just sit down to a test without studying. In this case, you will have done some reviewing (from superficial to in-depth), and your Practice Test will reflect this studying time. If, after reviewing the book and taking the practice test, your scores still indicate some weaknesses, you can then go back to the individual chapters and supplement your review with your texts.

Specific Information on the Step 2 Examination

The official source of all information with respect to the United States Medical Licensing Examination Step 2 is the National Board of Medical Examiners (NBME), 3930 Chestnut Street, Philadelphia, PA 19104. Established in

1915, the NBME is a voluntary, nonprofit, independent organization whose sole function is the design, implementation, distribution, and processing of a vast bank of question items, certifying examinations, and evaluative services in the professional medical field.

In order to sit for the Step 2 examination, a person must be either an officially enrolled medical student or a graduate of an accredited medical school. It is not necessary to complete any particular year of medical school to be a candidate for Step 2. Neither is it required to take Step 1 before Step 2.

In applying for Step 2, you must use forms supplied by NBME. Remember that registration closes *10 weeks* before the scheduled examination date. Some United States and Canadian medical schools require their students to take Step 2 even if they are noncandidates at the request of their school. A person who takes Step 2 as a noncandidate can later change to candidate status, and after payment of a fee, receive certification credit.

Scoring

You will receive two scores after completing Step 2. According to the information booklet provided by the National Board of Medical Examiners, a minimum score of 176 is recommended to pass Step 1, and 167 is recommended to pass Step 2. These two scores (from the three digit scale) equate to a score of 75 on the two digit scale. Keep in mind that the passing score for all three steps is determined on your proficiency of the examination content. Although the number of correct items to obtain these passing scores may change, the percentage of correct responses necessary to achieve them will fall between 55 and 65 percent.

Remember, there is no deduction for wrong answers, so even if you are unsure, you should answer every question.

Physical Conditions

The NBME is very concerned that all their exams be administered under uniform conditions in the numerous centers that are used. Except for several No. 2 pencils and an eraser, you are not permitted to bring anything (books, notes, calculators, etc.) into the test room. All examinees receive the same questions at the same session. However, the questions are printed in different se-

quences in several different booklets, and the booklets are randomly distributed. In addition, examinees are moved to different seats at least once during the test. And, of course, each test is policed by at least one proctor. The object of these maneuvers is to discourage cheating or even the temptation to cheat.

REFERENCES

Throughout this book, each question and chapter is referenced to two one-volume general psychiatry textbooks. Rather than list each textbook and its authors with each reference, they have been cited as 1 or 2 at the end of each answer explanation.

Reference 1:

Kaplan HI, Sadock BJ. *Synopsis of Psychiatry,* 6th ed. Baltimore, MD: Williams & Wilkins, 1991.

Reference 2:

Talbott JA, Hales RE, Yudofsky SC. *Textbook of Psychiatry.* Washington, DC: American Psychiatric Press, 1988.

In 1994, the Diagnostic and Statistical Manual IV (DSM-IV) will be published. The available reference textbooks are written according to DSM-III-R standards, and for the next few years, the examinations will continue to be prepared according to the DSM-III-R criteria. Gradually, however, the DSM-IV will become the standard for examinations.

Where there is a clear difference in the diagnostic nomenclature between DSM-III-R and DSM-IV, the difference is indicated by listing the two diagnostic terms one after the other. Undoubtedly this looks awkward, as in questions where the diagnosis is cited as "functional enuresis (DSM-III-R designation)" followed by the simpler "enuresis" (the DSM-IV term) given as "functional enuresis, enuresis." Similarly "elective mutism, selective mutism" and "simple phobia, specific phobia" give the two terminologies for the same syndrome.

The DSM-IV establishes the terminology for the next decade. Therefore, the reader should also learn the changed diagnostic terms and diagnostic criteria.

CHAPTER 1
Definitions
Questions

INTRODUCTION

Students may believe that definitions of psychological and psychiatric terms form a large part of any examination because such questions are easier to formulate and score, and undoubtedly this is true in part. There is another more important aspect. If students really understand these terms that they are asked to define, they have a very good comprehension of the way people develop, relate, and cope with life stresses, in health and in sickness.

To help their understanding and remembering, trainees should look for examples of these behaviors they will be asked to define in their own day-to-day living and in the interactions of people with whom they come in contact.

REFERENCES

1 Chapter 8,   Typical Signs and Symptoms of Psychiatric Illness Defined, pp 214–222
2 Appendix 2,   Excerpts from the American Psychiatric Glossary, pp 1239–1279

DIRECTIONS (Questions 1 through 31): Each of the numbered items or incomplete statements in this section is followed by answers or by completions of the statement. Select the ONE lettered answer or completion that is BEST in each case.

1. In a déjà vu situation the
    (A) subject feels a limb long since amputated
    (B) person, just falling asleep, has false sensory perceptions
    (C) subject incorrectly feels a new experience to be the repetition of a previous experience
    (D) patient uses intellectual reasoning to avoid dealing with an unacceptable feeling or idea
    (E) subject shows sleepwalking and stage 4 sleep

2. Blocking is the
    (A) deliberate resistance to sharing uncomfortable feelings
    (B) arrest of psychological development before full maturation
    (C) stoppage of the flow of thoughts or speech due to unconscious feelings
    (D) slowing down of physical and emotional activity due to depression
    (E) state of unusual calmness in response to adversity, seen in conversion disorder

3. Akathisia is the
    (A) marked reduction in frequency and amplitude of voluntary movements
    (B) unconscious falsification of memory where there are memory gaps
    (C) process of emotional defense where the opposite is stressed
    (D) inability to sit still or keep legs motionless
    (E) type of analytic psychotherapy where the patient is heavily sedated

4. When a person stresses the opposite of his true feelings, he is showing the defense of
    (A) rationalization
    (B) undoing
    (C) displacement
    (D) reaction formation
    (E) denial

5. Repression is the
    (A) return to earlier patterns of behavior
    (B) unconscious blocking out of disturbing feelings
    (C) stressing of opposite feelings
    (D) deliberate forgetting of distressing emotions

6. Paranoia involves the process of
    (A) introjection
    (B) regression
    (C) conversion
    (D) projection
    (E) isolation

7. Alexithymia is the
    (A) inability to read
    (B) false belief involving one's bodily feelings
    (C) inability to be aware of one's own emotions
    (D) state where patient seems to be asleep but ready to be aroused
    (E) dull, indifferent emotional state

8. Sensory experiences in the absence of external stimuli are called
    (A) projections
    (B) hallucinations
    (C) illusions
    (D) delusions
    (E) introjections

9. Regression
    (A) occurs commonly and normally with serious physical illness
    (B) usually indicates severe emotional disorder
    (C) is the unconscious blocking out of awareness of disturbing emotions
    (D) is mediated mainly through the autonomic nerves
    (E) occurs where there is underlying sexual conflict

10. Bulimia is
    (A) uncontrolled aggressive outbursts
    (B) hypersexuality in the female
    (C) chronic psychogenic constipation
    (D) recurrent compulsive intellectual rumination
    (E) a huge appetite with excessive gorging

11. The Halstead-Reitan battery is used to
    (A) measure galvanic skin resistance
    (B) assess impairment due to brain damage
    (C) differentiate infantile autism and childhood deafness
    (D) induce unilateral electroconvulsive therapy
    (E) provide negative reinforcement in operant conditioning

(E) arrest of emotional development before full maturity

12. In conversion

(A) feelings that are unacceptable when focused on one object are redirected to a more tolerable focus

(B) the subject has almost total memory loss for a significant period of his or her past

(C) emotional conflict is expressed in a single organ system controlled by the autonomic nerves

(D) the conflictual anxiety is symbolically manifested in a somatic symptom involving the special senses or voluntary nervous system

(E) an unacceptable drive is rechanneled into socially acceptable behavior

13. A delusion is

(A) a sensory experience in the absence of external stimuli

(B) a misinterpretation of actual perceptions

(C) a false belief not in accord with a person's intelligence or culture

(D) a manifestation of unacceptable feelings projected outward

(E) unconscious blocking of instinctual feelings

14. Delusions occur in all of the following except

(A) bipolar disorder, manic type

(B) amphetamine psychosis

(C) senile dementia

(D) paranoia

(E) schizoid personality disorder

15. Paranoid delusions are produced by the mechanism of

(A) displacement

(B) projection

(C) rationalization

(D) sublimation

(E) identification

16. The fetal alcohol syndrome includes all of the following *except*

(A) high birth weight

(B) mental retardation

(C) maternal alcoholism

(D) craniofacial abnormalities

(E) cardiac defects

17. In psychoanalysis, catharsis is the

(A) release of unconscious feelings with appropriate outward emotional expression

(B) investment of emotional energy in a specific purpose or object

(C) conscious or unconscious response of the psychotherapist to the patient

(D) process of knowing and learning

(E) defense whereby an unacceptable feeling is externalized

18. The collective unconscious was a concept introduced by

(A) E. Bleuler

(B) J. Breuer

(C) S. Freud

(D) H. S. Sullivan

(E) C. Jung

19. Transference is

(A) the transfer of feelings from an unacceptable object to a more acceptable focus

(B) a process whereby unacceptable thoughts and ideas are excluded from awareness

(C) a form of identification with a loved and feared parental figure

(D) a manifestation of early psychosis, especially in the adolescent or young adult

(E) the projection of feelings originally linked to nuclear early-life figures onto current objects

20. Somatization disorder is manifested by

(A) the misinterpretation of physical signs or sensations

(B) the voluntary, deliberate fabrication of symptoms

(C) the loss or alteration in physical function produced by emotional conflict or need

(D) the expression of emotions through physical symptoms

(E) none of the above

21. Psychosomatic reactions

(A) may be fatal

(B) are mediated through the voluntary motor system

(C) are produced solely by emotional problems

(D) should be treated only by psychotherapy

(E) do not occur in young children

Questions 22 and 23

A religiously devout woman learns of her husband's infidelity with initial anger. Her rage soon passes but she develops weakness of her right arm. No physical cause can be found for her illness and she remains remarkably complacent about her paralysis.

22. The arm weakness is a manifestation of

    (A) isolation
    (B) undoing
    (C) delusion
    (D) conversion
    (E) projection

23. Her seeming lack of concern can be considered as

    (A) autism
    (B) la belle indifference
    (C) malingering
    (D) rationalization
    (E) reaction formation

24. In spite of excellent emergency care, a middle-aged man dies suddenly of a myocardial infarction. The emergency room physician is quite upset when the shocked and grieving family become personally abusive to him. The doctor may take these comments less personally if he recognizes that he is the focus of the family's mourning anger, which is being

    (A) suppressed
    (B) sublimated
    (C) displaced
    (D) dissociated
    (E) denied

25. After he has been subjected to a long series of painful injections, a 7-year-old boy keeps telling everyone that he actually enjoys needles. The nurses may be able to manage him with more understanding when he starts parading around the ward with needles stuck under his skin, if they realize that much of his behavior is

    (A) compulsive
    (B) repressive
    (C) dissociative
    (D) counterphobic
    (E) negativistic

Questions 26 through 28

26. As she walks home at night, an elderly woman becomes convinced that those shadows moving under her neighbor's trees are really a watching man. Her belief is based on a(n)

    (A) hallucination
    (B) projection
    (C) illusion
    (D) reaction formation
    (E) rationalization

27. When she gets into her house, she prepares a meal but later phones the police to complain that the neighbors are poisoning her food. Her behavior now is a manifestation of

    (A) autism
    (B) dissociation
    (C) isolation
    (D) delusion
    (E) obsession

28. Several hours later she starts shooting wildly toward the neighboring house. She is sure that they are "coming to get her." Her belief that she is going to be attacked is an example of

    (A) dementia
    (B) denial
    (C) regression
    (D) displacement
    (E) projection

29. After he is severely reprimanded by his employer, a man goes home and is extremely nasty to his wife all evening. His behavior at home is an example of

    (A) sublimation
    (B) dissociation
    (C) displacement
    (D) rationalization
    (E) conversion

30. A middle-aged, experienced nurse notes a rapidly growing lump in her breast but does not seek medical treatment. When eventually the mass is noted at her annual physical examination, she says she thought the lump was quite normal near the time of menopause. Her response is an example of

    (A) dissociation
    (B) repression
    (C) sublimation
    (D) rationalization
    (E) projection

31. A previously shy 16-year-old teenager has his leg amputated following a car accident and is fitted with an artificial limb. Within a week of returning home, his physician learns that the boy has been out dancing every evening. This unusual social interest can be considered evidence of

   (A) dissociation
   (B) conversion
   (C) somatization
   (D) reaction formation
   (E) compulsion

DIRECTIONS (Questions 32 through 120): Each group of items in this section consists of lettered headings followed by a set of numbered words or phrases. For each numbered word or phrase, select the ONE lettered heading that is most closely associated with it. Each lettered heading may be selected once, more than once, or not at all.

Questions 32 through 35

   (A) socialization outside the family
   (B) identity resolution
   (C) training and control
   (D) establishment of basic trust

For each development phase, select the growth task.

32. Latency

33. Anal stage

34. Adolescence

35. Infancy

Questions 36 through 39

   (A) instinctual drives
   (B) conscience
   (C) reality testing
   (D) highest personal goal

For each psychoanalytic term, select the correct attribute.

36. Ego

37. Ego-Ideal

38. Superego

39. Id

Questions 40 through 44

   (A) unchanging repetition of behavior or speech
   (B) pathological imitation of another's movements
   (C) rigidity of posture with increase in tone
   (D) maintaining body position in which he has been placed
   (E) temporary loss of muscle tone

For each term, select the corresponding description of motor behavior.

40. Echopraxia

41. Stereotypy

42. Waxy flexibility

43. Catalepsy

44. Cataplexy

Questions 45 through 49

   (A) emotional response of the psychotherapist to the patient
   (B) return to earlier pattern of behavior
   (C) unconscious opposition to developing awareness
   (D) feelings from another relationship displaced onto the therapist
   (E) fellow-feeling with another person

Match the analytic name given below with the correct description.

45. Transference

46. Resistance

47. Empathy

48. Countertransference

49. Regression

Questions 50 through 54

    (A) sexual energy and drive

    (B) prelogical, egocentric thinking

    (C) feelings not usually in awareness but can be readily recalled

    (D) logical, consistent, reality-based thinking

    (E) investment of emotional energy

For each psychological term, select the correct definition.

50. Primary process

51. The preconscious

52. Libido

53. Secondary process

54. Cathexis

Questions 55 through 59

    (A) feelings of unreality and strangeness

    (B) feelings that are unacceptable to the individual

    (C) contradictory feelings toward the same person

    (D) normal range of feelings and mood

    (E) absence of pleasure

Select the most appropriate feeling state description for each term.

55. Anhedonia

56. Euthymia

57. Ego dystonic

58. Depersonalization

59. Ambivalence

Questions 60 through 63

    (A) feeling that insects are crawling in or on the skin

    (B) misinterpretation of real external sensory experience

    (C) false perceptions while awakening

    (D) false perceptions when falling asleep

    (E) sensation in one perceptual modality triggers a sensation in another sensory modality

Match the correct name with the description of perception.

60. Synesthesia

61. Illusion

62. Formication

63. Hypnagogic state

Questions 64 through 68

    (A) emphasis of opposite feelings and qualities

    (B) relating to people as all good or all bad

    (C) externalization of unacceptable personal feelings

    (D) unacceptable feelings and drives productively redirected

    (E) symbolic expression through physical symptoms

Match the defense mechanism with the appropriate description.

64. Projection

65. Reaction formation

66. Splitting

67. Sublimation

68. Conversion

Questions 69 through 73

    (A) irrelevant, over-inclusive speech but does get to the point

    (B) repetition of another's words

    (C) illogical jumble of words and phrases

    (D) connection of words based on sound, not on meaning

    (E) newly coined word or several words run together

Match the correct term with the speech process.

69. Echolalia

70. Clang association

71. Neologism

72. Circumstantiality

73. Word salad

Questions 74 through 78

    (A) deliberate forgetting of disturbing feelings or ideas

    (B) unconscious blocking out of unacceptable feelings

    (C) intellectualized justification

    (D) substitution of more acceptable focus for feelings

    (E) intolerable external reality is removed from awareness

Match the defense mechanism below with the description above.

74. Repression

75. Rationalization

76. Suppression

77. Displacement

78. Denial

Questions 79 through 83

    (A) exaggerated, inappropriate feeling of pleasure

    (B) falsification of memory to fill gaps

    (C) memory loss

    (D) abnormally repetitive response to different questions

    (E) sudden stopping of thought or feeling

For each symptom, select the correct description.

79. Amnesia

80. Euphoria

81. Perseveration

82. Confabulation

83. Blocking

Questions 84 through 87

    (A) personality disorder

    (B) senile dementia

    (C) mood disorder

    (D) autistic disorder

    (E) toxic psychosis

For each symptom, select the most likely diagnosis.

84. Anhedonia

85. Visual hallucinations

86. Antisocial behavior

87. Amnesia for recent events

Questions 88 through 92

    (A) misinterpretation of perceptual stimulus

    (B) false, fixed belief incompatible with culture

    (C) irrational fear

    (D) recurrent, intrusive, disturbing thought

    (E) false perception without reality stimulus

For each word listed below, select the correct definition.

88. Delusion

89. Obsession

90. Illusion

91. Hallucination

92. Phobia

Questions 93 through 97

    (A) tangentiality   (E) flight of ideas

    (B) perseveration   (F) blocking

    (C) glossolalia   (G) looseness of associations

    (D) circumstantiality   (H) neologisms

For each clinical description, select the correct term.

93. "He took a long time getting to the point but he did get there."

94. "I just could not follow his thinking. He just lost me."

95. "She was speaking in tongues."

96. "I could not get her to change the subject. She kept responding 'Dinner time'."

97. "My mind went blank."

Questions 98 through 102

    (A) achievement of sexual pleasure by inflicting pain

    (B) achievement of sexual gratification with a child partner

    (C) reaching sexual pleasure by watching the sexual organs or the sexual activities of others

    (D) attainment of sexual gratification by enduring inflicted pain

    (E) sexual relations between close members of the same family

For each paraphilia or sexual deviation, select the appropriate description.

98. Sadism

99. Masochism

100. Pedophilia

101. Voyeurism

102. Incest

Questions 103 through 107

    (A) psychological dependence

    (B) withdrawal symptoms that occur with physical dependence

    (C) habitual and compulsive need for drugs (with or without physical dependence)

    (D) declining effect of same dose of a drug with prolonged use

    (E) excessive drug intake unrelated to medical use

For each drug abuse term, select the appropriate definition.

103. Abstinence syndrome

104. Habituation

105. Drug abuse

106. Drug dependence

107. Tolerance

Questions 108 through 111

    (A) very rapid process of thinking, at times without obvious connections

    (B) urgent and compelling need to move: "restless" feet

    (C) sudden interruption in flow of thinking

    (D) acute anxiety in organic brain syndrome when patient becomes aware of handicaps

    (E) alternating periods of elation and depression

For each psychiatric term, select the correct description.

108. Thought blocking

109. Flight of ideas

110. Cyclothymia

111. Akathisia

112. Catastrophic reaction

Questions 113 through 120

    (A) assumption of new identity with amnesia for the old identity

    (B) compulsive pulling out of one's own hair

    (C) crying, sadness and rage

    (D) persistent eating of non-food materials

    (E) repeated chewing, swallowing, regurgitating and rechewing

    (F) rapid, involuntary, spasmodic motor movements

    (G) acute, episodic anxiety and dread

    (H) unrealistic interpretation of physical sensations

    (I) compulsive utterance of obscenities

    (J) continuous refusal to speak

Match each term below with the appropriate symptom.

113. Tic

114. Fugue

115. Pica

116. Affect

117. Rumination

118. Hypochondriasis

119. Coprolalia

120. Panic

Hallucinations Hypnagogic - just about to fall asleep.
Hypnopompic → just arousing from sleep.

Answers and Explanations

1. **(C)** In a *déjà vu* situation, the subject feels incorrectly that he or she has lived through the present experience at some time before. This feeling can occur in many emotional states and may also be part of an epileptic aura. *(1:221; 2:1248)*
A. When a subject senses or feels a body part that has been amputated or removed, this sensation is called a *phantom phenomenon*. *(1:220)*
B. *Hypnagogic hallucinations* may occur when a normal person is in the "in-between" stage of just falling asleep. Similar hallucinatory states can occur normally in the awakening *hypnopompic* state. *(1:220; 2:189)*
D. When intellectual reasoning is used to avoid dealing with unacceptable feelings, this would be considered *rationalization*. *(1:184; 2:1265)*
E. Sleepwalking *(somnambulism)* occurs usually during stages 3 and 4 of non-dreaming sleep. Sleep talking takes place during all stages of sleep. *(1:477; 2:749–50)*

2. **(C)** *Blocking, thought deprivation,* occurs in many situations but, when marked, is usually due to schizophrenia. *(1:219; 2:189)*
A. Deliberate resistance to sharing uncomfortable feelings is usually called *negativism*. In psychotherapy, *resistance* is the term given to unconscious attempts to avoid awareness. *(1:573–4; 2:140,173)*
B. *Fixation* is the arrest of psychological development before full maturation. *(1:174; 2:1252)*
D. *Psychomotor retardation* is the physical and emotional slowing seen in depression. *(1:367; 2:404, 1264)*
E. The pathological lack of concern about seeming misfortune, seen sometimes in patients with conversion disorder, was termed *la belle indifference* by Janet. This symptom is nonspecific and can occur in stoical persons and people who are emotionally healthy *or* ill. *(1:419; 2:539,1257)*

3. **(D)** *Akathisia*, the "restless leg" syndrome, occurs as a side effect with many psychotropic drugs and is likely to develop especially at the drug levels necessary to treat the psychotic patient. *(1:218; 2:779–80)*
A. With *akinesia*, the severe form of bradykinesia, the patient shows marked reduction in the frequency and amplitude of voluntary movements. *(1:618; 2:780)* Alcohol.
B. In Korsakoff's syndrome, *confabulation*, the unconscious falsification of memory, occurs to fill the gaps in recall produced by the illness. *(1:221; 2:323,1273)*
C. *Reaction formation* is the defense mechanism when the opposite emotion is stressed. *(1:184; 2:136)*
E. *Narcoanalysis* and *narcosynthesis* are the terms used for the procedure where narcotic drugs (most often barbiturates) are used to facilitate psychotherapeutic work. *(1:674–5; 2:565–6,1259)*

4. **(D)** In *reaction formation*, the opposite feeling is stressed—and the important word here is "stressed"—the opposite feeling is emphasized. *(1:184; 2:136)*
A. *Rationalization* is the unconsciously motivated use of logical explanations for behavior or feelings prompted by repressed feelings. *(1:184; 2:1265)*
B. *Undoing* is typically seen in obsessive compulsive disorder where the subject repetitiously and compulsively acts to prevent the feared and fantasized consequences of his or her recurrent obsession—the person repeatedly washes his hands in an effort to undo unacceptable feelings. *(1:184; 2:136)*
C. In *displacement* the emotion is unchanged but is directed to a more tolerable focus. When a child cannot comfortably be angry at a parent, the youngster may displace the anger and kick the cat or a younger sibling. *(1:184; 2:127,1249)*
E. In the process of *denial*, intolerable reality is blocked out of awareness by this unconscious mechanism. Approaching death may be denied because recognition of this reality produces unbearable anxiety. In *suppression*, on the other hand, the subject consciously shuts painful facts out of direct awareness. *(1:183; 2:137–8)*

5. **(B)** Regression is very different from *repression*. Repression occurs in emotional defense mechanisms where unacceptable or anxiety-arousing feelings are unconsciously blocked out of awareness. *(1:184; 2:136)*
A. *Regression* is the return to earlier patterns of behavior—the ill child may go back to thumb sucking or carrying an old worn doll. *(1:183; 2:136)*
C. In *reaction formation,* the intolerable feeling is kept out of awareness by the overemphasis of the opposite emotion or drive. The person who finds his or her angry or aggressive feelings too anxiety-provoking becomes overly sweet, friendly, and accepting. *(1:184; 2:136)*
D. In *suppression,* the individual consciously and deliberately shuts out disturbing feelings from awareness. The conscious decision is "I am not going to think about it." *(1:184; 2:1268)*
E. *Fixation* is the arrest of emotional development before full maturity and may occur at any stage of personality growth. *(1:174; 2:1252)*

6. **(D)** In *paranoia,* intolerable feelings are *projected* outward and ascribed to an external person or force. Rather than admit the reality of being inadequate, the subject may defend against anxiety by projection, by explaining away his inadequacies as being due to his employer's favoritism to others. *(1:183; 2:137)*
A. In *introjection,* the subject takes into his own personality make-up the totality of the perceived object. This is a primitive form of identification. *(1:183; 2:137)*
B. *Regression* is a return to earlier patterns of behavior and occurs in normal people under stress, especially physical illness. Severe and sustained regression is more likely to be a manifestation of emotional illness. *(1:183; 2:136)*
C. In *conversion,* the emotional conflict is kept out of awareness but is expressed ("converted") in a physical symptom. The wife who is angry enough to hit her husband, whom she also loves, solves the emotional conflict by developing an arm weakness. *(1:418–20; 2:537)*
E. In the defense mechanism of *isolation,* the subject can recall or discuss a disturbing idea or fact but the distressing feelings that usually accompany such recollections are blocked out of awareness, or isolated away.
Following a tragic car accident, a man may recall the events vividly, including the deaths of his loved family, but talk dispassionately. The emotion is isolated away in an emotional defense reaction to allow him to cope with the tragedy. *(1:184; 2:136)*

7. **(C)** *Alexithymia* is the inability to be aware of one's own feelings and may be characteristic of patients with somatization disorder. Some people express their feelings in physical sensations or symptoms. *(1:217,416–8; 2:1240)*
A. *Developmental reading disorder, dyslexia,* is the marked impairment of reading skills, not due to poor schooling, mental retardation, or physical handicap. *(1:711–3; 2:720–4)*
B. A *somatic delusion* is a false belief involving one's bodily functioning. *(1:219; 2:190)*
D. *Coma vigil* is the state when the patient seems to be asleep but ready to be aroused. The cause is usually due to an organic process. *(1:214)*
E. *Apathy* is the term for a dull, indifferent emotional state. *(1:217; 2:1242)*

8. **(B)** *Hallucinations* are sensory experiences in the absence of external stimuli. The schizophrenic hallucinates the voice of Christ; the delirium tremens patient hallucinates seeing animals moving. Hallucinations can occur in many normal situations—the mourner can hallucinate the presence of the departed, the lover can hallucinate the loved one. *(1:220–1; 2:189)*
A. In *projection,* unacceptable personal feelings or qualities are externalized—projected outward—onto other persons. *(1:183; 2:137)*
C. In an *illusion* the subject perceptually misinterprets a real external sensory stimulus. The fearful woman may see men standing in the shadows under a tree, when, in reality, she is misinterpreting empty shadows because of her fearfulness. *(1:221; 2:189)*
D. A *delusion* is a relatively stable false belief that is incompatible with the subject's intelligence, education, and culture.
The minority-group child may grow up believing that he is victimized by the majority culture. The personal belief, valid or otherwise, would not be considered a delusion because it is compatible with his upbringing and cultural environment. *(1:219; 2:190)*
E. *Introjection* is the process that is the opposite of projection. In introjection, the subject takes into his own personality external qualities or identities of the people around him. This is a more primitive, less selective form of personality development than *identification.* *(1:180; 2:137)*

9. **(A)** The unconscious blocking out of awareness of disturbing emotions is called *repression.* *(1:184; 2:136)*
A similar word, but with a very different meaning, *regression* may occur in the face of any stress, including sexual conflict, but sexual conflict in itself does not necessarily lead to regression. Regression is a behavioral reaction and is not mediated through any specific nerve pathway. Regression does not always indicate severe emotional disorder. Where regression is marked and long lasting, there is a likelihood of greater

causative stress or more profound preexisting emotional weakness.

Regression, however, does occur normally in the face of physical illness. The physically ill person takes to bed, allows himself to be cared for and nursed, and may become childishly demanding. *(1:183; 2:136)*

10. **(E)** *Bulimia* is the term for excessive gorging that goes with a huge appetite. The voracious eater may self-induce vomiting after an eating binge. Bulimia may precede or coexist with anorexia nervosa. *(1:746–8; 2:760)*

The other terms listed are self-explanatory.

11. **(B)** The Halstead-Reitan battery is a series of neuropsychological tests used to identify and localize brain damage. *(1:168–70; 2:240,1278)*

12. **(D)** In conversion disorders, *conversion* is the term used when the underlying emotional conflict is symbolically manifested outwardly in a symptom involving the special senses or the voluntary nervous system. The writer may be unable to face a lack of creativity but can blandly tolerate the physical incapacity of writer's cramp. *(1:418–20; 2:537)*
A. *Displacement* is the term to describe the mechanism whereby feelings that are intolerable when directed at one object or person are made more tolerable by redirecting these feelings toward another focus. In everyday experience, the father who "takes it out on" his family when he is frustrated by his work is displacing. *(1:184; 2:127,1249)*
B. When a subject has almost total memory loss for a significant part of his life, this would be considered *amnesia*. When this is part of a hysterical neurosis, this amnesia would be considered an example of *dissociation*. Amnesia may be produced by many organic syndromes. *(1:184,221; 2:293,560)*
C. In a *psychosomatic disorder* typically an emotional conflict is expressed in a single organ system controlled by the autonomic nerves. *(1:498; 2:493–6)*
E. When an otherwise unacceptable drive is rechanneled into socially acceptable behavior, *sublimation* has occurred. It may not be acceptable to an angry father to beat his children brutally but he can sublimate his rage by chopping wood or painting a wall. *(1:184; 2:138)*

13. **(C)** A false belief, not in accord with the individual's intelligence, age level, and culture, is a *delusion*. *(1:219; 2:190)*
A. A *hallucination* is a sensory experience in the absence of external stimuli—where the perception arises within the individual. *(1:220; 2:189)*
B. An *illusion* is a misinterpretation of actual perceptions where the quality of the misinterpretation is dictated by the subject's feelings. Because of

his suspiciousness and feelings of inadequacy, the individual has the illusion that waving branches are pointing fingers. *(1:221; 2:189)*
D. When unacceptable feelings are projected outward and ascribed to another person, this mechanism is called *projection*. *(1:183; 2:137)*
E. Unconscious blocking of any feelings, including instinctually based emotions, is labeled *repression*. *(1:184; 2:136)*

14. **(E)** Delusions do not occur in a subject who has a *schizoid personality*. These people are shy, oversensitive, vague, and often "different," but they are still in reasonable contact with reality. The schizoid personality is one example of a *personality disorder*. *(1:528–9; 2:190,629–30)*

The other syndromes listed are psychotic states where delusions can and do occur.

15. **(B)** Paranoid delusions are produced by the mechanism of *projection*, where unacceptable inner feelings are externalized outward and projected onto another person or group. *(1:183; 2:137)*
A. In *displacement*, the disturbing feelings are already being directed to an external object but the emotions are redirected (displaced) to a more acceptable object. *(1:184; 2:127,1249)*
C. When disturbing feelings or behavior are *rationalized* away, the subject comes up with a personally acceptable or tolerable intellectual reason for these distressing emotions. *(1:184; 2:1265)*
D. In *sublimation*, an emotion or urge that is personally or socially unacceptable becomes acceptable and often growth productive when it is rechanneled into socially approved behavior.

Where a youngster is intensely competitive with an older sibling, it is not acceptable to eliminate the elder child with an axe. It is very acceptable for the younger child to strive to beat the other child academically and athletically, often with the added reward of personal growth and enrichment. *(1:184; 2:138)*
E. In the process of *identification*, the individual integrates into her own personality selected qualities of significant people in her life. Identification has this quality of selection, integration, and ego work in the process. The more primitive forms of identification, incorporation, and introjection, are much less integrative or selective. *(1:180; 2:137)*

16. **(A)** Alcoholic women are more likely to have children born with the fetal alcohol syndrome, manifesting low birth weight, small size, craniofacial, limb, and cardiac abnormalities, and mental retardation.

It has been suggested that the relationship between childhood minimal brain damage and later antisocial behavior may be due primarily to the fetal alcohol syndrome. *(1:291; 2:317)*

17. **(A)** *Catharsis* is the psychoanalytic term for the release of previously unconscious feelings, with outward expressions of feelings, that comes usually with an appropriate interpretation in the course of treatment. *(1:586; 2:959)*
B. *Cathexis* is the analytic word for the investment of emotional energy in a specific purpose or object. Withdrawal of emotional investment is called *decathexis. (1:180; 2:128)*
C. The conscious or unconscious response of the psychotherapist to the patient is designated as *countertransference.* This concept emphasizes the two-way process in any psychotherapeutic interaction where the therapist must be aware of both the patient's transference feelings and also of his own logical and illogical feelings toward the patient. *(1:573; 2:172)*
D. In psychoanalytic practice, the process of knowing and learning is called achieving *insight.* *(1:586; 2:192)*
E. When an unacceptable feeling is externalized and ascribed to an external person, the process is called *projection. (1:183; 2:137)*

18. **(E)** The *collective unconscious* was a concept introduced by *Carl Jung* early in his career. It implied the common unconscious that is inherent in human beings, a species-specific unconscious that is then integrated with other aspects of the unconscious that are individual and social. *(1:188; 2:153–4)*

19. **(E)** When feelings originally linked to significant or nuclear early-life figures are projected on, or transferred to, a current-life person, *transference* has occurred—and this process occurs in everyday relationships as well as in psychotherapeutic relationships. *(1:573; 2:139–40,171–2)*
A.. *Displacement* is the mechanism whereby feelings are transferred from an unacceptable to a more acceptable object. *(1:184; 2:127,1249)*
B. When unacceptable thoughts and ideas are unconsciously excluded from awareness, they are said to have been *repressed. (1:184; 2:136)*
C. Identification implies internalization, the taking into the personality significant aspects of a parent–child relationship. In transference, externally directed feelings are transferred to a new external object. *(1:180; 2:137)*
D. Transference is in no way indicative of early psychosis, though an illogical transference or a transference unduly acted out may indicate a psychotic process.
A woman may naturally feel initial dislike for bald, middle-aged men because her brutal father was bald—as part of an understandable transference reaction that is not psychotic. However, if she assaulted these bald men, her behavior would indicate a psychotic break with accepted reality. *(1:573; 2:139–40,171–2)*

20. **(D)** A patient who has a *somatization disorder,* expresses feelings by having physical symptoms or complaints. This is an automatic or unconscious process. *(1:416–8; 2:544–6)*
In *hypochondriasis,* the patient misinterprets real physical signs or sensations. *(1:422–4; 2:547–9)*
When the individual has a loss or change in physical function produced by an emotional conflict or need, this is designated a *conversion disorder. (1:418–20; 2:535–7)*
The malingering patient deliberately and consciously fabricates symptoms for some recognizable personal gain. *(1:548; 2:552–4)*

21. **(A)** Psychosomatic reactions, such as peptic ulcers or ulcerative colitis, may indeed be fatal.
B. They are predominantly mediated through the autonomic nervous system. Conversion disorders affect the voluntary motor system and the special senses.
C. Psychosomatic reactions are not produced solely by emotional problems. Usually there is a strong physical, constitutional predisposition and often other etiological factors.
D. Psychosomatic reactions should be treated by all means necessary, usually by more than psychotherapy alone. A child in status asthmaticus requires prompt effective medical and psychiatric treatment. Psychotherapy has little effect on a dead child.
E. Psychosomatic illness occurs in young children, even in the neonate. *(1:498–524; 2:493–532)*

22. **(D)** This history outline points out how a good, caring woman finds herself angry at the husband she loves. She deals with the emotional conflict of love–rage by repressing (and undoubtedly also suppressing) the anger. This unacceptable feeling of anger, however, is converted into a physical symptom, the right-arm paralysis. The symptom has a symbolic meaning—if her right arm is paralyzed, she cannot use it to hit out at her unfaithful spouse. The symptom is a manifestation of *conversion. (1:418–20; 2:535–40)*

23. **(B)** Since this physical symptom does relieve her conflict, she can indeed be relatively unconcerned, manifesting the classical *la belle indifference* of the hysteric. *(1:419; 2:539)*

24. **(C)** In normal mourning, the grieving relatives must face their sadness and anger at the loss, and they must reinvest emotionally. Often in Western society, mourners find it difficult to deal with the normally felt anger at this pain and separation. It is difficult to be angry at the deceased and it is not acceptable to be angry at God. This mourning anger may be *displaced* onto the nurse or physician—the emotion retains the same quality but is

focused on a more acceptable target. *(1:184; 2:127, 1249)*

25. **(D)** Whistling through the graveyard and singing cheerily while walking down dark deserted alleys are the kind of *counterphobic* reactions seen in normal people. The adolescent and childhood games of "daring" and playing "chicken" have a strong counterphobic quality. In order to avoid admitting or facing fears about a situation, the subject actively seeks out or repetitiously engages in the experience.

    With the natural pride of a seven-year-old, this young man finds it difficult to admit just how scared he is of painful needles—and rightfully scared. He copes with his fear by the *counterphobic* measure of seeking out and actively engaging in the feared behavior. Many counterphobic behaviors raise tension in observers who can sense the subject's overreaction and underlying anxiety. *(1:400–1; 2:1247)*

26. **(C)** Due to her fearfulness, the subject misinterprets actual perceptual stimuli. The shadows are actually there, but she interprets her perceptions to see, in these shadows, a watching man. This form of misperception is termed an *illusion*. *(1:221; 2:189)*

27. **(D)** When she phones the police to complain that the neighbors are poisoning her food, she is manifesting a false belief that probably is inconsistent with her intelligence and cultural background—she is manifesting a *delusion*. She is now externalizing her inner insecurities and directing these feelings toward her neighbors. *Projection* is occurring. *(1:183; 2:136)*

28. **(E)** The *projection* becomes more fixed and stronger. She can now justify taking action against these neighbors, in a way that endangers them, under the paranoid justification of her delusion. *(1:183; 2:190)*

Answers 26 through 28 describe the development of a paranoid delusion to the point of illogical action. Frequently, however, a paranoid delusion forms around a core of reality. In this instance, the lady's paranoid delusion may be based not only in her own inner conflicts and insecurity but also on the fact that the neighbors were uncooperative, unfriendly, or distressing. (1:812–3; 2:1124–8)

If this elderly woman then claimed that her food—for instance the milk—had a bitter taste of poison and no one else could detect this taste, she would be showing a *gustatory hallucination*. Much more frequent are taste illusions where a taste is misinterpreted—everyone can taste a chalky flavor in the milk but the subject interprets this as being due to strychnine. *(1:220; 2:189)*

29. **(C)** The man is naturally angry, anxious, and sensitive at being reprimanded by his employer. He has found it difficult to express his feelings toward the disturbing person, the employer, possibly because he could be dismissed or because the employer was fully justified in the reprimand. The man continues feeling upset. He cannot or does not suppress or repress the anger. He does not sublimate his tension in more forceful work. He displaces his anger onto a safer target, his wife. This is an example of *displacement,* an everyday, normal (though unproductive), reaction. *(1:184; 2:127,1249)*

30. **(D)** This middle-aged nurse very readily would have diagnosed the possible seriousness of this breast lump in anyone else. In reality, she did realize the potential threat of this growing mass to her physical integrity and continued existence, but the thought was so disturbing that she blocked it out of awareness. She *denied* the reality. *(1:183; 2:137–8)*

    When she could not avoid facing this reality, she explained away her seemingly illogical behavior with intellectual reasons; she *rationalized.* *(1:184; 2:1265)*

31. **(D)** When Hamlet's mother pointed out to him "The lady doth protest too much, methinks," *(Hamlet,* Act 3, Sc. 2.242), she was highlighting an example of *reaction formation.* For a young man who had been socially backward to become suddenly prominent would necessitate quite a reversal of behavior. A leg amputee would not usually consider dancing the easiest activity. Reasonably he might want to work up gradually to this form of social interaction. The patient described here is handling his understandable anxiety about his amputation by emphasizing the opposite behavior to his fears.

    All normal people show reaction formation in some of their activities. This defense is reality distorting—this boy naturally, as an amputee, would find it more difficult to dance well—and this form of emotional reaction takes a great deal of psychologic energy to maintain and tends to make other people uneasy or anxious. *(1:184; 2:136)*

32. **(A)** In Freudian theory, *latency* follows the resolution of the *phallic phase* of development and is the time when the youngster first moves outside the family and should become adapted to wider society. This approximates the grade school or elementary school period. *(1:37–8; 2:106–7,129)*

33. **(C)** The *anal stage* follows the *oral stage* and is the time of initial training and control within the family according to psychoanalytic theory. *(1:35–6; 2:129)*

34. (B) Erikson characterized adolescence as the period when the growing child establishes his or her unique individual *identity,* a sense of personal integrity, compatible with community values and goals. *(1:42–3; 2:145–6)*

35. (D) According to Erikson, *basic trust* should be established during infancy, during the Freudian oral stage. *(1:34; 2:145–6)*

Answers 35 through 39 refer to psychoanalytic concepts. The id, ego, ego-ideal, and the superego are components of the psychic structure.

36. (C) The *ego* is the coordinating, organizing part of the personality, the part that perceives and evaluates reality. *(1:180–1; 2:132–5)*

37. (D) The *ego-ideal,* a less frequently used concept, is the idealized self-image, the private, personal optimal goal. *(2:134,1251)*

38. (B) The *superego,* the conscience part of the personality, is derived largely from significant relationships where standards and models, good and bad, have been set. *(1:180; 2:132–5)*

39. (A) The *id,* according to Freudian theory, is instinctual drives with which the infant is born. *(1:180; 2:132–5)*

Answers 40 through 44 deal with changes in the way the patients present.

40. (B) *Echopraxia* is the pathological imitation of the movements of another person. *Echolalia* is the repetition of another person's words or phrases. These symptoms may be seen in patients with organic brain damage or schizophrenia. *(1:217; 2:1250)*

41. (A) *Stereotypy* is the unchanging (stereotyped) repetition of behavior or speech, a repetitive constant pattern. *(1:218; 2:365,1268)*

42. (D) *Waxy flexibility* (*cerea flexibilitas*), is the syndrome where the patient can be placed in a posture or position and will maintain this stance for a lengthy period. Psychiatry textbooks used to have rather grotesque pictures of patients who maintained unusual postures for periods of days or months. *(1:217; 2:365,1245)*

43. (C) *Catalepsy* is a general term referring to an increase in tone with rigidity of posture. *(1:217; 2:1245)*

Catalepsy should be clearly differentiated from cataplexy.

44. (E) *Cataplexy* is a sudden, transient attack of marked general muscle weakness, often precipi-

tated by laughing or other emotional reactions. *(1:218; 2:747–8)*

Answers 45 through 49 focus on the psychotherapy process.

45. (D) *Transference* is the process whereby feelings initially directed to an earlier significant person are *transferred* onto a person in an immediate present relationship. In psychoanalytic psychotherapy, transference toward the therapist or analyst is allowed and then becomes a major focus of the psychotherapy. *(1:573; 2:171–2)*

46. (C) *Resistance* in psychotherapy is the conscious and unconscious opposition to bringing to awareness previously unconscious feelings. *(1:573–4; 2:173)*

47. (E) *Empathy* is a fellow feeling for another human being; this is contrasted with *sympathy,* where the feeling is subjective. *(1:586; 2:1251)*

48. (A) *Countertransference* is the conscious and unconscious emotional response of the psychotherapist to the patient in treatment. Many psychotherapists use these reactions elicited by the patient as further diagnostic and therapeutic tools. *(1:573; 2:172)*

49. (B) *Regression* implies a return to earlier patterns of behavior; this may be a normal reaction to severe stress, as in serious physical illness, or may be a manifestation of emotional disorder. *(1:183; 2:136)*

This set of answers (50 through 54) deals with concepts that were developed early in the evolution of psychoanalytic theory.

50. (B) *Primary process* thinking is associated with the unconscious and is pre-logical or illogical, accepting contradictions, without time boundaries and seeking wish fulfillment. *(1:179; 2:126–7)*

51. (C) *The preconscious* is that part of the mind where ideas and feelings are just out of awareness but, with effort, can be recalled. *(1:179; 2:125–6)*

52. (A) *Libido* specifically is the sexual instinctual forces and drives: "sexual" is used in the widest sense of life-directed and living. *(1:174,178; 2:129, 131)*

53. (D) *Secondary process* thinking is logical, reality-based, and consistent. *(1:179; 2:127)*

54. (E) *Cathexis* is the psychoanalytic term for the investment of emotional energy in an object, goal, or drive. *(1:180; 2:128)*

Questions 55 through 59 define different feeling states.

55. **(E)** *Anhedonia* is the withdrawal from and loss of interest in activities and interests that are usually pleasurable for the individual. Anhedonia is an important symptom of schizophrenia and depression. *(1:217; 2:366,404–8)*

56. **(D)** *Euthymia* is the normal range of mood, not unduly depressed or elated. *(1:217)*

57. **(B)** When feelings or ideas are *ego-dystonic,* they are not a fully acceptable part of the individual's personality—and thus liable to cause anxiety or discomfort. A comparable term is ego-alien. *(1:401; 2:624,1251)*

58. **(A)** *Depersonalization* is the feeling that one's body has become unreal and strange. Brief episodes of depersonalization occur normally, especially during adolescence but this feeling may occur as a symptom in many psychiatric and organic disorders. *(1:433–5; 2:189)*

59. **(C)** *Ambivalence* is the emotional state where the individual feels contradictory and conflicting feelings toward the same object. Ambivalence is part of every normal mature relationship, but the healthy person usually prefers to respond to one side of the ambivalence. In schizophrenia, ambivalence may be marked, and the schizophrenic may act or express both aspects of the ambivalence. *(1:405; 2:475)*

Questions 60 through 63 deal with perceptual variations.

60. **(E)** *Synesthesia* is the state where a stimulus in one sensory modality results in a sensation in another sensory modality. In a hallucinogen-induced psychosis, a sound may cause a visual sensation. *(1:221; 2:344)*

61. **(B)** *Illusions* are misinterpretations of real external sensory stimuli. Because she is afraid, the old lady misinterprets the shadow she sees in a corner and believes that a man is waiting there. *(1:221; 2:189)*

62. **(A)** *Formication* is an example of a haptic (tactile) hallucination where the subject has the feeling that insects are crawling in or on the skin. This symptom may occur with an amphetamine psychosis. "Cocaine bugs" are a long recognized manifestation of a cocaine-induced toxic psychosis. *(1:220,304; 2:364)*

63. **(D)** A *hypnagogic state* is the experience of illusions and hallucinations that often occur to normal people during the period of falling asleep. The comparable awakening experience is the *hypnopompic state* (C). *(1:202; 2:189)*

Answers 64 through 68 deal with mental mechanisms and emotional defenses.

64. **(C)** In *projection,* personally unacceptable inner feelings and impulses are externalized and ascribed to another person. The defense in this process is the externalizing intolerable emotions and drives and then blaming another person for the exact same feelings and intentions. *(1:183,527; 2:137)*

65. **(A)** In *reaction formation,* the subject defends unconsciously against an anxiety-arousing feeling by outwardly stressing the opposite emotion. This defense is not merely repression of one feeling; it involves the emphasis of just the opposite. *(1:184,405; 2:136)*

66. **(B)** *Splitting* is the mechanism whereby external relationships and experiences are divided into "all good" and "all bad." Splitting, like other defenses, is used by emotionally healthy people but is used more actively and extensively by patients with certain personality disorders. *(1:183,188–9,527; 2:138)*

67. **(D)** In *sublimation,* unacceptable drives and feelings are repressed, but the energy of these emotions is rechanneled in socially acceptable and sometimes growth-productive ways. The naturally competitive young boy cannot destroy his father physically but he can learn to beat him in chess or in football, both good sublimations. *(1:184; 2:138)*

68. **(E)** When a disturbing emotional conflict is repressed and manifested through a physical symptom, usually involving the special senses or the voluntary muscles, this mechanism is termed *conversion.* Conversion is a term that implies a process but this process has never been proved. *(1:418–20; 2:537)*

Questions 69 through 73 focus on speech symptoms.

69. **(B)** When a subject repetitiously and word-for-word repeats the words and phrases that are said to him, this symptom is called *echolalia* and may be a manifestation of an organic brain disorder or schizophrenia.

Question: "What is your name, Sir?"
Response: "Name Sir. Name Sir."
Question: "Where are you now?"
Response: "You now, you now."
Echopraxia is the comparable symptom where the other person's movements are automatically imitated. *(1:218; 2:366,1273)*

70. **(D)** Where there is a *clang association*, the individual's train of thought follows the sound of the words rather than their meaning. *(1:219; 2:365, 1245)*

71. **(E)** A *neologism* is a newly coined word or a series of words run together to form a seemingly nonsensical word. Typically neologisms occur in schizophrenia or acute manic states. *(1:218; 2:365,1259)*

72. **(A)** When the subject rambles and digresses but eventually gets to the point, he could be described as manifesting *circumstantiality*. *(1:218; 2:365, 1245)*

73. **(C)** A *word salad* is an incoherent jumble of words and phrases, sometimes with neologisms. *(1:218; 2:1271)*

Answers 74 through 78 also deal with mental mechanisms and defenses.

74. **(B)** *Repression* is the unconsciously motivated blocking out of unacceptable feelings from conscious awareness and is a factor in most, if not all, emotional defense mechanisms. *(1:184; 2:136)*

75. **(C)** *Rationalization* is the defense where intellectual, seemingly logical reasons are presented to justify feelings or behaviors. This defense is motivated by unconscious factors.

    A father rationalizes his sudden eruption of rage at his son because he was overtired—a lame excuse that everyone uses. In reality, the father's anxiety and anger arose when he sensed his son was superior to him intellectually and physically—and recognized momentarily his declining capability. *(1:184; 2:1265)*

76. **(A)** The deliberate conscious forgetting or blocking out from immediate awareness of disturbing feelings or ideas is called *suppression*. This blocking out is conscious ("I will not think about it") as opposed to the unconsciously motivated *repression*. *(1:184; 2:1268)*

77. **(D)** In *displacement*, the feelings remain the same but they are redirected (displaced), to a more tolerable or acceptable object. After the junior employee is reprimanded by a supervisor, the employee goes out and kicks a passing innocent cat. *(1:184; 2:127,1249)*

78. **(E)** When external reality is too disturbing, the individual may continue to cope by blocking out this reality from awareness—by *denial*. In a fatal illness, the patient may continue to function productively only by denying, by blocking this aware-

ness from reality. Since denial is a reality-distorting defense, this denial may be more difficult to maintain as the reality of approaching death becomes more obvious. The denial may suddenly give way, leaving the dying patient to face his or her loneliness, anxiety, and anger. *(1:183; 2:137–8)*

The next four questions, 79 through 83, deal with a range of symptoms.

79. **(C)** *Amnesia* is loss of memory and may be total or partial, reversible or permanent. Usually total amnesia is due to organic causes, but partial amnesia is a frequent symptom of emotional illness. *(1:221,254–6; 2:293,560)*

80. **(A)** *Euphoria* is an exaggerated, somewhat inappropriate feeling of pleasure. In states of unusual happiness and excitement, normal people experience euphoria, which also is seen frequently in hypomanic and manic states. *(1:217; 2:1252)*

81. **(D)** *Perseveration* is an abnormally repetitive response to different questions and is seen most often in senile dementia, after injury to brain speech centers, or in catatonia. *(1:218; 2:286,1273)*

82. **(B)** Classically, *confabulation* occurs in *Korsakoff's syndrome* and is the unconscious falsification of memory where the recall is impaired. Confabulation is a type of *paramnesia*. *(1:203,221; 2:293,323)*

83. **(E)** *Thought deprivation* or *blocking* is the sudden stoppage of the flow of thought or feeling. Normal people occasionally have thought blocking—"My mind just went blank"—but severe blocking is usually symptomatic of schizophrenia. *(1:183,219; 2:189)*

Answers 84 through 87 focus on symptoms of emotional illness.

84. **(C)** *Mood* or *affective disorder*. Anhedonia, the loss of interest in pleasurable activities and sometimes the active withdrawal from enjoyable pursuits, is a common symptom of depression and schizophrenia. In affective or mood disorders, the symptoms are caused by the disabling intensity of mood (affect). *(1:217; 2:366,404–8)*

85. **(E)** *Toxic psychosis*. Visual hallucinations occur early in a toxic psychosis. In a schizophrenic psychosis, definite visual hallucinations occur late when many other psychotic and regressed symptoms are present. *(1:220; 2:249)*

86. **(A)** *Personality disorder*. Patients with personality disorders show recurrent, inflexible maladap-

tive patterns of behavior that typically cause distress to other people. Antisocial behavior is an example of maladaptive, anxiety-arousing behavior seen in some types of personality disorder. *(1:525–42; 2:621–48)*

87. **(B)** *Senile dementia.* In senile dementia, the patient characteristically has great difficulty recalling recent events but often can remember childhood happenings in great detail (anterograde amnesia). Patients with senile dementia may try very hard to remember but still be unable to recall recent events; depressed patients may just lack the energy and the wish to try to remember and may present with a *pseudo-dementia. (1:246; 2:284–8)*

Questions 88 through 92 match symptoms with the definition.

88. **(B)** A false belief that is inconsistent with a subject's intelligence, level of maturity, and social background is called a *delusion. (1:219; 2:190)*

89. **(D)** An *obsession* is a recurrent, intrusive, disturbing thought. The subject may have a repetitive intrusive thought that she is going to die or may attack someone. The sufferer is quite aware that the thought is illogical and finds the obsession distressing.

    A *compulsion* is an illogical act that the subject feels forced to carry out repetitiously. In *obsessive–compulsive disorder,* recurrent thoughts are obsessions, recurrent acts are compulsions—both are illogical, repetitive, and intrusive. *(1:218,404–9; 2:473–4)*

90. **(A)** An *illusion* is a misinterpretation of an actual perceptual stimulus. The quality of the misinterpretation is a reflection of the subject's emotional state. The confused, frightened senile patient may misinterpret the chatter of the nursing staff in the distance as a plan to kill her. *(1:221; 2:190)*

91. **(E)** A false perception without an actual reality stimulus is termed a *hallucination.* The schizophrenic may hear voices where there are no external auditory stimuli. This is different from the illusion described in question 90, where an external auditory stimulus is present but is misinterpreted. *(1:220–1; 2:190)*

92. **(C)** A *phobia* is a persistent irrational fear. The subject knows that this fear is illogical but cannot prevent the recurrent intrusion of the phobia into his or her thinking. In phobias, the fear is focused on a defined target: fear of germs—mysophobia; fear of open spaces—agoraphobia; fear of heights—acrophobia. *(1:220; 2:458–9)*

In questions 93 through 97, definitions are matched with brief clinical statements.

93. **(D)** *Circumstantiality* is manifested by rambling and digressions by a speaker who eventually gets to the point. We all know many very normal people who are circumstantial, even though this symptom may be evidence of a developing thought disorder. *(1:218; 2:189)*

94. **(G)** *Looseness of associations* is present in thought disorders where there is no obvious connection in the thinking process—there is no clear train of thought for the listener to follow. Looseness of associations indicates a defect in thought processing. *(1:219,330; 2:189)*

95. **(C)** *Glossolalia* is "speaking in tongues," the verbal expression that may appear strange and unintelligible to the observer. In some religious groups this is a way of sharing personal revelation. In other situations, glossolalia may be a manifestation of a thought disorder. *(1:219; 2:1253)*

96. **(B)** *Perseveration* is the inflexible repetition of the same verbal or motoric response to different stimuli or questions. This symptom occurs most often in patients with organic disorders. *(1:218; 2:286,1273)*

97. **(F)** Thought *blocking*, the sudden interruption in the train of thought, occurs in many normal and pathological situations. Many students have experienced thought blocking in the stress of an oral examination—"My mind just went blank when he asked me the question"—but thought blocking can be a sign of a more serious thought disorder. *(1:219; 2:189)*

    Tangentiality is present when the patient in his speaking or thinking goes off on all kinds of tangents and never gets to the point. *(1:218; 2:189)*

    Flight of ideas is a very rapid flow of speech and ideas that appears increasingly disconnected and outwardly illogical as the flow becomes faster. *(1:219; 2:189)*

    Neologisms are words made up by the patient. Sometimes the underlying thoughts and intent are apparent from the structure of the neologisms, in other instances the neologism is totally idiosyncratic. Neologisms tend to be pathognomonic of schizophrenia. *(1:218; 2:189)*

Answers 98 through 102 define various paraphilias, sexual deviations. (1:443–465; 2:592–5)

98. **(A)** *Sadism* is the achievement of sexual pleasure by inflicting pain on the sexual object. Sadism is named after the author de Sade. *(1:445; 2:642–3)*

99. **(D)** *Masochism* is the achievement of sexual pleasure by enduring inflicted pain. Masochism is named after Sacher-Masoch, an Austrian writer. *(1:445–6; 2:592–5)*

100. **(B)** In *pedophilia*, the paraphiliac achieves sexual gratification through some form of contact with a child. Pedophilia is usually applied to the relationship of an adult, at least 16 years old, with a child, at least 5 years younger, and does not refer to activities between children. *(1:444–5; 2:592–5)*

101. **(C)** *Voyeurism* or *Scopophilia* is the pattern of achieving sexual pleasure by watching sexual organs or the sexual activities of others. A "Peeping Tom" is a *voyeur*. *(1:446; 2:592–5)*

102. **(E)** *Incest* is the occurrence of sexual relations between close members of the same family. For incest to be present a blood relationship is not necessary. A sexual relationship between a stepfather and stepchild would usually be considered incestuous. *(1:463–4)*

Various terms dealing with drug dependence are considered in answers 103 through 107. (1:278–83)

103. **(B)** An *abstinence* or *withdrawal syndrome* is a term for the physical and emotional symptoms that occur on the withdrawal of a drug to which the subject has been addicted. *Addiction* implies dependence on the drug with the presence of physical withdrawal symptoms. *(1:279; 2:324–5.339–40)*

104. **(A)** *Habituation* is the psychological dependence on a drug because of its pleasurable or tension-relieving effect. Habituation or *habit formation* implies only emotional dependence with periodic or continuous craving; where there is also physical dependence, a *withdrawal syndrome* with physical symptoms occurs on stopping the drug. *(1:279)*

105. **(E)** The term *drug abuse* (*substance abuse*), as defined by the World Health Organization, is the use of drugs, persistently or sporadically, for other than acceptable medical purposes. *(1:279)*

106. **(C)** *Drug dependence*, with the qualifying phrase specifying the drug or type of drugs involved, implies a state of psychological dependence, with or without physical dependence, on that drug or drug type. *(1:279)*

107. **(D)** Where there is *tolerance* to a drug, the individual finds a decreasing effect from the same dose of the drug and has to increase the drug dosage to produce the same desired effect. *(1:279; 2:315)*

Questions 108 through 120 match different terms with their definitions.

108. **(C)** Where there is *thought blocking*, there is a sudden interruption in the flow of thinking. This *thought deprivation* or blocking can occur in normal people or in less serious emotional disorders. Where blocking is marked, the symptom usually indicates a schizophrenic illness. *(1:219; 2:189, 365)*

109. **(A)** Where an individual manifests a very rapid process of thinking, at times without obvious connection between thoughts, he is said to be showing a *flight of ideas*. This symptom is most characteristic of the manic state. *(1:219; 2:189, 404–5)*

110. **(E)** *Cyclothymia*, mood swings, is a state of alternating periods of depression and elation and is sometimes considered to be a mild form of bipolar disorder. Many well functioning people have a mild form of cyclothymia. *Kretschmer* suggested that cyclothymia typically occurs in people with *pyknic* constitutional build—with well developed trunk and somewhat short limbs. *(1:386–8; 2:414–5)*

111. **(B)** *Akathisia*, the "restless leg" syndrome, is a side effect of many neuroleptic drugs, especially of the piperazine and butyrophenone group. The patient may feel restless and unable to keep still, and may complain that his or her feet are restless. Even though the patient may not feel anxious, akathesia symptoms may superficially mimic some of the motoric symptoms of anxiety. *(1:218; 2:779–80)*

112. **(D)** A *catastrophic reaction* is the acute eruption of anxiety that occurs in patients with organic brain syndromes when the subject becomes unavoidably aware of his or her mental handicaps. The patient may present with a wide range of disruptive symptoms. *(1:167,246; 2:285)*

113. **(F)** A *tic* is a rapid, involuntary, spasmodic movement of functionally related muscle groups. Though tics are involuntary, they can usually be suppressed for periods of time. Some children with tics are able to suppress tics in the classroom and then allow tic discharge in the privacy of the school restroom. *(1:756–63; 2:684–8)*

114. **(A)** A *fugue* is a form of dissociative disorder in which the patient assumes a new identity with amnesia for the old identity. The syndrome is uncommon and most often occurs in situations of severe personal stress. In most cases, the fugue state is brief, recovery is spontaneous and recurrence infrequent. *(1:430–1; 2:566–9)*

115. **(D)** *Pica* is usually defined as the persistent eating of non-food materials—clay, paint chips, plaster, hair, and other non-nutritious materials. Pica is more common in certain cultural groups. In some Southern communities it is very common for pregnant women to eat starch or clay at some time during the pregnancy. *(1:740–1; 2:679–81)*

116. **(C)** *Affect* is the external expression of emotions as opposed to *mood* which is the inner experience of emotions. Affect is the part of emotions that can be observed—crying, sadness, and rage, and other outward expressions of emotion. *(1:214,363; 2:188)*

117. **(E)** *Rumination* is the repeated chewing, swallowing, regurgitating, and rechewing of food. This rare and potentially fatal syndrome is most often seen in mentally retarded infants but can also be seen in adults. *(1:741–2; 2:681–3)*

118. **(H)** *Hypochondriasis* is manifested by an unrealistic interpretation of physical sensations, a preoccupation with bodily functions and fears of possible diseases. These fears are not delusional but may be disabling; typically these concerns persist in spite of repeated reassurance. *(1:422–4; 2:547–9)*

119. **(I)** *Coprolalia*, the compulsive utterance of obscenities, may be part of a tic disorder, a paraphilia symptom or a manifestation of other disorders. Kopros is the Greek word for dung so "copro-" at the beginning of a word usually indicates filth, feces or obscenity; coprophagy is the eating of feces, sometimes a manifestation of pica. *(1:447, 756; 2:686)*

120. **(G)** *Panic* typically occurs in episodic acute attacks of extreme anxiety and dread with fear of dying, going crazy or losing control. The patients show marked physical signs of anxiety. *(1:394–400; 2:443–58)*

Trichotillomania is the compulsive pulling out of one's own hair. The hair is often chewed or swallowed, sometimes producing a *hair ball (trichobezoar)* in the stomach. *(1:491–3; 2:617–9)*

Mutism is the continuous refusal to speak. Elective mutism, selective mutism, is one of the few childhood syndromes that is more common in girls than in boys. *(1:218, 772–3; 2:694–7)*

CHAPTER 2

Psychological Testing
Questions

INTRODUCTION

For many examinations and certainly for general clinical practice, the professional trainee will need more information about psychological testing than is given in standard psychiatry textbooks. It is difficult, if not impossible, to learn the purpose and the usefulness of psychological testing from books, lectures, or seminars. The student should take every opportunity to see the actual test materials, to watch testing in different settings, and to discuss the validity of testing with the professionals who administer, interpret, and use the tests.

REFERENCES

1. Chapter 5,   Psychology and Psychiatry: Psychometric and Neuropsychological Testing, pp 155–170

   Chapter 31,   Child Psychiatry: Assessment, Examination and Psychological Testing. Developmental and Psychological Testing, pp 681–4

2. Chapter 8,   Psychological Assessment: Tests and Rating Scales, pp 225–46.

   Table of Psychological Tests, pp 1277–9

DIRECTIONS (Questions 1 through 17): Each of the numbered items or incomplete statements in this section is followed by answers or by completions of the statement. Select the ONE lettered answer or completion that is BEST in each case.

1. Which test would be most helpful in evaluating the emotional boundaries and appreciation of reality in an adult patient?

    (A) Stanford–Binet
    (B) Vineland
    (C) Bender–Gestalt
    (D) Rorschach
    (E) Halstead-Reitan

2. The scoring of the Rorschach test takes into account all of the following *except*

    (A) use of color and shading
    (B) response to the whole blot
    (C) ability to copy designs
    (D) popular and unusual responses
    (E) use of the white areas

3. All of the following statements are valid about intelligence testing *except*

    (A) affected by the subject's motivation
    (B) culturally biased
    (C) tend to emphasize verbal ability
    (D) high scores are incompatible with psychosis
    (E) measures skills enhanced by traditional education

4. The Galvanic Skin Resistance is a measure often used in psychophysiological studies. It reflects

    (A) skin warmth
    (B) blood flow through the superficial tissues
    (C) heart rate and output
    (D) sweat gland activity
    (E) muscle tension

5. All of the following statements apply to the Minnesota Multiphasic Personality Inventory (MMPI) *except*

    (A) subjects may be able to predict acceptable answers from the nature of the questions
    (B) it may be given to a group at one time
    (C) it requires a high level of professional skill to administer and score
    (D) questions may arouse or increase the subject's anxiety
    (E) it places a high emphasis on verbal comprehension

6. Some indication of the inner fantasy of a nine-year-old child may be given by all of the following tests *except*

    (A) modeling clay
    (B) Children's Apperception Test
    (C) Bender–Gestalt Test
    (D) finger painting
    (E) toy soldier play

7. All of the following statements apply to the Thematic Apperception Test *except*

    (A) blank card included in the test series
    (B) includes three colored cards towards the end of the series
    (C) made up of ambiguous pictures
    (D) usually reflects the subject's mood and quality of emotions
    (E) prompts sharing of feeling about family relationships

8. The Draw-a-Person Test, the Sentence Completion Test, and the Thematic Apperception Test are similar in that they

    (A) all require the subject to draw
    (B) are projective tests
    (C) measure intelligence
    (D) diagnose sensory-motor incoordination
    (E) can be machine scored

9. The Word Association Test was first used by

    (A) S. Freud
    (B) A. Adler
    (C) K. Horney
    (D) C. Jung
    (E) H. Rorschach

10. Psychological testing can reasonably be requested for all of the following *except*

    (A) localizing a lesion in the brain
    (B) comparing present intelligence capabilities with previous functioning
    (C) differentiating psychotic and organic disorders
    (D) measuring vocational aptitude
    (E) evaluating suitability for psychotherapy

11. The validity of a psychological test refers to the

    (A) ability of the test to measure what it is supposed to measure
    (B) consistency the test shows on test–retest results
    (C) absence of cultural bias

(D) test usefulness in predicting outcome

(E) lack of examiner bias

Questions 12 and 13

You are evaluating an eight-year-old girl from an innercity school. Her school report states she has an 80 Intelligence Quotient.

12. When you are asked the significance of this intelligence rating, you should state that

(A) the child is in the borderline retarded range

(B) the youngster is probably above average in basic intelligence

(C) until you know the type and circumstance of the testing, you do not know

(D) ghetto girls are normally more advanced than boys

(E) all testing at this age level has poor predictive value

13. You learn that this intelligence quotient is based on one group test. You can state that all of the following are true *except*

(A) this would most likely have been a paper-and-pencil test

(B) the test result was strongly influenced by verbal and reading skills

(C) biased by sociocultural factors

(D) affected by individual motivation

(E) cannot exclude severe retardation

14. All of the following statements apply to the Bender–Gestalt Test *except*

(A) test cards have geometric designs

(B) subject is asked to copy designs

(C) used in eliciting psychotic responses

(D) useful in diagnosing brain damage

(E) evaluates perceptual-motor coordination

15. The ratio of the Mental Age over the Chronological Age multiplied by 100 is the

(A) rating of mental retardation

(B) Intelligence Quotient

(C) Social Maturity Rating

(D) Rorschach F score

(E) performance rating on the Weschler Intelligence Scale

16. The Cattell Infant Intelligence Scale

(A) can be used up to grade school age

(B) predicts intelligence level in childhood and adult life

(C) measures neuromuscular development

(D) cannot detect mental retardation

(E) is based largely on parental reporting

17. Group psychological tests are less reliable than individual tests due to all of the following *except*

(A) they are dependent on reading ability

(B) they test speed more than other factors

(C) anxiety interferes with reading speed

(D) they are valid only with adults

(E) individual motivation is less easily measured

DIRECTIONS (Questions 18 through 24): Each set of matching questions in this section consists of a list of five to eight lettered options followed by a set of numbered words or phrases. For each numbered word or phrase, select the ONE lettered option that is most closely associated with it. Each lettered heading may be selected once, more than once, or not at all.

Questions 18 through 22

(A) ambiguous pictures

(B) geometric designs

(C) identifying body parts

(D) inkblots

(E) sentence completion

(F) clerical speed and accuracy

(G) reports of social functioning

(H) positive and negative responses

Match the test named below with the description listed above.

18. Rorschach

19. Thematic Apperception

20. Bender–Gestalt

21. Minnesota Multiphasic Personality Inventory (MMPI)

22. Vineland Scale

Questions 23 through 25

    (A) verbal and performance scale scores

    (B) reading readiness scores

    (C) mechanical aptitude scores

    (D) pre-kindergarten motor and language scores

    (E) health and physical development scores

    (F) select from multiple choices to complete picture

Match the test named below with the description listed in column one.

23. Gesell Developmental Schedule

24. Weschler Intelligence Scale for Children

25. Raven's Progressive Matrices

Answers and Explanations

1. **(D)** In the *Rorschach Test*, the subject is presented with ambiguous stimuli (inkblots) for which the subject must supply the structure. Where the person being examined lacks a definite sense of individual reality and firm personal boundaries, it is impossible for the subject to give clearly defined, reality-based responses to these unstructured stimuli. *(1:159–60; 2:234–5,241)*
A. The *Stanford–Binet Test,* developed from the first intelligence tests published by Binet, was used extensively for intelligence testing of children and adults. Child psychologists still find it especially useful in evaluating mental retardation and for testing preschool children. *(1:683; 2:98,703)*
B. The *Vineland Social Maturity Scale* determines the patient's *Developmental Quotient* based on social function as noted by observers, usually parents. This rating is not based on direct clinical observation. *(1:682; 2:703–4)*
C. The *Bender–Gestalt Test* is used in testing perceptual-visual-motor coordination and immediate visual recall. Though it has been used by some psychologists as a form of projective test, this use needs much more extensive validation. *(1:166; 2:301,1277)*
E. The *Halstead-Reitan Battery* is composed of ten tests which together help to differentiate brain-damaged from neurologically intact patients. *(1:168–9; 2:239–40)*

2. **(C)** In the *Rorschach Test,* the patient does not copy the designs (as is done with the Bender–Gestalt geometric designs). Several of the cards present color stimuli and all show shadowing tones. The subject's ability to respond to the whole card is significant, as are responses to the white or unshaded areas of the card. Each inkblot has responses that are usual, common, or popular, but the range of unusual responses is limitless and all reflect the personality of the subject. *(1:159–60; 2:234–5)*

3. **(D)** Many psychotic patients can score well on intelligence tests. Paranoid patients are especially good on these tests: high scores in intelligence tests are in no way incompatible with psychotic illness.
Testing results are highly affected by the patient's motivation and level of energy at the time of testing. If the patient does not try or does not wish to cooperate, the scores will be lowered.
Most intelligence tests tend to emphasize verbal ability and often reading ability also—especially group paper-and-pencil tests, on which many school intelligence ratings are based. Intelligence tests tend to be biased against minority groups or lower socioeconomic populations. They emphasize skills learned in traditional education rather than survival ability, the capacity for productive action, or nonverbal skills. Intelligence testing may set up a self-fulfilling prophecy. A minority group child may test at a low score level because the test is culturally biased. The child's educational program is often geared to the level of his or her test score, to meet the needs only of a less capable child. Intellectually, the youngster may then be stunted by an insufficiently stimulating or an unrewarding academic program, thus leading to equally low or lower intelligence test scores later. *(1:155–7,683; 2:238–9)*

4. **(D)** The *galvanic skin resistance (GSR)* is a manifestation of changes in skin resistance to the passage of a weak electric current and is largely responsive to sweat gland activity. This measure has often been used in the evaluation of the physical aspects of emotion. *(1:594)*

5. **(C)** One of the most useful attributes of the *Minnesota Multiphasic Personality Inventory (MMPI)* is that it can be administered and scored by a relatively untrained person. The final evaluation of the score should be done by a professional clinician. Response C is thus incorrect.
A reasonably alert subject can guess from many of the questions what is likely to be the expected and acceptable answer. The MMPI is frequently given as a group paper-and-pencil test. Both the group test and the individual test require that the subject read and understand the long se-

ries of questions. Because of the nature of the questions and the directness of each question, the individual may be made quite anxious. *(1:157–8; 2:229–30)*

6. **(C)** When children are *modeling clay* or *finger painting* on blank paper, they are forced to express themselves to give form, integration, and quality to their activities. With *toy soldiers,* the stimulus is more specific but still allows for freedom of self-expression and the use of inner fantasy. The *Children's Apperception Test (CAT)* is merely a more formal way of presenting ambiguous stimuli on which children must express (project) themselves and show their own personalities and inner fantasies. *(1:684; 2:1003,1277)*

   The *Bender–Gestalt Test* measures visual motor coordination and immediate visual recall; this test is not usually used to elicit a child's fantasy. *(1:166; 2:1277)*

7. **(B)** The *Thematic Apperception Test* does not have any colored cards. Answer B is wrong.

   The test is a series of ambiguous picture scenes that are planned to bring out the subject's mood and feelings. Many of the pictures show situations that are easily perceived as family interaction and thus prompt the expression of feelings about family relationships. The card series has one blank card that may be given to the subject, who is asked to make up a story completely without external stimuli. *(1:160–2; 2:241)*

8. **(B)** The *Draw-a-Person Test,* the *Sentence Completion Test,* and the *Thematic Apperception Test* are all similar in that they require subjects to express themselves and to project feelings and ideas in order to do or to complete the test. Thus they are all projective tests.

   Only the Draw-a-Person Test requires the subject to draw. None of these three tests specifically measure intelligence though they are all strongly affected by the subject's motivation, intelligence, and academic and cultural background.

   On the Draw-a-Person Test, sensory-motor incoordination may be apparent but this is better measured by other tests.

   None of the three tests can be machine scored. *(1:160–3; 2:229,241,1277–9)*

9. **(D)** *Carl Jung* (1875–1961), the Swiss analyst, developed the use of the *Word Association Test* to demonstrate emotional drives and conflicts. *(1:163; 2:153–4)*

10. **(A)** Psychological testing results are too nonspecific to give more than a very gross localization of a *brain lesion.* In the hands of a few specialized testers, localization may be fairly good, but in general clinical practice other localizing techniques are much more efficient.

   Psychological testing is clinically useful in comparing past and present intellectual functioning, to differentiate psychotic and organic states, to measure vocational aptitude, and to evaluate suitability for psychotherapy. *(1:163–72; 2:239–40)*

11. **(A)** The validity of a psychological test refers to the level of accuracy with which it measures what it is supposed to measure. The validity of intelligence testing has been shown by the way these scales accurately assess mental retardation levels. The reliability of a test refers to its ability to show consistent test–retest results or when used by different examiners. *(1:137–8; 2:227–8)*

12. **(C)** The clinician does not know the significance of any *intelligence quotient score* of any person until he or she knows the circumstances of the testing, the tests given, and the subject's social and academic background. In the situation described there is not sufficient information.

   Unfortunately, many children are labeled "borderline retarded" solely on the basis of an Intelligence Quotient rating. *(1:155–7,683; 2:238–9,706)*

13. **(E)** Because a *group test* is most often a paper-and-pencil test, strongly influenced by verbal and reading skills, biased by sociocultural factors, and markedly affected by individual motivation, you can indeed state that a youngster who scores even moderately well is unlikely to be severely retarded. With all these factors weighing against a high score, you can accept the fact that the child's intelligence level is not below the scored IQ 80— that is, the test result does indeed exclude severe retardation. *(1:155–5, 683; 2:706)*

14. **(C)** Although the subject may show psychotic responses to the *Bender–Gestalt Test,* this test is not used specifically to elicit psychotic responses.

   The subject is usually asked to copy geometric designs from test cards and then sometimes by memory. The test measures perceptual motor coordination and visual recall and is thus useful in diagnosing brain damage. *(1:166; 2:1277)*

15. **(B)** $$\frac{\text{Mental age}}{\text{Chronological age}} \times 100 = \text{Intelligence Quotient}$$

   Mental retardation can be rated as an intelligence quotient level. *(1:685–6; 2:238)*

   The *Vineland Adaptive Behavior Scales* measure social maturity behavior based on parent interview and teacher rating. *(1:682; 2:703–4)*

   The *F score* on the *Rorschach Test* is the measure of good or poor form responses to the inkblots. *(1:159–60; 2:240–1)*

The *Performance Scale* on the *Weschler Intelligence Scale* is a summation of the five nonverbal tests. The *Verbal Scale* measures the verbal subtests. *(1:156–7; 2:238–9)*

16. **(C)** The *Cattell Infant Intelligence Scale* primarily measures *neuromuscular ability,* the ability to grasp, sit, stand, walk, talk, self-feed, and self-care in children from 3 to 36 months. The test can detect moderate degrees of mental retardation that are usually evident in the child's slower neuromuscular development. The test does not go beyond three years of age, after which the Stanford–Binet is used. This test, while it can detect moderate to severe retardation, has no predictive ability to indicate the level of intelligence the child may attain in later life. Infant tests are notoriously poor at predicting.

The Cattell Scale is based on direct child testing; the Vineland Scale uses parental observations. *(1:682–3; 2:1277)*

17. **(D)** *Group psychological tests* are used extensively with *children* as well as with *adults.* Most routine school psychological tests are given in group situations.

The other statements are reasons why group tests are less reliable. They are dependent on verbal and reading ability. They do place high emphasis on speed. Anxiety can markedly interfere with reading and writing speed. In individual testing, motivation is much more easily evaluated. *(1:155, 683)*

18. **(D)** The *Rorschach Test* uses *inkblots* as the unstructured stimuli to produce personality projection. The *Holtzman Test* also uses inkblots. *(1:159–60; 2:234–5)*

19. **(A)** In the *Thematic Apperception Test,* the subject is asked to respond to a set of cards showing *ambiguous pictures.* *(1:160–2; 2:241)*

20. **(B)** The subject is asked to copy a series of *geometric designs* in the *Bender–Gestalt Test* with the original in front of him and sometimes also from memory. *(1:166; 2:1277)*

21. **(H)** In the *Minnesota Multiphasic Personality Inventory (MMPI),* the subject is asked to respond "true," "false," or "cannot say" to a long series of questions. From the *positive, negative,* and *uncertain* responses, the inventory is scored. *(1:157–8; 2:229–30)*

22. **(D)** The *Vineland Social Maturity Scale* is most often used with children. From reports of the child's functioning, usually from parents and teachers, the youngster's social development is evaluated and her *Developmental Quotient* measured. *(1:682; 2:703–4)*

23. **(D)** The *Gesell Developmental Schedule* gives scores on social, motor, language and adaptive skills for pre-kindergarten-age children, based on direct observations and reports from caretakers. *(1:683; 2:92–3,99–100)*

24. **(A)** The *Weschler Intelligence Scale for Children - Revised* (the WISC-R) is the most widely used intelligence test for school-age children. This test provides verbal and performance scale scores and a full-scale Intelligence Quotient score. *(1:683; 2:238)*

25. **(F)** *Raven's Progressive Matrices* present the patient with an increasingly complex sequence of designs that the subject is expected to complete. This test, which does not use language and is relatively culture fair, can be used to measure intelligence and to detect impaired visual-constructive ability and posterior hemisphere brain damage. *(1:166)*

Child and Adolescent Psychiatry
Questions

INTRODUCTION

Most examinations have questions on how to manage the child as a member of the family. Often the questions are awkwardly stated but they are trying to elicit some principle. The answers required may seem rigid or dogmatic because only one response is sought when usually there are various possibilities that are correct to different degrees.

REFERENCES

1. Chapters 31–44, Child and Adolescent Psychiatry, pp 678–806

2. Chapter 21,   Disorders Usually First Evident in Infancy, Childhood or Adolescence, pp 649–735

   30,   Treatment of Children and Adolescents, pp 985–1020

DIRECTIONS (Questions 1 through 38): Each of the numbered items or incomplete statements in this section is followed by answers or by completions of the statement. Select the ONE lettered answer or completion that is BEST in each case.

1. You get a phone call from a mother whose four-year-old son has just asked, "Mommy, where do I come from?" You should advise her to

   (A) pretend she did not hear the question
   (B) find out what the child wants to know
   (C) demonstrate on herself and the child's father the differences between boys and girls
   (D) punish him for asking such a nasty question
   (E) bring the child in for the next available appointment when you will teach him simple biology

2. A worried mother asks you how to manage her four-year-old son, who she says is stealing. Apparently he keeps bringing home toys that belong to other children. You should advise her to

   (A) take the toys back herself, without any fuss, and buy him similar toys
   (B) tell him that if he stops stealing, he will have a reward every weekend
   (C) point out that this is stealing and spank him
   (D) make sure he has enough toys and see that he returns the toys to the owners
   (E) ignore the whole affair; this is a developmental phase that will soon pass

3. The hospital attendants find a confused sixteen-year-old girl wandering in the hospital parking lot where apparently her friends have left her.

   She seems physically normal and allows you to do a thorough physical. Periodically she asks you to be quiet as she listens to sounds that no one else can hear and to look at the little animals "like rabbits or small dogs" that she sees running around the emergency room. All of the following are applicable except

   (A) she is likely to be suffering from an acute toxic psychosis due to drug abuse
   (B) you reassure, reorient, and support
   (C) reduced sensory stimulation may be helpful
   (D) after these symptoms clear, she may have recurrent hallucinatory episodes ("flashbacks") even without further drug use
   (E) you can be sure that she will recover fully from the episode

4. A sixteen-year-old diabetic teenager insists on a weekly physical checkup but nevertheless does not cooperate in his necessary medical treatment. He is probably showing manifestations of

   (A) schizophrenia, disorganized type
   (B) organic mental disorder
   (C) malingering
   (D) obsessive-compulsive disorder
   (E) oppositional defiant disorder

5. A teenage boy in psychotherapy says to his psychotherapist, "Nobody cares for me." The therapist knows the adolescent is receiving at least the usual amount of family love and attention. The doctor should respond

   (A) "Of course your family cares for you."
   (B) "I wonder why that should be so."
   (C) "I care for you."
   (D) "How much caring do you need?"
   (E) "Maybe you are not worth caring for."

Questions 6 through 9

6. In classical school phobia, the problem typically arises because the

   (A) child has been a scapegoat in school
   (B) teacher is rigid, punitive, and overly demanding
   (C) parents have unreasonably high academic standards
   (D) child is mentally retarded
   (E) child has difficulty separating from the parents

7. Separation anxiety disorder is seen

   (A) only in boys
   (B) only in kindergarten or first-grade children
   (C) where the Oedipus complex is not resolved
   (D) at every age level in childhood and adolescence
   (E) mainly in unusually intelligent, sensitive children

8. To prevent school refusal, parents should

   (A) make sure children know the sexual facts of life
   (B) encourage the gradual development of independence from early childhood
   (C) convince children that they will always have their parents to care for them
   (D) point out how unwise they are to be afraid of school
   (E) make sure they are protected from frustrations and anxiety as they grow

9. The optimum treatment for school refusal is

   (A) immediate assignment of a homebound teacher
   (B) family therapy for the parents and child
   (C) return the child to school and then work on the underlying problem
   (D) arrange for a change of teacher or school, with family therapy
   (E) hospitalize the child to evaluate his or her functioning when separated from the family

10. A previously normal four-year-old boy is hospitalized for an emergency appendectomy. When he returns from the hospital, he is irritable and demanding. He starts to suck his thumb and, after he has wet his bed several nights in succession, his mother brings him for pediatric examination. The pediatrician will tell the mother that

   (A) these symptoms may be the early signs of severe personality pathology and should be further evaluated
   (B) his behavior is an outward manifestation that the boy is working through his Oedipal conflict
   (C) these regressive symptoms indicate undue psychological dependency and suggest the need for greater independence training
   (D) this is a normal transient reaction to a stressful situation, and with care and support the child should soon revert to his preoperative behavior
   (E) this infantile behavior suggests the possibility of operative anoxia and the child should have further neurological and psychological examination

11. In Tourette's Disorder all of the following are applicable *except*

   (A) multiple tics
   (B) compulsive swearing
   (C) childhood onset
   (D) haloperidol therapeutic
   (E) grandiose delusions

12. Autistic disorder

   (A) occurs more frequently in urban ghetto residents
   (B) may show symptoms similar to those seen with congenital deafness
   (C) is less severe in girls than in boys
   (D) does not occur in African-American children
   (E) was first described by Bleuler

13. All of the following symptoms tend to occur in autistic disorder *except*

   (A) insistence on sameness
   (B) hallucinations
   (C) twirling
   (D) fascination with moving objects
   (E) walking on toes

14. After a visit to the physician, two five-year-old children play "hospital" all afternoon. Their behavior is a manifestation of

   (A) projection
   (B) identification
   (C) rationalization
   (D) displacement
   (E) dissociation

15. As part of an adjustment disorder in adolescence, all of the following symptoms may be present *except*

   (A) school failure
   (B) delinquency
   (C) paranoid delusions
   (D) depression
   (E) stomach and head pains

Questions 16 and 17

When the supermarket checker does not charge for a can of peas, the parents are delighted. Later that evening at the movie theater, they claim their thirteen-year-old daughter is only 11 so that they pay less. Next day they are most upset when their eight-year-old son is caught stealing from lockers in school.

16. The parents' attitude at the supermarket and movie theater is evidence of their

   (A) reaction formation
   (B) intellectualization
   (C) superego lacunae
   (D) undoing
   (E) repression

17. They should remember that their eight-year-old develops his conscience by all of the following mechanisms *except*

   (A) introjection
   (B) projection
   (C) imitation
   (D) internalization
   (E) identification

Questions 18 and 19

In the course of a routine physical examination, a mother mentions that her 4 1/2-year-old son has been sleeping with her and her husband for the past two weeks. The little boy had been having scary dreams of ghosts and witches and felt much safer with his parents.

18. The pediatrician should

    (A) inquire gently about the mother's sexual feeling toward her son
    (B) anticipate that time and family sensitivity will take care of the problem
    (C) assume that the parental marital relationship is unstable
    (D) recommend firmly that the little boy be required to sleep in his own bed
    (E) all of the above

19. The doctor appreciates that

    (A) the little boy is showing early identity confusion
    (B) scary dreams are an early sign of future emotional problems
    (C) the father must be evaluated also
    (D) scary dreams are often part of the normal four- to five-year-old's maturation experience
    (E) none of the above

20. An adjustment reaction in childhood may include all of the following symptoms *except*

    (A) autism
    (B) phobias
    (C) nail biting
    (D) bed wetting
    (E) nightmares

21. On Intelligence Quotient scales, average intelligence is taken as

    (A) 50
    (B) 60–80
    (C) 80–100
    (D) 90–110
    (E) 100–120

22. In which age group is the highest incidence of mental retardation diagnosed?

    (A) infant
    (B) preschool
    (C) kindergarten
    (D) adolescent
    (E) adult

23. The social group with the highest reported incidence of mental retardation is

    (A) urban ghetto residents
    (B) second-generation immigrants
    (C) Jews of Eastern European origin
    (D) blond-haired, blue-eyed Scandinavians
    (E) drug addicts

Questions 24 through 27

24. When you are asked to see an eight-year-old patient with enuresis, you anticipate that the child is likely to be

    (A) a girl
    (B) a boy
    (C) mentally retarded
    (D) autistic
    (E) obsessive-compulsive

25. As you take the history, you recognize that

    (A) enuresis usually has encopresis as an accompanying symptom
    (B) both parents have typically been toilet trained early
    (C) a family history of enuresis is more common
    (D) diurnal enuresis is more common than nocturnal
    (E) usually an organic defect of the urinary tract is an important cause

26. Enuresis occurs

    (A) during all stages of sleep
    (B) primarily during non-REM sleep
    (C) most often when the child has just wakened
    (D) when the child is asleep and hungry
    (E) more often during weekends and vacation periods

27. In the treatment of enuresis, you may wish to use all of the following *except*

    (A) psychotherapy for the child
    (B) imipramine
    (C) conditioning device
    (D) parental counseling
    (E) barbiturates

28. The following statements are applicable to petit mal, absence seizures, *except*

    (A) onset usually in childhood
    (B) disappear before adulthood
    (C) characteristic EEG pattern

(D) usually associated with borderline mental retardation

(E) treated with trimethadione

29. X-rays of long bones of children suffering from chronic lead poisoning show

(A) increased thickness and density at zones of provisional calcification

(B) multiple poorly healed fractures

(C) calcified periosteal hemorrhages

(D) cupping and fraying of the distal ends with generalized reduction in shaft density

(E) premature closure of epiphyses

30. The child with attention deficit hyperactivity disorder

(A) grows out of the symptoms by the end of adolescence

(B) may benefit from treatment with stimulants

(C) is most likely to be a grade-school girl

(D) frequently develops a convulsive disorder

(E) commonly becomes an adolescent schizophrenic

31. At 4:00 AM you are called by the mother of an eleven-year-old asthmatic boy who has had recurrent severe asthma for three years. She is strongly convinced about the emotional basis for asthma. She has read about asthma being called a "cry for mother." The boy is in the midst of an acute asthmatic attack. The mother thinks you should see him now so you can begin to deal with his basic emotional problems. Considering the above course of events, you should

(A) make an appointment to see the mother and the boy in your office that morning at 9:00 AM

(B) tell the mother that this is a case for a pediatrician

(C) tell the mother you will be willing to help the boy but only in conjunction with close pediatric care

(D) see the boy an hour later in your office for his first psychotherapy session

(E) realize that this early morning call must be prompted by the mother's over-anxiety so you arrange to see her alone in your office the next morning

32. The normal child can appreciate that death is irreversible when the youngster is

(A) two years old

(B) three years old

(C) five years old

(D) seven years old

(E) twelve years old

33. Sleepwalking

(A) tends to run in families

(B) is most common in preschool children

(C) is caused by emotional tension

(D) episodes are remembered later

(E) occurs during the latter part of night sleep

34. A four-year-old boy is brought to the pediatric emergency room because he is frantically trying to run away from monsters he sees coming to eat him. Even in the examining room he tries to escape from the monsters. His symptoms are most likely a manifestation of

(A) moderate mental retardation

(B) autistic disorder

(C) toxic psychosis

(D) panic disorder

(E) childhood schizophrenia

35. About 50% of children will have physical and/or mental defects if the mother has rubella

(A) during her adolescence

(B) in the first month of pregnancy

(C) in the fourth month of pregnancy

(D) in the sixth month of pregnancy

(E) just before delivery

36. In diagnosing phenylketonuria, you might find all of the following except

(A) musty odor to urine

(B) hydrocephalus

(C) retardation in siblings

(D) dermatitis

(E) blond hair, blue eyes

37. School refusal is usually a manifestation of

(A) mental retardation

(B) infantile autism

(C) separation anxiety

(D) malingering

(E) attention deficit hyperactivity disorder

38. The childhood syndromes of fire-setting, functional enuresis, and autistic disorder are similar in that they

(A) are much more common in boys

(B) should be treated in a hospital setting

(C) respond to imipramine

(D) were first described by Leo Kanner

(E) lead to childhood schizophrenia

DIRECTIONS (Questions 39 through 80): Each set of items in this section consists of a list of lettered headings followed by several numbered words or phrases. For each numbered word or phrase, select the ONE lettered option that is most closely associated with it. Each lettered option may be selected once, more than once, or not at all.

Questions 39 through 43

    (A) urine with musty odor
    (B) reversal of letters and words
    (C) lead poisoning
    (D) separation from mother in second six months of life
    (E) more common in girls than in boys

For each clinical syndrome, select the associated clinical statement.

39. Pica

40. Phenylketonuria

41. Anaclitic depression

42. Elective mutism, selective mutism

43. Strephosymbolia

Questions 44 through 47

    (A) autosomal recessive inheritance
    (B) butyrophenones therapeutically effective
    (C) more frequent with elderly mother
    (D) imipramine symptomatically effective treatment

For each of the diagnoses listed, select the appropriate clinical statement.

44. Down's syndrome

45. Functional enuresis, enuresis

46. Phenylketonuria

47. Tourette's Disorder

Questions 48 through 52

    (A) coprolalia
    (B) fecal soiling
    (C) short stature, webbed neck
    (D) twirling
    (E) hair pulling and baldness

For each diagnosis, select the appropriate symptom.

48. Encopresis

49. Tourette's Disorder

50. Trichotillomania

51. Turner's syndrome

52. Autistic disorder

Questions 53 through 55

    (A) Klinefelter's Syndrome
    (B) Tay-Sach's Disease
    (C) Turner's Syndrome
    (D) Wilson's Disease
    (E) Down's Syndrome
    (F) Tourette's Disorder
    (G) Korsakoff's Syndrome

For each chromosome listing below, select the correct syndrome or disease.

53. XXY-47 chromosomes

54. 45 chromosomes

55. trisomy 21

Questions 56 through 58

    (A) 2 months
    (B) 6 months
    (C) 10 months
    (D) 2 years
    (E) 3 years

For each motoric task listed below, select the normal age when this is achieved.

56. Reach for and grasp a toy

57. Ride a tricycle

58. Pick up a small object using thumb and index finger

Questions 59 through 61

    (A) 2 months
    (B) 5 months
    (C) 6 months
    (D) 12 months
    (E) 18 months

From the age levels listed above, select the correct age when the following social skills are shown.

59. Smiles

60. Holds out arms to be held

61. Says two or three words

Questions 62 through 64

(A) 1 month
(B) 2 months
(C) 4 months
(D) 6 months
(E) 10 months

Match each level of development with the appropriate age level.

62. Begins to hold up head

63. Sits for brief periods

64. Stands without support

Questions 65 through 69

(A) neurofibroma, optic glioma
(B) cerebral angioma, convulsions, retardation
(C) ovarian dysgenesis, sexual infantilism, XO-45 chromosomes
(D) retardation, brain glioma, pulmonary and renal cysts
(E) progressive intellectual and motor deterioration, hepatic cirrhosis

Match the physical findings with the appropriate syndrome.

65. Facial "port wine stain"

66. Adenoma sebaceum of the face

67. Café au lait spots and skin polyps

68. Greenish-brown ring in the iris

69. Short stature, webbed neck

Questions 70 through 74

(A) 47 chromosomes, XXY pattern
(B) lack of phenylalanine hydroxylase
(C) Jewish infants of Eastern European extraction
(D) Rh incompatibility between mother and fetus
(E) chromosome 5, short arm deletion

Match the syndrome with the predisposing or etiologic factor.

70. Progressive weakness, cherry-red spot on macula, early death

71. Severe retardation, dermatitis, convulsions, blonde hair, blue eyes

72. Marked retardation, microcephaly, catlike cry in childhood

73. Mild retardation, asthenic build, testicular atrophy, gynecomastia

74. Retardation, choreo-athetosis, deafness, yellow-pigmented basal ganglia

Questions 75 through 77

(A) pimozide
(B) calcium disodium versenate
(C) pemoline
(D) carbamazepine

Match the childhood illness with the appropriate treatment.

75. Attention deficit hyperactivity disorder

76. Tourette's Disorder

77. Lead poisoning

Questions 78 through 80

(A) trichotillomania
(B) Munchausen's Syndrome
(C) tardive dyskinesia
(D) Tourette's Disorder
(E) autistic disorder
(F) elective mutism, selective mutism

For each patient description, select the most likely diagnosis.

78. An eight-year-old boy who has recurrent shoulder shrugging and makes periodic "shi. . shi. . . " and throat clearing noises

79. A six-year-old girl who has patches of baldness and no eyebrows

80. A seven-year-old girl who can be heard talking to her cat but does not speak to her parents or her teacher

Answers and Explanations

1. **(B)** This question highlights the fact that the supportive parent should answer the child's curiosity in a fashion the youngster can use productively.

   To answer a question, the parents need to know what the child really wants to know. The four-year-old in this example may just want to know whether he comes from Detroit or Philadelphia. By the nature of his question the inquiring youngster indicates what he is seeking and also what information he can usefully integrate. There is no point in overwhelming (or in this case overstimulating) the youngster with information he is not seeking. *(1:36–7; 2:105–6,112)*

2. **(D)** This question deals with the level of comprehension that usually can be expected from a four-year-old child. This is the age period when the child's conscience (superego) is being established and the parental model is especially important.

   A four-year-old finds it difficult to grasp the abstract concept of stealing. His sense of time is still limited so he cannot usefully integrate the idea of a reward after a week. The parents need to know why the child is taking toys from other children. The child should understand that taking other people's possessions is not acceptable. The youngster can be starting to be responsible for his behavior and this can be emphasized by his returning the toys himself, with gentle parent support. *(1:36–7; 2:134)*

3. **(E)** The sixteen-year-old girl presents the symptoms of an *organic mental disorder,* most likely due to one of the hallucinogens. It is not uncommon for such patients to be brought in to the hospital emergency room by the police who have found them wandering, or for these patients to be dropped off near a treatment center by friends or relatives who hesitate to be more closely involved for fear of legal difficulties.

   If the patient is in contact with her surroundings, her anxiety may be relieved by constant reassurance, reorienting, and support. If the girl is out of contact, her symptoms are more likely to improve in an environment of reduced sensory stimulation.

   The patient may indeed have recurrent *flashbacks* after the acute episode is over.

   One of the major hazards of hallucinogen use is the fact that the outcome of the reaction is never totally predictable. A good or a bad "trip" cannot totally be foreseen. The disturbing effects of a drug trip may hang on unexpectedly, and the user has no guarantee that the next trip may not result in a more prolonged disturbed or psychotic state. *(1:280–1; 2:343–5)*

4. **(E)** This teenage diabetic is showing both an insistent dependency and a constant resistance, symptom patterns that together are typical of the *oppositional defiant disorder.*

   In reality, most adolescents are scared, angry, and bitter when they suffer from a chronic illness such as diabetes or epilepsy. They have no prospect of getting well. They may not have control over their own bodies. They are different, possibly handicapped. Often they manifest both their anger and their anxiety in passive–aggressive behavior—behavior that is sometimes self-destructive.

   This patient shows no manifestations of delusional or hallucinatory behavior usually seen in the disorganized (hebephrenic) schizophrenic teenager. He is not deliberately feigning illness, as would be seen in *malingering*. He is not manifesting the memory loss or emotional lability of the patient with an organic mental disorder, which would be a very late development in diabetes due to arteriosclerosis.

   Though his behavior has some of the repetitiveness of the *obsessive compulsive,* this teenager is not compelled to carry out these acts nor does he feel personal anxiety at his recurrent behaviors; others feel the pain. *(1:730–2; 2:641–2,670–2)*

5. **(B)** Many examinations have questions about the process needed to facilitate psychotherapy. The task in psychotherapy is to help the patient understand why he feels the way he does. This means that concrete answers, even socially appropriate answers, may have to be delayed.

   In the psychotherapy relationship, especially

with an adolescent, the response of the psychotherapist is often factual and direct. To facilitate the teenager's introspection and self-awareness, the appropriate response is "I wonder why that should be so." *(1:787–92; 2:1002–4)*

School phobia, or school refusal, as it is sometimes called, is often a manifestation of separation anxiety disorder in children. This is a favorite examination topic. The answers sought by the examination are often much more specific than is possible or reasonable in clinical practice.

6. **(E)** Classically, *school phobia* arises because the child has difficulty separating from the parents—and the parents from the child.

   All the other reasons listed in this question will indeed make the school experience more anxiety-arousing to the child and, in some situations, become major factors in causing and maintaining school refusal. *(1:733–6; 2:673–7)*

7. **(D)** *Separation anxiety disorder* can occur whenever there is a significant emotional separation from previously gratifying and supportive relationships. Separation anxiety can occur throughout life. "Homesickness" is one form of separation anxiety with which most people cope reasonably well.

   Separation anxiety is more liable to occur where the youngster is less mature and more dependent, at the time of first leaving home and going to school. When school phobia, *separation anxiety disorder,* manifests in older children or adults, it suggests a level of emotional vulnerability indicative at that age of more severe psychopathology.

   The correct response is that school phobia can occur at every age level in childhood and adolescence (and in adult life). *(1:733–6; 2:674–5)*

8. **(B)** The optimum way to minimize or prevent *separation anxiety disorder* and *school refusal* is to encourage the gradual development of the child's independence over the years, from early childhood onward. Overprotection may lead to the stunting of growth; overloading with responsibility or with "facts" may overwhelm the youngster. *(1:733–6; 2:673–7)*

9. **(C)** Once the child has left the school or been removed from school, it is usually more difficult to get him or her back into school. With a clear separation, the child's fears become less easily reversible. The longer the child is out of school, the harder it is to go back. The school peers and teachers tend to grow away (socially) from the phobic child who is no longer at school.

   If at all possible the child should be returned to school and maintained there, even in a tenuous fashion—eg, sitting or studying in the counselor's office—while the underlying factors producing the school refusal are defined and handled. In clinical practice it may not be possible to keep the child in school due to factors in the school, the family, and the child—in which case the other measures may be indicated. *(1:733–6; 2:676–7)*

10. **(D)** In this *adjustment disorder* the little boy is showing more regressed behavior; he is acting like a younger child.

    Regression is a return to earlier patterns of behavior. At times of illness we all normally tend to regress. We allow ourselves to be cared for, and we are likely to act in a more self-centered, childlike fashion.

    Regression is a normal response in childhood to the stress of separation, hospitalization, and the trauma of operation. With extra caring and support, the child should soon return to his more mature preoperative behavior. *(1:494–7; 2:605–11,672)*

11. **(E)** The symptoms of *Tourette's Disorder* usually begin in early childhood, most often in the grade school years. Many children present with symptoms of attention deficit hyperactivity disorder before tics appear. In the full-blown syndrome, patients have *multiple tics,* compulsive swearing *(coprolalia),* and often *echolalia.* Patients with less severe manifestations of the disorder are being more frequently diagnosed.

    Patients do not manifest delusional thinking. *(1:760–3; 2:686–8)*

12. **(B)** *Autistic Disorder, Infantile Autism* is rare, occurring in probably less than five in every 10,000 preadolescent children. The syndrome is important to diagnose early and is extremely significant in research into early personality development and the etiology of emotional illness.

    Infantile autism was first described as occurring mainly in intellectual middle- and upper-class families—this was probably due to the initial patient referral base. Further research has shown that this disorder occurs just as frequently in other socioeconomic groups.

    Autism was described as one of the cardinal symptoms of schizophrenia by Bleuler; it was *Leo Kanner* who first defined the syndrome of infantile autism in a classical article which delineated most of the basic symptoms.

    Girls with autistic disorder tend to be more severely affected than boys. Boys are affected three to five times more often than girls. Patients with autistic disorder frequently develop seizures before age twenty.

    Children who are born with or develop early severe hearing loss are likely to develop symptoms very similar to infantile autism. *(1:699–704; 2:711–7)*

13. **(B)** *Hallucinations* do not occur in autistic disorder. If hallucinations are present in a child

younger than age seven or eight, a toxic or organic disorder is likely to be present. *(1:699–704; 2:712–4)*

14. **(B)** *Identification* in these five-year-old children could be an attempt to imitate someone they admire or an effort to cope with their anxiety about someone they fear. *(1:180–1; 2:111–3)*

   Projection is the emotional defense whereby conflictual and anxiety-provoking feelings are externalized and projected onto another person or group. *Rationalization* is a means of intellectually explaining away the otherwise anxiety-causing reality. In *displacement,* the feeling is directed at a more acceptable object or target, and in *dissociation,* disturbing feelings are split off from the rest of the personality. *(1:183–4; 2:135–8)*

15. **(C)** An *adjustment disorder* at any age is a temporary, transitional period of maladaptation in response to unusual stresses.

   Paranoid delusions, or delusions of any kind, would be such a major disruption of reality contact as to indicate more serious psychopathology than implied in the diagnosis of adjustment disorder.

   The other symptoms—school or job failure, delinquency or antisocial behavior, depression or emotional discomfort, and somatic symptoms—all indicate a personality under stress, but stress from which recovery can reasonably be expected with appropriate management, support, and understanding. *(1:494–7; 2:605–11)*

Answers to 16 and 17 are concerned with conscience development.

16. **(C)** Question 16 portrays the kind of *conscience defects (superego lacunae)* that are present in normal parents and families—the conscience lapse that is almost socially acceptable—in avoiding payment at the movie or cheating the income tax authorities, but is not socially tolerable when acted out in other settings—like stealing from other children in school. Children learn from parental examples. *(1:36–7,44; 2:112–3,134–5)*

17. **(B)** The growing child develops a conscience by taking into her personality the qualities and the models she sees in the significant people in her life.

   Introjection, imitation, internalization, and *identification* are all ways the child has of taking in, of internalizing, and of establishing her conscience.

   Projection, on the other hand, is a pushing out, or extruding, and attributing to someone else feelings that are otherwise unacceptable. *(1:36–7, 180;2:134–5)*

18. **(D)** The pediatrician should recommend that the boy sleep in his own bed. Gently but firmly, the

youngster must be taught to tolerate reasonable separation. The parents should support and reward healthy age-appropriate independence. If the parents find it difficult to allow the boy to grow up, time may not take care of the situation.

   When a child routinely sleeps in the parental bed, the parents' sexual activities are likely to be curtailed. In some situations, a child may be encouraged to stay in the parental bed to help perpetuate sexual distance. However, this should not be the first assumption of the physician.

   In any clinical situation, it is best to look for the common patterns of behavior adaptation and maladaptation. It is premature to ask about the mother's sexual feelings toward her son. *(1:36–9; 2:111–3)*

19. **(D)** Scary dreams and even nightmares are often part of normal four- and five-year-old growing up. At this age, the maturing child understands that he is a separate, unique individual and also is a very small being in a very big world. At night, this awareness of vulnerability may lead to frightening dreams that the youngster gradually outgrows.

   As in any family evaluation, the father should be interviewed. But it is even more important to recognize that the child's behavior is not pathologic or evidence of serious identity, developmental, or emotional problems. *(1:38–9; 2:111–3)*

20. **(A)** *Phobias, nail biting, bed wetting,* and *nightmares* can all be transitional reactions to stress in a child who basically is emotionally healthy—temporary regressive symptoms often seen as part of an *adjustment disorder.*

   Autism and autistic behaviors are not temporary regressive phenomena and indicate a much more serious and pervasive emotional disorder. *(1:474–7; 2:605–11)*

21. **(D)** Average intelligence is usually taken as the Intelligence Quotient levels 90–110 or 85–115, with 100 the mean, plus or minus 10 or 15.

   None of the other ranges equally overlap the intelligence mean. *(1:155–6; 2:238,702–3)*

22. **(D)** The *highest incidence* of diagnosed or recognized *mental retardation* is in the adolescent age group when the growing youngster is faced with the responsibility of more complicated social and academic tasks.

   The *borderline retarded person,* who may not be diagnosed as being intellectually limited until the teenage years, often adapts productively to society and, in later adult years, is no longer recognized or thought of as being retarded. *(1:685–6; 2:705–9)*

23. **(A)** The highest incidence of reported mental retardation is among urban ghetto residents.

Complex cultural factors play a profound role in producing intellectual stunting in children who may already be at risk intellectually and medically.

In culturally biased tests, these children will tend to test at a lower score level. *(1:685–94; 2:705–9)*

The diagnosis and treatment of enuresis is referred to in answers 24 through 27.

24. (B) An enuretic child is more apt to be a boy with a *family history* of enuresis. Autistic children are often relatively easy to toilet train, while obsessive–compulsive children are typically overtrained. Mentally retarded children may be slower at being trained. The enuretic child is much more likely to be intellectually normal than retarded. *(1:765–7; 2:690–2)*

25. (C) *Encopresis, psychogenic soiling,* is relatively uncommon but, when present, often coexists with enuresis. Enuresis, a common symptom, only rarely has coexistent encopresis.

There is frequently a parental history of enuresis rather than early toilet training.

Nocturnal enuresis is more common than *diurnal incontinence.* Organic defects of the urinary tract are demonstrated in only a small percentage of enuretics. *(1:764–7; 2:690–2)*

26. (A) Enuresis occurs in all stages of sleep and not specifically in one stage though incontinence may be more common in non-REM deep sleep. *(1:766; 2:691)*

27. (E) A wide range of treatments has been used in enuretics with varying success. It does appear that many enuretic children are emotionally damaged more by being shamed, abused, and overtreated than by the enuresis itself. In the total treatment of the child in the family, *psychotherapy* for the child and *counseling* for the parents is often beneficial especially where there is parent–child tension. With the cooperation of the child, a *conditioning device* is often effective. Low dose *imipramine* may produce symptomatic improvement but tolerance to the medication effect often develops with recurrence of the bed wetting.

Barbiturates have no beneficial effect and would not be indicated. *(1:765–7; 2:692)*

28. (D) *Petit mal, absence seizures,* is not associated with borderline mental retardation. Absence seizures usually begin in *childhood,* can be treated with *trimethadione, ethosuximide* or *valproic acid,* nearly always disappear before *adulthood,* and have a characteristic three-per-second spike and wave EEG pattern. *(1:263–6)*

29. (A) Lead poisoning still occurs frequently in children from deprived social environments and the clinician should be able to recognize the symptoms and laboratory signs. X-rays in cases of *lead poisoning in children* may show increased thickness and density at the zones of provisional calcification of the long bones. However, lead poisoning may be present even in the absence of radiologic signs.

Other diagnostic features would be basophilic stippling of the red cells with hypochromic anemia, coproporphyrinuria, and excessive concentrations of lead in the urine and the blood. Multiple poorly healed fractures might indicate a *battered child,* a severe nutritional deficiency, or a hypoparathyroid syndrome. Calcified periosteal hemorrhages would suggest healing lesions of *scurvy.*

Severe vitamin D deficiency, *rickets,* would lead to cupping and fraying of the epiphyseal ends with generalized reduction in shaft density.

Premature closure of the epiphyses may be due to one of the endocrine syndromes producing *premature sexual development. (1:692,740; 2:680–1)*

30. (B) The child with *attention deficit hyperactivity disorder* may benefit from treatment with stimulants, amphetamines or, more commonly, methylphenidate.

The youngster with this diagnosis is much more likely to be a boy. The symptoms tend to start in the preschool years but the syndrome is often not diagnosed until grade-school years.

Increasingly it is being recognized that many of these children do not grow out of their symptoms in adolescence or adulthood. However, in adolescence and adulthood the patient may learn to control, hide, or channel the symptoms more efficiently. *(1:725–30; 2:651–64)*

31. (C) The youngster with an acute asthmatic attack (and his family) need immediate treatment. Unless you are competent to handle all pediatric medical treatment, you should plan any treatment program in the closest association with a pediatrician who can treat the boy intensively from the medical aspect.

It is relatively useless to begin psychotherapy in the midst of a life-threatening asthmatic attack. The immediate reality must be handled therapeutically and efficiently before the underlying factors can be elucidated and managed.

Since the mother called you for help, you have the responsibility to see that she and her son have all the assistance they need—and they need it at once, not at an appointment the next day. You must join with her in getting the necessary total treatment and evaluation, medical and psychiatric.

Asthma was at one time considered to be a "cry for mother" or "cry for help." It is now agreed that this is much too simplistic an explanation of an illness with multiple etiological factors. Emotional symptoms in asthmatic patients may be a result of this life-threatening illness rather than the cause. *(1:505; 2:505)*

32. **(D)** To understand the irreversibility of death, the child must be aware of the continuity of time, be able to fantasize, and have a solid sense of his or her own individuality. This level of maturity usually comes between the ages of six and ten years. The child is typically seven or eight years old when he begins to understand the basic irreversibility of death. *(1:58; 2:106–7)*

33. **(A)** Sleepwalking does tend to run in families. Emotional tensions do not appear to cause sleepwalking. In children who sleepwalk, there is usually no evidence of increased psychopathology. Sleepwalking tends to occur during the first half of the night, during non-REM stage 3–4 sleep, and the subject is amnestic for the episode later. Sleepwalking is most common in the 6- to 12-year age group. *(1:477; 2:749–50)*

34. **(C)** When a child presents with florid visual hallucinations, the most common cause is a *toxic psychosis* caused by endogenous toxin such an infection or an endocrine dysfunction, or an exogenous toxin, including legal and illegal drugs, over-the-counter remedies, and many household agents. Hallucinations do not occur in patients with an autistic disorder, a panic disorder, or uncomplicated moderate mental retardation. Visual hallucinations do occur in childhood schizophrenia but this syndrome is extremely rare. *(1:256–7; 2:282–4)*

35. **(B)** When the mother has *rubella* in the first month of pregnancy, the risk of *congenital defects* in the child is 50%. The frequency of congenital malformations due to rubella decreases inversely with the duration of pregnancy at the time of the disease.

As a prophylactic measure, before rubella immunization was available, teenage girls were encouraged to contract rubella prior to marriage. *(1:687; 2:707)*

36. **(B)** Children with *phenylketonuria* tend to have head measurements smaller than normal. Hydrocephalus is not a typical finding.

These patients quite often have *blond hair* and *blue eyes*. They frequently have *dermatitis* or *eczema. Convulsions* are common. Other siblings may be affected by this disorder, which is transmitted as a simple recessive trait. The musty odor of the urine was the initial finding that led to the demonstration of this syndrome. *(1:688–92; 2:707–9)*

37. **(C)** *School refusal* is usually a manifestation of *separation anxiety*. Both the child and the caring person often have difficulty separating from each other. To treat separation anxiety effectively, often both partners in the relationship need help and support to separate in a way both can tolerate.

The *mentally retarded* child who is more dependent on the parent may have greater difficulty in becoming separate and independent, but school phobia is not specifically associated with retardation.

The *autistic child* who is markedly egocentric often separates easily. He may, however, become upset because his routine has been disturbed.

Malingering is relatively rare in childhood but malingering by proxy is becoming increasingly recognized. The parent or care-giving person gains some benefit by presenting the child as being ill— the parent who brings the child for treatment for some complaint in order to collect increased security payments. *Attention deficit disorder* and school refusal are not directly interrelated. *(1:733–6; 2:673–7)*

38. **(A)** *Fire-setting, enuresis,* and *autistic disorder* are all more common in boys.

Enuresis certainly does not need to be treated in hospital. Inpatient care may be needed for the other two syndromes.

Enuresis may respond to *imipramine* but the syndromes of fire-setting or autistic disorder are not affected by this drug. *Leo Kanner* first described infantile autism.

Fire-setting and enuresis are usually not precursors to childhood schizophrenia. Autistic disorder is clearly a different syndrome than childhood schizophrenia and does not lead to schizophrenia. *(1:490–1,699–704,765–7; 2:612–3,690–2,711–7)*

39. **(C)** *Lead poisoning* should always be considered as a possible complication of childhood *pica*, caused by chronic ingestion of lead-containing paint, plaster, and soil. *(1:740–1; 2:680–1)*

40. **(A)** *Phenylketonuria* was first recognized by the musty smell of the urine of these children—due to phenylalanine and its derivatives. Early diagnosis and supervised dietary treatment can prevent development of retardation. *(1:688–92; 2:707)*

41. **(D)** *Anaclitic depression,* a form of reactive attachment disorder of infancy, is the withdrawn, overwhelmed, "depressed" condition that can develop in infants who are separated from the mothering person in the second six months of life—that is, after the infant has developed an emotional bond to the caretaker. *(1:35,107,774–7; 2:697–9)*

42. **(E)** *Elective mutism, selective mutism,* the selective refusal to talk in certain social situations is one of the few childhood syndromes that is commoner in girls. *(1:772–3; 2:694–7)*

43. **(B)** *Strephosymbolia* means specifically reversal of letters and words and is one manifestation of dyslexia *developmental reading disorder.* Characteristically the child sees *b*'s for *d*'s, *p*'s for *g*'s, *was* for *saw*. *(1:711–3; 2:722–4)*

44. **(C)** *Down's syndrome, mongolism,* is more common in children born to older mothers and possibly also to older fathers. Down's syndrome patients show abnormal chromosome types, the most common being trisomy 21. *(1:687–8; 2:708)*

45. **(D)** With patients with *functional enuresis,* low dose imipramine is still often used. Benefit tends to be time limited. The clinician should be alert to the potential cardiotoxic effects on children of this not innocuous drug. *(1:767; 2:994–5)*

46. **(A)** *Phenylketonuria* is an autosomal recessive metabolic deficiency syndrome that, untreated, can lead to severe mental retardation and convulsions. *(1:688–92; 2:707)*

47. **(B)** Butyrophenones can be used to treat *Tourette's Disorder* (multiple tics, explosive grunting noises, and coprolalia) but may cause impaired learning, annoying early side effects and possible long-range tardive dyskinesia. Withdrawal from the butyrophenones may cause acute symptomatic worsening. *(1:760–3; 2:998)*

48. **(B)** *Functional encopresis, enuresis,* is the syndrome of psychogenic *fecal soiling.* The symptom may be due to fecal leakage in a state of chronic constipation or it can be a manifestation of a lack of bowel training and control. Encopresis is a symptom that is socially very self harming. Functional encopresis is commoner during the day whereas enuresis is more common at night. *(1:764–5; 2:688–90)*

49. **(A)** In *Tourette's Disorder,* the patient—more often a boy—shows multiple tics, recurrent compulsive swearing *(coprolalia),* and sometimes *echolalia.* The disease, which usually begins before puberty, may respond to haloperidol, pimozide, or clonidine. *(1:760–3; 2:686–8)*

50. **(E)** *Trichotillomania* is the syndrome, usually seen in children and more common in girls, where the patient compulsively pulls out her (or his) hair, sometimes leading to patchy baldness. These bald areas are in scalp regions accessible to the favored hand. The hair may be chewed or swallowed. *(1:491–3; 2:617–9)*

51. **(C)** *Turner's syndrome, gonadal dysgenesis,* occurs in females with 45,XO chromosomes. These patients are typically short-statured, with webbing of the neck. Without replacement hormone therapy they do not develop sexually at puberty; they are infertile. *(1:754; 2:58)*

52. **(D)** Patients with *autistic disorder* show many unusual body movements and postures, often stereotypic and repetitive—sometimes called *autisms.* Twirling was one of the repetitive movements described early in the descriptions of the syndrome—some severely autistic patients could be started twirling round and round and would continue this movement. This symptom is not commonly noted, but occasionally it is still an examination topic. *(1:699–704; 2:712–3)*

Chromosome labeling (karyotyping) is becoming increasingly important in psychiatry, especially in understanding the retardation syndromes. The trainee must be acquainted with the more common syndromes.

53. **(A)** *Klinefelter's syndrome,* a sex chromosome increase syndrome, is found in XXY,47 chromosome males. Characteristically these males are tall and thin, with small testes and mild gynecomastia in adolescence. There is a higher incidence of mild mental retardation and emotional disorders in these patients. *(1:754; 2:58)*

54. **(C)** *Turner's syndrome,* female gonadal dysgenesis, is manifested by females with the 45 chromosome XO pattern.
These patients are short, somewhat stocky, with webbing of the neck. These girls do not show secondary sexual development at puberty without hormone replacement therapy. *(1:754; 2:58)*

55. **(E)** *Trisomy 21* is associated with Down's syndrome. The trisomy may be associated with 46 or 47 chromosomes, depending on the underlying chromosome defect. *(1:687–8; 2:57–8)*

The student must know the basic developmental milestones. A few of these are indicated in the answers to questions 56 through 64. (1:31–4; 2:99–100)

56. **(B)** The normal child reaches for and can *grasp* a toy at *six months* of age. *(1:32; 2:99)*

57. **(E)** The growing youngster has adequate muscular coordination and balance to ride a *tricycle* at *three years.* *(1:32; 2:99)*

58. **(C)** The average child can *pick up a small object* with thumb and forefinger by *ten months of age.* *(1:32; 2:99)*
In the Cattell Infant testing the child is ex-

pected to pick up a pellet with a "scissor" grasp at nine months and a "pincer" grasp at eleven months. *(1:682–3; 2:1277)*

59. **(A)** The growing child *smiles* preferentially and cries tears by about *two months* of age. *(1:32; 2:99)*

60. **(C)** At *six months,* the average infant will be *holding out his or her arms* to be taken and held.

61. **(D)** By *twelve months,* the young child should be saying *two or three words* like "Mama" and "Dada" communicatively. *(1:33; 2:99)*

62. **(C)** At *four months,* the child usually starts to *hold up his or her head. (1:32; 2:99)*

63. **(D)** Normal youngsters can *sit for brief periods* at *six months* of age. They can sit for longer times when they lean forward, supporting themselves on their hands. *(1:32; 2:99)*

64. **(E)** At *ten months,* the growing youngster can stand without support. *(1:32; 3:99)*

Congenital or hereditary syndromes are discussed in answers 65 through 74. (1:687–94; 2:706–9)

65. **(B)** In the *Sturge–Weber–Dimitri syndrome,* classically, the child has a large facial telangiectasis or *port wine stain* involving the trigeminal distribution in the face, most often the ophthalmic division. Associated with this stigma are *intracranial angioma* with resultant focal *seizures* and *paralyses.* Many other symptoms coexist and *mental retardation* is common. *(1:691)*

66. **(D)** In *tuberous sclerosis,* the disorder may be first manifested by *adenoma sebaceum* over the nose and cheeks. These patients often have hemangioma, *cysts,* or tumors of the kidney, liver, spleen, and lungs, and *glioma* of the brain (which may become calcified).

These patients tend to present with *mental retardation* and *seizures. (1:691)*

67. **(A)** In *neurofibromatosis* (von Recklinghausen's disease), the syndrome tends to be first recognized by the multiple *café au lait spots* and the cutaneous and subcutaneous *neurofibromata* along the nerves. Many of these fibroma become pedunculated.

Meningiomata and optic and acoustic glioma are not uncommon. These patients may present with normal intelligence or with varying degrees of retardation. Epilepsy is a frequent presenting symptom. *(1:690)*

68. **(E)** The *Kayser–Fleisher ring,* a greenish-yellow ring near the margin of the iris, is characteristic of *Wilson's disease, hepatolenticular degeneration,* where, due to inborn metabolic copper metabolism defect, there is progressive intellectual and motor deterioration with gradually developing hepatic cirrhosis.

In these patients there is increased urinary excretion of copper. The illness can be treated by penicillamine. *(1:73; 2:290)*

69. **(C)** In *Turner's syndrome,* the young girl is short-statured with neck webbing or extra neck skin. At puberty there is no development of secondary sex characteristics and the child shows persistent sexual infantilism unless replacement hormonal therapy is given for the ovarian dysgenesis. On chromosome testing, the subject shows the 45 chromosome XO pattern. *(1:754; 2:58)*

70. **(C)** The *infantile cerebral lipoidosis, Tay-Sach's disease,* is most common in young children of *Eastern European Jewish* origin. These infants present with progressive hypotonic weakness and lack of development. On examination, they show the bilateral *cherry-red spot* on the macula. Death usually occurs in one to three years.

Prenatal diagnosis is possible from culture of amniotic cells. *(1:693)*

71. **(B)** In *phenylketonuria,* the patients are deficient in phenylalanine hydroxylase.

Frequently these children have blond hair and blue eyes, with dermatitis or eczema. Often they develop convulsions. Untreated they become severely retarded. *(1:688–92; 2:707)*

72. **(E)** The *cri-du-chat syndrome, "cat cry" syndrome,* occurs in children with a *deletion of the short arm of the 5 chromosome.* The subjects are usually markedly retarded and microcephalic with craniofacial anomalies. *(1:688; 2:58)*

73. **(A)** In *Klinefelter's syndrome,* the subject is an XXY,47-chromosome male, usually of asthenic build. He tends to have small or underdeveloped testes and, commonly after puberty, gynecomastia. Mild mental retardation is quite common. *(1:754; 2:58)*

74. **(D)** In *bilirubin encephalopathy, kernicterus,* due to Rh incompatibility between mother and fetus, yellow pigmentation of the basal ganglia, cerebellum, and brain stem can be shown on autopsy. These lesions lead to cerebral palsy, deafness, choreoathetosis, and retardation in children who survive.

This reaction also occurs where there is incompatibility of other blood factors between mother and fetus. *(2:707)*

The answers to questions 75 through 77 deal with psychopharmacology in childhood disorders. Increasingly childhood emotional disorders are being treated with medication, sometimes in high doses even though there are few well controlled research studies on the effect of medications on children and on the long-range effects.

75. **(C)** *Attention deficit hyperactivity disorder* is most often treated first with *amphetamines* or *methylphenidate*. If these medications are symptomatically ineffective in adequate doses or cause distressing side effects, magnesium pemoline may be used. *(1:729; 2:660–3)*

76. **(A)** *Pimozide* is presently an effective symptomatic treatment for the *Tourette's Disorder* (multiple tics, coprolalia, and echolalia) and may cause less cognitive sluggishness than haloperidol. Clonidine is used especially with Tourette's Disorder children who have attention deficit hyperactivity disorder. *(1:638,798; 2:688)*

77. **(B)** Chronic *lead poisoning* in children is usually treated with calcium disodium versenate. *(1:740; 2:680–1)*

78. **(D)** Characteristically, *Tourette's Disorder* begins in the grade-school years, more often in boys, and is manifested by recurrent motor and vocal tics which wax and wane over weeks or months. The vocal tics may be repeated throat clearing, grunts, coughs, and complete or incomplete expletitives. *(1:760–3; 2:686–8)*

79. **(A)** *Trichotillomania,* compulsive pulling out of one's own hair is more often seen in girls, usually in childhood. Any body hair areas may be affected. Sometimes the patients chew or swallow the loose hair, occasionally causing a stomach hair ball. Trichotillomania in adults is more often associated with psychosis. *(1:491–3; 2:617–9)*

80. **(F)** *Elective mutism, selective mutism,* is the selective refusal to talk in certain social situations. The symptom is commoner in girls. These children are more likely to have delayed speech development or a language or speech disorder. *(1:772–3; 2:694–7)*

CHAPTER 4

Adult Psychopathology
Questions

INTRODUCTION

Examination questions dealing with adult psychopathology may be focused on a discrete symptom, syndrome, or treatment, but often one question touches on a wide variety of loosely related concepts. The candidate should not assume that topics included in the same questions are necessarily associated.

REFERENCES

For this chapter the reader must be prepared to use the whole range of the standard textbook.

DIRECTIONS (Questions 1 through 64): Each of the numbered items or incomplete statements in this section is followed by answers or by completions of the statement. Select the ONE lettered answer or completion that is BEST in each case.

1. The drift hypothesis is one theory to explain

   (A) the higher incidence of schizophrenia in urban ghetto areas
   (B) the occurrence of Rorschach contamination responses in schizophrenia
   (C) the frequency of illusions in senile dementia
   (D) recurring flashbacks after hallucinogen intake
   (E) the incidence of twin autism

2. Typically, a cocaine-induced psychosis is preponderantly

   (A) paranoid
   (B) depressive
   (C) grandiose
   (D) confusional
   (E) manic

3. In depression all of the following occur *except*

   (A) early morning awakening
   (B) chronic tiredness
   (C) loss of appetite
   (D) flattened affect
   (E) low self-esteem

4. The highest suicide rate is likely to occur in

   (A) adolescent black girls
   (B) elderly white males
   (C) middle-class menopausal women
   (D) adolescent white males
   (E) married teenage females

5. The acutely depressed patient may be treated with one or a combination of the following *except*

   (A) monoamine oxidase inhibitors
   (B) electroconvulsive therapy
   (C) imipramine
   (D) propanolol
   (E) psychotherapy

6. A serious suicide attempt is more likely in patients who

   (A) are quietly depressed
   (B) threaten suicide
   (C) have made previous serious attempts
   (D) have received bad news
   (E) are given inadequate antidepressant medication

7. A suicide attempt may be a manifestation of

   (A) self-punishment
   (B) a wish to rejoin loved ones
   (C) angry retaliation
   (D) an effort to end a painful situation
   (E) all of the above

8. Bleuler described all the following as fundamental symptoms of schizophrenia *except*

   (A) autism
   (B) affect inappropriate
   (C) aggression uncontrolled
   (D) ambivalence
   (E) associations loosened

9. All of the following are true about obesity *except*

   (A) more common in lower socioeconomic groups
   (B) diagnosed when body weight is above 120% standard weight
   (C) women show higher prevalence of obesity than men
   (D) weight reduction more effective where obesity started in childhood
   (E) group self-help treatment programs are often most helpful

10. In the cerebrospinal fluid of suicidal patients, which of the following neurotransmitters has been shown more likely to be reduced?

    (A) histamine
    (B) Serotonin
    (C) GABA (gamma aminobutyric acid)
    (D) cortisol
    (E) norepinephrine

11. A 27-year-old medical student is finding it increasingly difficult to sit through lectures. Over the past six months, she has had repeated episodes of heart pounding, difficulty breathing, light headedness and tremor. During these episodes, she feels "like I am going to die—it feels awful." Your most likely diagnosis is

    (A) somatization disorder
    (B) hypochondriasis
    (C) panic disorder
    (D) dissociation disorder
    (E) phobia

12. Barbiturates affect REM sleep by

    (A) increasing REM periods
    (B) reducing REM sleep time
    (C) increasing REM sleep and producing frightening dreams
    (D) increasing REM sleep to as much as 50% of sleep cycle
    (E) no change of REM cycles but rise in arousal threshold

13. When barbiturates are withdrawn from chronic users, there is

    (A) increased REM time, often with nightmares
    (B) temporary abolition of REM sleep
    (C) increased REM sleep without disturbing dreams
    (D) unchanged REM cycles but production of nightmares
    (E) no change in REM activity but lowering of arousal threshold

14. All of the following traits are characteristic of the anal character *except*

    (A) punctuality
    (B) dependency
    (C) neatness
    (D) miserliness
    (E) obstinacy

15. Three times in the past month, a 42-year-old married woman has arrived unexpectedly for consultation after the doctor's regular office hours. She has complained of abdominal pain but no specific physical findings can be discovered. The next time she arrives to see the doctor when he is working alone in the evening, he should

    (A) tell her firmly that there is nothing wrong with her and she should see a psychiatrist
    (B) point out that she needs careful, thorough evaluation and give her the next available appointment during scheduled office hours
    (C) sit down and have a long heart-to-heart talk with her
    (D) show her that she has many things to be thankful for and should pull herself together
    (E) refuse to answer the office doorbell

16. An 18-year-old girl comes to see the physician. Soon after she begins talking, she starts to cry. Usually the doctor should

    (A) comfort her and put her at ease by gently patting her arm or shoulder
    (B) quickly apologize for causing her stress
    (C) reassure her that everything will soon be all right
    (D) ignore her crying and continue the history taking
    (E) acknowledge her crying but try to find out what led the girl to cry

17. The chronic emotional handicapping produced by severe maternal deprivation has been shown most clearly by

    (A) Harlow's studies of primates
    (B) Freud's "Little Hans" study
    (C) Piaget's investigation of growing children
    (D) Kallmann's twin studies
    (E) Hollingshead's and Redlich's social studies

18. The following are examples of dissociation *except*

    (A) multiple personality
    (B) fugue state
    (C) psychogenic amnesia
    (D) waxy flexibility
    (E) automatic writing

19. The following patterns are all common in obsessive–compulsive disorder *except*

    (A) intellectualization
    (B) magical thinking
    (C) recurrent obtrusive thoughts
    (D) repetitive rumination
    (E) dissociation

20. All of the following are correct about depression *except*

    (A) psychomotor retardation common
    (B) tends to be more common in men
    (C) frequent loss of appetite and weight
    (D) frequent sleep difficulties
    (E) males may become impotent

21. Cross-cultural studies of emotional disorders have shown greatest agreement on prevalence of

    (A) psychosomatic disorders
    (B) phobias
    (C) psychoses
    (D) personality disorders
    (E) paraphilias

22. All of the following characteristics are typical of the oral personality *except*

    (A) dependency
    (B) narcissism
    (C) inability to delay gratification
    (D) obstinacy
    (E) greed

23. All of the following are associated with REM sleep *except*

    (A) respiration rate decreases
    (B) peak plasma testosterone levels
    (C) penile erection
    (D) skeletal muscle tone decreases
    (E) dreaming

24. All of the following are associated with delirium tremens *except*

    (A) visual and tactile hallucinations
    (B) irregular flapping tremor of arms
    (C) uncommon before age 30
    (D) disoriented for time and place
    (E) marked motor restlessness

25. In the management of the elderly patient, the following are useful *except*

    (A) nighttime diazepam for insomnia
    (B) vitamin supplements
    (C) well-lighted, simplified home environment
    (D) hospital care if markedly confused or agitated
    (E) counseling for the family

26. Electroconvulsive treatment is most specifically therapeutic for

    (A) delirium tremens, alcohol withdrawal delirium
    (B) senile dementia
    (C) major depression
    (D) schizophrenia, residual type
    (E) obsessive–compulsive disorder

27. The evidence for genetic factors in the etiology of schizophrenia is most clearly demonstrated by

    (A) adopted away studies
    (B) studies on borderline personality disorder
    (C) infant-rearing primate research
    (D) studies on infant deprivation
    (E) Freud's Schreber study

28. The prognosis in schizophrenia is liable to be unfavorable when all of the following factors are present *except*

    (A) insidious onset
    (B) lack of obvious precipitating factors
    (C) previous schizoid personality
    (D) clearly apparent anxiety
    (E) parental and familial psychopathology

29. A depressed patient is most likely to commit suicide when

    (A) the depression is most profound
    (B) the patient is starting to recover from the depression
    (C) the patient receives bad news or a disappointment
    (D) the patient becomes physically ill
    (E) the patient has completed a course of electroconvulsive treatments

30. A 25-year-old service man is being considered for disciplinary procedures because he has been found for the second time sleeping on duty. He had been examined several months previously after complaining about having difficulty getting out of bed in the morning. To confirm your diagnosis, you will want to ask specifically whether

    (A) he has had sudden loss of muscle tone with muscle weakness when emotionally excited
    (B) his work is too stressful and he is actively seeking his discharge
    (C) he is depressed, anorexic, and possibly suicidal
    (D) he had petit mal episodes during childhood
    (E) he has been sexually propositioned by his roommate and is having difficulty dealing with his feelings

31. Sensory deprivation is a causative factor in each of the following *except*

    (A) factory assembly line accidents
    (B) psychosis in coronary care patients
    (C) psychotic states in body-cast patients
    (D) absence seizures
    (E) highway accidents

32. Freud postulated that paranoia was a manifestation of

    (A) unresolved dependency needs
    (B) identification with the aggressor
    (C) an anaclitic depressive reaction
    (D) repressed homosexual impulses
    (E) introjection and symbolization

33. Weight loss, early morning awakening, and general tiredness are usually symptomatic of

(A) paranoia

(B) schizophrenia

(C) obsessive–compulsive disorder

(D) depression

(E) phobic disorder

34. Folie à deux is

(A) mercury poisoning

(B) psychotic reaction seen in Malayans

(C) form of senile dementia

(D) result of infant maternal deprivation

(E) communicated psychosis

35. The largest single group of hospitalized psychiatric patients in North America have the diagnosis

(A) bipolar disorder

(B) schizophrenia

(C) dementia of the Alzheimer's type

(D) alcoholism

(E) substance abuse

36. In treating posttraumatic stress disorder, acute combat neurosis, which of the following management plans is least likely to lead to long-term disability?

(A) remove immediately to base hospital for intensive psychotherapy

(B) handle in front-line station with brief, firm support and temporary sedation

(C) return to home country for rehabilitation

(D) insist that the soldier remain in front-line duty and continue as part of his troup

(E) none of the above

37. A 37-year-old man complains of chronic lower back pain. Repeated physical, laboratory, and radiological examinations are negative. The doctor should

(A) tell the patient that he is absolutely healthy and should forget the pain

(B) tell the patient that the pain is psychological in origin and he needs to learn to relax

(C) tell the patient that such pain usually indicates personal or family problems

(D) ask the patient about his individual, family, and work situations

(E) prescribe medication to relax his back muscles

38. In using the muscle relaxant succinylcholine during electroconvulsive therapy, the physician must be alert to the rare complication in which the

(A) relaxant may potentiate the convulsive effect

(B) patient may constitutionally lack succinylcholinesterase and so stay apneic

(C) succinylcholine may precipitate a toxic psychosis

(D) muscle relaxant may cause acute hemolysis

(E) patient is resistant to the succinylcholine

39. An idiot savant is a(n)

(A) intellectually superior person who has one limited, clearly defined, area of retardation

(B) basically retarded individual who has a very limited, specialized area of superior functioning

(C) mentally defective person with a mental age of three to seven years

(D) adolescent or young adult, diagnosed as retarded in school, but now functioning as an acceptable member of society

(E) socially deprived youngster who scores low on standard intelligence testing

40. In the treatment of acute mania, all of the following may be appropriate except

(A) lithium carbonate

(B) chlorpromazine

(C) electroconvulsive therapy

(D) hospitalization

(E) imipramine

41. All of the following statements are true about obesity except

(A) more common in lower socioeconomic groups

(B) more common in women, especially after age 50

(C) those affected commonly have oral, demanding personalities

(D) individual psychotherapy usually unsuccessful over the long term

(E) juvenile-onset obesity tends to persist

42. In law, criminal responsibility may be determined on the basis of all the following guidelines except

(A) M'Naghten rule

(B) Durham Decision

(C) irresistible impulse test

(D) testamentary capacity

(E) right and wrong test

43. In addicts using morphine, heroin, or methadone, an abstinence syndrome may be precipitated by

(A) naloxone

(B) meperidine

(C) codeine

(D) chlorpromazine

(E) methadone

44. With chronic dependency, convulsions may occur on sudden withdrawal from

    (A) marijuana
    (B) amphetamines
    (C) lysergic acid diethylamide
    (D) meprobamate
    (E) monoamine oxidase inhibitors

45. Chronic amphetamine use may lead to a clinical syndrome similar to

    (A) manic–depressive illness, manic type
    (B) schizophrenia, paranoid type
    (C) schizophrenia, disorganized type
    (D) delirium tremens, alcohol withdrawal delirium
    (E) catastrophic reaction

46. Tricyclic antidepressants should be avoided where there is

    (A) senile dementia
    (B) urinary retention
    (C) sleep disturbance
    (D) weight and appetite loss
    (E) myopia

47. Hypnosis would be therapeutically useful in treating

    (A) schizophrenia, residual type
    (B) dysthymic disorder
    (C) conversion disorder
    (D) senile dementia
    (E) bipolar disorder, manic type

48. The risk for suicide in the elderly is associated with all of the following *except*

    (A) chronic illness
    (B) male
    (C) minority group
    (D) divorced
    (E) alcoholism

49. Patients taking monoamine oxidase inhibitors should be warned to avoid

    (A) cholesterol
    (B) butter
    (C) polyunsaturated fats
    (D) cheese
    (E) salt

50. Electroconvulsive therapy is most useful in treating

    (A) hypochondriasis
    (B) major depression
    (C) schizophrenia, residual type
    (D) senile dementia
    (E) autistic disorder

51. A 17-year-old giggling, weeping, schizophrenic girl is brought to your office because "her head is turning to one side." Your best initial procedure would be

    (A) immediate electroconvulsive therapy
    (B) intramuscular benztropine
    (C) intramuscular amobarbital
    (D) oral propanolol
    (E) intramuscular haloperidol

52. Stressful life events have been shown to lead to increased incidence of physical and psychiatric illness. The life event found to be most stressful is

    (A) death of a close family member
    (B) marriage separation
    (C) death of a husband or wife
    (D) retirement
    (E) personal injury

53. Hallucinations may occur in all of the following *except*

    (A) bipolar disorder, manic type
    (B) cyclothymia
    (C) schizophrenia, disorganized type
    (D) major depression
    (E) delirium tremens

54. In psychoanalytic theory, the major factor in producing depression is

    (A) projection
    (B) sublimation
    (C) introjection
    (D) dissociation
    (E) displacement

55. The work of grief or mourning is the

    (A) continued absence of obvious feelings following the death of a loved one
    (B) lengthy prolongation of sadness after a loss
    (C) emotional process of adapting to a loss and reinvesting in others
    (D) denial that is necessary to shield the bereaved from awareness of loss
    (E) accentuated grief reactions due to guilt or ambivalence

56. All of the following are characteristic of delirium *except*

(A) impulsive behavior

(B) labile mood changes

(C) neologisms

(D) disorientation

(E) memory loss

57. Peripheral neuropathy is most liable to occur with chronic use of

(A) reserpine

(B) chloral hydrate

(C) disulfiram

(D) thioridazine

(E) paraldehyde

58. Systematic desensitization is most often therapeutically beneficial in

(A) passive–aggressive personality disorder

(B) conversion disorder

(C) depression

(D) agoraphobia

(E) attention deficit hyperactivity disorder

59. All of the following statements about Acquired Immune Deficiency Syndrome (AIDS) are incorrect *except*

(A) a negative test for AIDS after possible exposure means you are immune to AIDS

(B) the presence of positive HIV antibodies means that you have developed resistance to the disease and will not develop AIDS

(C) infants can develop AIDS through infection from HIV positive mothers through breast milk

(D) people who are HIV positive do not spread the infection until they develop active AIDS

(E) after exposure to possible AIDS, the absence of HIV antibodies after 12 weeks means that you have escaped infection

60. A mother asks her fifteen-year-old daughter where she is going this evening. The daughter hesitates. When she does tell, her mother is very likely to respond "I don't know why you need to ask my permission all the time. You're a big girl now!" On the other hand, when she does not tell in extensive detail, her mother will complain loudly that she is not being loved, appreciated, and respected. This situation is an example of

(A) Von Domarus Principle

(B) double-bind

(C) superego lacunae

(D) reaction formation

(E) folie à deux

61. A black physician has a series of patient deaths in spite of his meticulous treatment. He is depressed by his clinical results but begins to be less guilt ridden; he now feels that his patients were probably poisoned by the hospital pharmacy staff so he would not be so obviously better than his white colleagues. He has now developed a

(A) dissociative reaction

(B) delusional disorder

(C) sublimation

(D) reaction formation

(E) phobia

Questions 62 and 63

A 26-year-old woman is hospitalized at the request of her husband. In recent weeks she has refused to leave home, saying that her neighbors were trying to kill her. She has twice tried to telephone the President to offer her assistance in preventing the spread of AIDS. When her husband tries to reason with her, she tells him that her special "messages" tell her what to do.

62. The probable diagnosis is

(A) paranoid personality disorder

(B) schizophrenia, disorganized type

(C) social phobia

(D) histrionic personality disorder

(E) schizophrenia, paranoid type

63. The most appropriate treatment is

(A) amphetamines

(B) imipramine

(C) haloperidol

(D) phenobarbital

(E) methylphenidate

64. A 24-year-old married man comes for marital counseling. At his request, the counselor gives fairly specific advice. The patient does not attempt to carry out certain suggestions and even seems to be acting directly counter to other directions of the counselor. The patient may be showing which of the following personality disorders?

(A) antisocial

(B) histrionic

(C) compulsive

(D) passive–aggressive

(E) schizoid

DIRECTIONS (Questions 65 through 117): Each group of items in this section consists of four to eight lettered options followed by a set of numbered words or phrases. For each numbered word or phrase, select the ONE lettered option that is most closely associated with it. Each lettered option may be selected once, more than once, or not at all.

Questions 65 through 68

(A) general neurone lipid deposition
(B) frontoparietal cortical atrophy
(C) congestion and hemorrhage around third ventricle and aqueduct and in mammillary bodies
(D) cavity formation in basal ganglia

For each pathology description, select the most likely diagnosis.

65. General paresis (paralysis)

66. Wilson's disease

67. Wernicke's encephalopathy

68. Tay-Sach's disease

Questions 69 through 73

(A) stupor, excitement, negativism, automatisms
(B) shallow, apathetic, moody, vague, illogical
(C) aloof, distrustful, suspicious, grandiose, sometimes assaultive
(D) silly, giggling, hallucinating, regressed
(E) bizarre ideas with depression and elation, anxious

For each clinical description select the most appropriate psychosis diagnosis.

69. Residual schizophrenia

70. Disorganized schizophrenia

71. Paranoid schizophrenia

72. Catatonic schizophrenia

73. Schizoaffective disorder

Questions 74 through 78

(A) episodes of REM sleep
(B) three-per-second spike and wave
(C) diffuse slow activity on electroencephalogram
(D) temporal lobe EEG foci
(E) increased REM sleep with nightmares

For each electroencephalogram description select the most likely associated clinical state.

74. Following alcohol withdrawal

75. Absence seizures

76. Psychomotor epilepsy

77. Narcolepsy

78. Delirium

Questions 79 through 83

(A) up to 50% sleep cycle is REM sleep
(B) suppression of REM sleep
(C) rebound increase in REM sleep with nightmares
(D) non-REM stage 4 sleep
(E) alpha rhythm declines with increasing slow-wave activity

For each electroencephalographic statement, select the appropriate clinical state.

79. After barbiturate withdrawal in chronic users

80. Newborn

81. During sensory deprivation

82. Chronic amphetamines use

83. Sleepwalking

Questions 84 through 88

(A) basophilic stippling
(B) neurofibrillary tangles and cortical plaques
(C) elevated urine porphobilinogen
(D) lowered serum ceruloplasmin
(E) lowered basal ganglia dopamine

Match the laboratory results with the most likely associated syndrome.

84. Acute intermittent pophyria

85. Hepatolenticular degeneration

86. Chronic lead poisoning

87. Parkinsonism

88. Alzheimer's disease

Questions 89 through 93

    (A) more organized delusions of persecution and grandiosity

    (B) loss of interest and drive; aimless, apathetic; illogical

    (C) suspicious, fearful and vague hallucinations; later tearful and hopeless

    (D) grinning, grimacing and silly; hallucinations

    (E) mutism, posturing, rigidity, stupor

Match the clinical descriptions with the types of schizophrenia.

89. Schizophrenia, residual

90. Schizophrenia, disorganized type

91. Schizophrenia, paranoid type

92. Schizophrenia, catatonic type

93. Schizoaffective disorder

Questions 94 through 98

    (A) conversion disorder

    (B) Korsakoff's syndrome

    (C) bipolar disorder, manic type

    (D) Ganser syndrome

    (E) transvestism

Match the syndromes listed above with the characteristic symptoms listed above.

94. Confabulation

95. Cross dressing

96. La belle indifference

97. Approximate answer

98. Flight of ideas

Questions 99 through 103

    (A) marked impairment of reality contact, often with severe personality disorganization

    (B) stable, maladaptive patterns of interaction during developmental years

    (C) temporary acute reaction to identifiable life stress

    (D) maladaptive reaction to conflict or stress without severe reality distortion or personality disorganization

    (E) chronic fixed maladaptive behavior patterns

Match the clinical description with the most appropriate diagnosis.

99. Psychosis

100. Anxiety disorder

101. Conduct disorder

102. Adjustment disorder

103. Personality disorder

Questions 104 through 108

    (A) sexual gratification from an inanimate object

    (B) desire to change to the opposite sex

    (C) pathological sexual interest in children

    (D) dressing in clothing of opposite sex

    (E) sexual gratification through self-exposure

Match the clinical description with the appropriate paraphilia.

104. Pedophilia

105. Transvestism

106. Fetishism

107. Transsexualism

108. Exhibitionism

Questions 109 through 113

    (A) acute agitation in brain-injured person unable to solve problem

    (B) unacceptable feelings repressed but symbolized in physical symptoms

    (C) obsessive overeating

    (D) compulsive chewing and grinding

    (E) illusion of previous experience

Select the most likely term for the clinical situation described above.

109. Conversion

110. Déjà vu

111. Catastrophic reaction

112. Bruxism

113. Bulimia

Questions 114 through 117

    (A) agoraphobia

    (B) psychogenic fugue

    (C) multiple personality disorder

    (D) cocaine delusional disorder

    (E) generalized anxiety disorder

    (F) conversion disorder

    (G) somatization disorder

    (H) adjustment disorder

For each clinical vignette, select the most likely diagnosis.

114. Julie, a 23-year-old woman, comes to see you. She is unmarried and happy in her job. Recently she was driving in a nearby city and stopped for gasoline. The people there called her "Mary" and talked as if they knew her well. Somehow they seemed familiar.

115. You are called to the emergency room to see a 28-year-old woman who has lost her voice. You find her sitting upright on the examining table with her mother and husband by her side. They fear that she might have had a stroke. Earlier in the evening, her husband came home late again and mildly drunk. "She began to fuss at him when suddenly her voice went."

116. You are asked to see a 23-year-old man because he is upset. He is slender, slightly unkempt, restless, and periodically preoccupied. He tells you that he and his wife developed lice—and they have always been clean people. At his request the Public Health Inspector came to their house "but they refused to do anything." Now the man is certain that the Public Health staff told their neighbors about the lice problem because the neighbors "are looking at us funny."

117. A 29-year-old secretary begins to be absent from her work. When you call her at home, tearfully she tells you that it is more and more impossible for her to travel on the bus to work. When she is in the bus, she finds it hard to breathe, she feels suffocated, and she is scared she is going to "pass out."

Answers and Explanations

1. **(A)** The *drift hypothesis* is one theory to explain the higher rates of schizophrenia in populations that are disorganized or highly mobile. The theory postulates that schizophrenics stay in the lower socioeconomic groups or drift into these groups due to social and vocational dysfunction. *(1:321; 2:382)*

2. **(A)** A *cocaine-induced psychosis* is typically paranoid in nature and may resemble a paranoid schizophrenic reaction, though the subject usually shows less thought disorder. *Cocaine bugs* are tactile hallucinations (*formication*) of insects crawling on or in the skin. *(1:303–305; 2:339)*

3. **(D)** In *depression* there is an increase in depressive affect. In schizophrenia there may be a flattening of all affect. The other symptoms, early morning awakening, chronic tiredness, loss of appetite, and low self-esteem, are characteristic of depression. *(1:366–71; 2:404)*

4. **(B)** The highest *suicide rate* is likely to occur in elderly white males. *(1:551–4; 2:1023–5)*

5. **(D)** Propanolol may cause depression as a side effect and would not be indicated with the acutely depressed patient. In the treatment of acute depression, *electroconvulsive therapy* has the most prompt therapeutic effect but the *monoamine oxidase inhibitors* or the *imipramine*-related antidepressant drugs are often tried first. *Psychotherapy* is helpful in all phases of the illness. *(1:378–82,628; 2:427–41,833–5)*

6. **(C)** When an individual has allowed himself to cross the crucial personal and social prohibition barrier and makes a serious *suicidal* attempt, that restraining barrier is much weaker on subsequent occasions. The person who has made a previous serious suicide attempt is more liable to make a further serious attempt and to succeed in killing himself or herself. Any suicide gesture, comment, or tendency must be taken very seriously in all patients. *(1:554–5; 2:1021–35)*

7. **(E)** Suicide and suicidal behaviors are symptomatic manifestations of many feelings, drives, and conflicts. Quite commonly a suicide attempt is a form of self-hurting or self-punishment as an expiation for guilt. Following the death of a loved person, suicide may be an attempt to rejoin the dear departed. In the immature and the childish, a suicide attempt may be an angry retaliation akin to "I will eat worms and die—and you will be sorry."

   Suicide is always one way to bring pain to an end or to settle an intolerable problem. *(1:551–8; 2:1023–35)*

8. **(C)** In his book *Dementia Praecox or the Group of Schizophrenias*, Eugen Bleuler lists the fundamental symptoms of *schizophrenia* as loosened *associations*, inappropriate *affect*, persistent, pervasive *ambivalence*, and a pathological predominance of the subject's inner life, *autism*—these symptoms are sometimes called the four A's, with a fifth A, the *accessory symptoms*, under which Bleuler included all the symptoms he thought arose from the fundamental symptoms. These accessory symptoms are hallucinations and delusions. *(1:320; 2:358–9)*

9. **(D)** Obesity, diagnosed when the body weight is greater than 120% of the standard body weight listed in height–weight tables, is more common in women and, in both sexes, is more prevalent in lower socioeconomic groups.

   Group self-help programs, such as TOPS (Take Off Pounds Sensibly), provide what is often the most effective therapeutic approach available.

   The prognosis for effective weight reduction is especially poor when obesity has been present from childhood. *(1:506; 2:763–6)*

10. **(B)** In the cerebrospinal fluid of patients who have made suicide attempts, especially by violent means, *serotonin* has been found to be decreased. *(1:93; 2:1027)*

11. **(C)** *Panic* disorder is manifested by periodic, intense, spontaneous episodes of acute anxiety. An episode usually builds up in intensity for 5 to 15

minutes, lasts typically 20 to 30 minutes and rarely persists for more than an hour. During the attack, the victim often fears dying, going crazy, or losing control. Agoraphobia is frequently associated with panic attacks. *(1:394–400; 2:443–58)*

12. **(B)** *Barbiturates* reduce *REM sleep* time. *(1:292–5)*

13. **(A)** When *barbiturates* are *withdrawn* from chronic users, the electroencephalogram shows an increase in *REM sleep,* a "rebound" phenomenon. Often this increased REM sleep is accompanied by *frightening nightmares. (1:294; 2:328–30)*

14. **(B)** In psychoanalytic theory, the person with an *anal character* (due to fixation at the anal training stage of psychosexual development) is characteristically punctual, neat, tidy, somewhat miserly, and has a marked tendency to be obstinate or stubborn.

　　Dependency is more a characteristic of the oral character. *(1:526; 2:129)*

15. **(B)** This question presents the problem of managing the seductive patient. While the clinician must be aware of, and sensitive to, the seductive patient, he must also give her the medical and psychological care she needs. To maintain a therapeutic clinical distance, the doctor should set up an appointment during office hours when he can have his nurse in attendance. If the physical examination is still negative, it would be appropriate to suggest that her symptoms might be a sign of stress, strain, or difficulty. A psychiatrist then might be called in consultation.
A. If there is "nothing wrong with her," she does not need to see a psychiatrist either. This is an example of poorly sublimated anger on the physician's part.
C. To sit down and have a heart-to-heart talk with her, alone after office hours, would mean that the doctor was allowing himself to be seduced. He has become vulnerable and he may or may not then be able to help the patient in this relatively unstructured intimacy.
D. This woman is hurting somewhere, somehow. She feels pain. She is seeking closeness. The "pull yourself together, woman" approach may ask her to use emotional strengths she does not have and leave her feeling more inadequate and guilty when she cannot fulfill the physician's demands.
E. To refuse to answer the doorbell is personally rude and unprofessional, the bluntest form of rejection. When a patient is in pain and asking for help, the doctor should not refuse to respond. *(1:11–2; 2:171–83)*

16. **(E)** The doctor does not really know why the patient is crying. A pat on the arm or shoulder may appear seductive, threatening, or intrusive to the patient. The physician must learn to cope with pain and not apologize in the presence of pain, physical or emotional—he or she can be empathetic but not apologetic. It is presumptuous to assure a patient that everything will be all right when this may be totally untrue. If the situation is indeed dreadful, by this comment the physician will have made it more difficult for the patient to share the anguish and the cause of the anguish. Too many physicians take this path of steadfastly reassuring because they find it difficult to tolerate anxiety or uncertainty. To ignore the patient's crying would be totally unrealistic and insensitive and probably would reflect the doctor's own discomfort.

　　The correct approach is quietly to recognize with the patient that she is crying and then try to find out with her why she is so bothered. *(1:1–13; 2:174–83)*

17. **(A)** *Harlow's primate studies* at the University of Wisconsin have most clearly shown the chronic emotional handicapping produced by severe *maternal deprivation. (1:125–63; 2:95,101)*
B. In his *"Little Hans" study,* using the father as intermediary, *Freud* evaluated and treated the phobia of a five-year-old boy. *(1:400; 2:462–3)*
C. *Piaget's* investigation of *normal growing children,* starting with his own family, has led to an extensive theory of child development. *(1:104–6; 2:98–101)*
D. *Kallman's twin studies* suggest a genetic basis for schizophrenia and for homosexuality. Later studies have challenged the significance of Kallmann's findings. *(1:327,842; 2:47)*
E. *Hollingshead's and Redlich's studies* pointed out the different incidence of emotional illness in different socioeconomic groups and the varying availability of care. *(1:135; 2:80)*

18. **(D)** *Waxy flexibility (cerea flexibilitas),* is the motor symptom where the patient maintains a posture in which he or she has been placed. Typically, waxy flexibility occurs in catatonic schizophrenia. *(1:329; 2:371)*
　　Multiple personality, fugue states, psychogenic amnesia (somnambulism), and *automatic writing* are all examples of *dissociation. (1:428–37; 2:557–85)*

19. **(E)** *Dissociation,* the splitting off of part of the emotions and personality to avoid conflict, is a manifestation of dissociative disorders. *(1:184; 2:558)*
　　Intellectualization, magical thinking, recurrent obtrusive thoughts, and *repetitive rumination* are all typical symptoms of an *obsessive–compulsive* disorder. *(1:404–9; 2:472–9)*

20. **(B)** Depression tends to be more common in women. Psychomotor retardation, loss of appetite and weight, sleep difficulties, and male impotence are common symptoms of depression. *(1:366–8; 2:407–8)*

21. **(C)** Across cultures, it is easiest to define what is intolerable, crazy, hospitalized, or, in modern terms, psychotic. *Cross cultural studies* of emotional disorders have shown greatest agreement on the incidence of psychoses.

The definition of paraphilias and personality disorders varies from culture to culture. Phobias are more difficult to measure, as they are not hospital directed. There is still much discussion about the etiology and syndrome definition of the psychosomatic disorders. *(1:129; 2:1103–4)*

22. **(D)** In psychoanalytic theory, an *oral personality* or a person with an *oral character,* fixated at the *oral phase* of psychosexual development, is primarily dependent, narcissistic and self-centered, greedy, demanding, and unable to delay gratification.

Obstinacy is more characteristic of the *anal* personality, a fixation at the training phase. *(1:526; 2:129)*

23. **(A)** Respiration rate (and pulse rate and blood pressure) increases during REM sleep.

Plasma testosterone increases during sleep with maximum levels during REM phases. During REM sleep stages dreaming predominantly occurs; there is reduction in skeletal muscle tone. Phasic penile erections tend to precede REM sleep phases by several minutes. *(1:466–7; 2:727–41)*

24. **(B)** In *delirium tremens, alcohol withdrawal delirium,* a coarse tremor of the hands, lips, and face is a common symptom. An *irregular flapping tremor* of the extended arms is an ominous sign of *hepatic failure* and is not part of the delirium tremens syndrome.

Delirium tremens, alcohol withdrawal delirium, is relatively uncommon in young adults under age thirty. The typical delirium tremens patient shows visual and tactile hallucinations, disorientation for time and place, and often a marked motor restlessness that may exhaust the patient. *(1:288–9; 2:323)*

25. **(A)** In *elderly* patients, repeated use of nighttime *diazepam* is likely to cause anterograde amnesia, worsen existing memory impairment, cause insomnia and produce confusion. *(1:813, 816–7; 2:1135)*

In the general management of the elderly, it is necessary to ensure a *good balanced diet,* with *vitamin supplements* as indicated. The family may be helped by *counseling* in the management of elderly relatives. To prevent the development of confusional states, a *well-lighted, simplified home environment* is often beneficial. If the geriatric patient

does become markedly confused and agitated, it will help the patient and the family to suggest *hospital care. (1:807–19; 2:1136–7)*

26. **(C)** *Electroconvulsive therapy* is the most specific therapy for major depression. This treatment is ineffective or contraindicated in delirium tremens, senile dementia, schizophrenia, residual type, or obsessive–compulsive neurosis. *(1:669–73; 2:836–841)*

27. **(A)** The evidence for *genetic factors* in the etiology of *schizophrenia* is clearly demonstrated by adopted away studies. *(1:327–8; 2:46–9)*
B. *Kernberg* used the term *borderline personality* state for patients with identity diffusion, primitive emotional defenses (especially splitting) and recurrent primary process thinking. *(1:188,533–5; 2:636–7)*
C. *Harlow's* primate studies focused on the effect of mother–child separation and infant deprivation. *(1:29,125–6; 2:101)*
D. *Spitz* did early research on the effects of human mother–child separation and of institutionalization. *(1:29–30; 2:108–10)*
E. In the study of the *Schreber case, Sigmund Freud* outlined his theoretical concepts for the development of paranoid thinking. Freud postulated that unconscious homosexual impulses are denied and projected in the form of paranoid feelings. This theory has not been clinically proven. *(1:344; 2:630)*

28. **(D)** The *prognosis* in *schizophrenia* is less favorable when the onset of the illness is *insidious,* with no obvious *precipitating factors,* in a person with a previously *schizoid* personality coming from a family with a high incidence of *psychopathology.*

Where the schizophrenic patient is clearly anxious and distressed, the prognosis is more optimistic. *(1:332; 2:369–70)*

29. **(B)** When the depression is most profound, the depressed patient is more likely to be immobilized by the absolute depth of the depression. When beginning to recover from the depressive apathy, he or she is still profoundly depressed but is more mobile and active, and can act out the depression in *suicide.*

Bad news, disappointment, and physical illness can certainly deepen the depression of a patient already depressed.

A course of electroconvulsive treatments should symptomatically have alleviated the depression. *(1:551–9; 2:1021–35)*

30. **(A)** The most common symptom of *narcolepsy* is the occurrence of *sleep attacks,* when the subject cannot stop himself from falling asleep. More than half these patients also suffer from *cataplexy,* sud-

den episodes of loss of muscle tone which may be focal, manifesting as head or jaw drop or knee weakness, or may be general. Cataplexy is often precipitated by emotional stimuli such as laughing. These patients show other abnormalities of sleep including hypnagogic and hypnopompic phenomena and brief sleep paralysis on morning awakening. *(1:475; 2:747–8)*

31. **(D)** *Sensory deprivation* is not a specific causative factor in producing *absence seizures, petit mal seizures.* Sensory deprivation does lead to accidents on the highways (highway hypnosis) and on monotonous factory assembly line work. Sensory deprivation may be a contributory factor leading to psychotic reactions in coronary care patients and in patients immobilized in body casts. *(1:125–7; 2:242)*

32. **(D)** Freud postulated that *paranoia* was a manifestation of unresolved *homosexual* conflicts (Schreber case). *(1:344; 2:630)*

33. **(D)** Weight loss, early morning awakening, and general tiredness are usually symptomatic of *depression. (1:366–8; 2:404)*

34. **(E)** *Folie à deux* is a form of *communicated psychosis* where a submissive or passive person takes on the psychosis, most often paranoid, of the dominant partner, relative, or friend. *(1:214; 2:393)*

     Chronic mercury poisoning, which used to be an occupational disease of hatters and is depicted in the Mad Hatter in *Alice in Wonderland,* may lead to irritability, depression, and sometimes hallucinations. *(1:241–9; 2:283)*

     Latah is a profound startle reaction or sudden eruption of bizarre behavior seen in Malaysian women due to acute disruptive anxiety or an exacerbation of more serious underlying psychopathology. Koro and Amok are other Malayan syndromes. *(1:132,758; 2:1104–5)*

     Children seem to be most vulnerable to *maternal deprivation* between the ages of six and twenty-four months. Separation from the mother leads to a wide range of infant symptoms and may predispose to the development of serious psychopathology in later life. *(1:27–30,107; 2:101)*

35. **(B)** The largest group of *hospitalized psychiatric patients* in North America have the diagnosis of schizophrenia. *(1:324; 2:378)*

36. **(B)** In treating the soldier with an *acute combat neurosis* (posttraumatic stress disorder), the patient should be treated promptly and firmly with strong psychological support, temporary sedation as needed, and early return to duty if possible. Withdrawal from duty and hospitalization tend to accentuate or perpetuate emotional disability. *(1:409–12; 2:610)*

37. **(D)** Before making any diagnosis, including a psychiatric diagnosis, the physician must show by examination that the condition does exist. Just because an organic illness cannot be proved at that time does not allow the physician to diagnose a psychiatric illness. Neither medical nor psychiatric illnesses are diagnosed merely by excluding the other. In order to verify whether an emotional illness does exist, the doctor should make the requisite examination, which, in this case, could begin by asking about the patient's life situation.

     To prescribe medication for a symptom without a clearly defined etiology is dubious medical care that may lead to concealment of a serious disorder, medical or psychiatric. *(1:510–11; 2:527–9)*

38. **(B)** When using the muscle relaxant *succinylcholine* during electroconvulsive therapy, the anesthetist must be cautious lest the patient is one of the rare people who lack active *succinylcholinesterase.* These patients are deficient in their ability to break down the drug so the induced apnea may continue for an extended period. *(1:671–2; 2:839–41)*

39. **(B)** An *idiot savant* is a *retarded* individual who has a very *limited specialized talent.* Such a person may have an unusual ability to memorize mathematical details, a special artistic talent, or a unique vocational skill. *(1:703; 2:712)*

40. **(E)** *Imipramine* would have little benefit in the treatment of *acute mania* where the patient (and society) needs rapid relief from the patient's symptoms. Antidepressants may worsen mania.

     These patients need *hospitalization* where they may be treated with *lithium carbonate, antipsychotics including the sedating neuroleptic chlorpromazine, carbamazepine, clonazepam,* or *electroconvulsive therapy. (1:382; 2:430–2)*

41. **(C)** No one specific personality pattern has been shown to lead to obesity. Obesity is indeed more common in the poor and in women, especially older women. Obese children tend to become obese adults, and early onset obesity is especially difficult to treat.

     Long-term results with individual psychotherapy of patients for treatment of their obesity have been poor. *(1:506; 2:763–5)*

42. **(D)** *Testamentary capacity* is the legal capacity to make a will. *(1:825–6; 2:1069–70)*

     The *Durham Decision* stated that the patient was not responsible for his or her behavior if this behavior was a product of a mental illness. In 1972, the Courts discarded this rule. *(1:828)*

     Under the *irresistible impulse test,* the person is not responsible for behavior that is the result of an irresistible impulse. *(1:828)*

The *M'Naghten rule* or the *"right and wrong test"* states that persons cannot be held responsible for their behavior if they did not know the nature or quality of their behavior or if they could not appreciate that their actions were wrong. *(1:827–8; 2:1064)*

43. **(A)** *Naloxone* may precipitate an *abstinence syndrome* in chronic users of *morphine, heroin,* or *methadone.* In chronic opioid abusers, withdrawal symptoms precipitated by naloxone, naltrexone, or nalorphine can be severe. (1:297–301; 2:331–6)

44. **(D)** Convulsions may occur in *chronic meprobamate users* who are suddenly withdrawn from the drug (and also with chronic users of benzodiazepines, barbiturates, or alcohol). *(1:288,294, 296,612; 2:324,328)*

45. **(B)** *Chronic amphetamine use* may lead to a clinical syndrome similar to *paranoid schizophrenia* but usually with less thought disorder and often with visual hallucinations. *(1:306–7; 2:342–3)*

46. **(B)** *Tricyclic antidepressants* may produce *urinary retention* due to their anticholinergic side effects, so should not be used in patients who already have this tendency. Other anticholinergic side effects include dry mouth, constipation, erectile dysfunction and visual blurring. *(1:666; 2:798–9)*

47. **(C)** *Hypnosis* is often effective in producing a symptomatic cure of *conversion disorder.* Under hypnosis the conversion disorder patient may be instructed to regain use of a paralyzed limb or recover sight or hearing lost as part of a conversion disorder. *(1:599–601; 2:907–28)*

48. **(C)** The risk of *suicide* is higher in elderly males, in those who are divorced, chronically ill, or suffer from alcoholism, but the suicide rate is higher in the elderly white population than in minority groups. *(1:551–4; 2:1023–31)*

49. **(D)** Patients taking *monoamine oxidase inhibitors* should be warned about the hypertensive effects they could suffer due to the dietary tyramine in cheese, beer, wine, chicken liver, and beans. *(1:657–8; 2:802–3)*

50. **(B)** Electroconvulsive therapy is most useful in treating *major depression.* This treatment has little beneficial effect in *hypochondriasis, schizophrenia, residual type,* or children with *autistic disorder.* Patients with *senile dementia* who have a severe depression will have relief of the depression after a course of electroconvulsive therapy but the dementia will not be improved and may be temporarily worsened. *(1:669–73; 2:836–41)*

51. **(B)** Intramuscular benztropine. Extrapyramidal drug side effects can be mistaken for the bizarre movements and posturing of the schizophrenic patient and vice versa. Drug-induced dyskinesias will be quickly and dramatically reduced or relieved by intramuscular antiparkinsonian drugs such as benztropine, which, however, will have no effect on psychotic mannerisms. Some patients, however, enjoy the emotional lift they get from benztropine or trihexyphenidyl and may fake extrapyramidal symptoms to get the medication.

Amobarbital would sedate the patient and possibly make her confused but with no symptomatic relief. Electroconvulsive therapy and oral propanolol are not indicated. *(1:643–4; 2:779)*

52. **(C)** In the social readjustment scale of Holmes and Rahe, the death of a spouse is rated as most stressful and thus most likely to cause disruption of healthy adaptation.

Divorce, marital separation, and being jailed also rate high as stress factors. *(1:499–500; 2:496)*

53. **(B)** *Hallucinations* do not occur in patients who suffer from *cyclothymia.* These patients experience mood swings, with depression often more marked. Psychotic symptoms such as hallucinations are not present.

Bipolar disorder, manic type, disorganized schizophrenia, major depression, and *delirium tremens* are all psychotic states where hallucinations may occur. In manic states, hallucinations are relatively uncommon and are more illusionary. *(1:386–8; 2:414–5)*

54. **(C)** In psychoanalytic theory, the major factor in producing *depression* is *introjection* of hostile feelings once directed against others but now inwardly directed. *(1:366; 2:424–6)*

55. **(C)** The *work of grief or mourning* is the emotional process of adapting to a loss and of reinvesting in other people and other goals.

The continued absence of obvious feelings following the death of a loved one would be an example of *denial.* The lengthy prolongation, more than six months, of acute sadness following a loss is *pathological mourning.* In all mourning there is some denial to allow gradual adaptation to the loss and to permit individual repression of intolerable feelings. Accentuated grief reactions due to guilt or ambivalence are further examples of pathological mourning. *(1:58–61; 2:299–300)*

56. **(C)** In *delirium,* disorientation, memory loss, labile mood changes, and impulse behavior are common symptoms. *(1:241–5; 2:282–4)*

Neologisms, the forming of new idiosyncratic words, are most often found in schizophrenia. *(1:68,218,330; 2:189,365)*

57. **(C)** Disulfiram (Antabuse), used to treat alcoholics, may produce confusion, sleepiness, and worsening of schizophrenic symptoms. With chronic use, it may produce delirium, parkinsonism, and peripheral neuropathy. *(1:291–2; 2:326)*

58. **(D)** *Agoraphobia* is often benefitted therapeutically by *systematic desensitization. (1:399; 2:892–4)*

59. **(C)** Infants can develop AIDS through transmission in the breast milk from an HIV infected mother.

A negative AIDS test after exposure means only that the subject may have been lucky this time but no one appears to be immune to the AIDS infection. The presence of positive HIV immune antibodies indicates that the subject is now infected with the AIDS virus. Subjects who are infected with the AIDS virus can infect others at any time, even before seroconversion and certainly before the development of active AIDS. While most people who are infected with the AIDS virus develop HIV antibodies within twelve weeks of exposure, some patients do not seroconvert until six to twelve months after being infected. *(1:270–77; 2:252,290)*

60. **(B)** The classical message of the *double-bind* situation is "Get away closer." The subject is faced with two equally imperative contradictory messages and, in the schizophrenogenic situation, cannot escape. *(1:328; 2:943)*

The *Von Domarus Principle* points out that the normal person accepts similarity of identity on the basis of identical subjects, but the primitive thinker—in this case the schizophrenic—accepts similar identity on the basis of predicates.

The schizophrenic can think, "Jesus Christ is a man. I am a man. Jesus Christ and I are both men, therefore I am Jesus Christ," or "Grass is green. Money is green. Therefore grass is money."
C. *Superego lacunae,* or *conscience defects,* allow the subject to act in an antisocial fashion. Superego lacunae in parents may be one factor leading to delinquency in their children who identify with them: parents consciously and unconsciously convey their own basic conscience standards to their children. *Reaction formation* is an emotional defense whereby the individual stresses the opposite of his or her underlying basic feelings. Unlike the situation presented in the question, both opposing feelings or messages are not outwardly apparent in reaction formation; the feeling intolerable to the subject is unconsciously suppressed as he or she emphasizes the opposite.

Folie à deux, induced psychotic disorder, is a form of communicated psychosis where a psychosis, usually paranoid, is communicated or imposed by a dominant individual on a more passive or submissive partner. *(1:214,357–9; 2:393)*

61. **(B)** The brief history given outlines the development of a *delusional disorder,* in this case a paranoid delusional disorder. Because it is intolerable to this perfectionistic physician to feel that he has been therapeutically unsuccessful, he represses this feeling of inadequacy and failure and unconsciously externalizes his blame. Rather than blame himself, he projects the blame outward and blames an external agency for what he feels to be failures.

As in many cases of *paranoia,* there is likely to be a kernel of truth in the subject's suspiciousness. As a minority-group member, this doctor is likely to have been treated differently from his majority peers in the past. *(1:343–50; 2:391–6)*

62. **(E)** This lady has a well-integrated delusion of persecution and of grandeur. She feels she is being specially victimized by her neighbors and she is important enough to ally herself with the President. Her delusional thinking and her hallucinations reinforce her psychosis.

Socially, her behavior is not markedly bizarre, disorganized, or disruptive.

This is the clinical picture of *schizophrenia, paranoid type.* (1:334–5; 2:371)
A. A patient with a *paranoid personality* disorder might be suspicious or grandiose but would not have psychotic symptoms such as auditory hallucinations. *(1:527–8; 2:630–1)*
B. The *disorganized (hebephrenic) schizophrenic* fits the layman's concept of "craziness." These patients are more openly inappropriate, socially bizarre, uncontrolled, and regressed. *(1:332–4; 2:371)*
C. An individual with a *social phobia, social anxiety disorder,* has a fear of failure, humiliation, or embarrassment in some public activity—such as speaking, eating, urinating in the presence of others—a fear which he or she realizes is illogical. These patients do not have delusional or hallucinatory thinking. *(1:400–4; 2:461–2)*
D. *Histrionic personalities* are theatrical, self-centered, demanding, and excitable. They seek attention by overreacting, by demanding, and sometimes by lying, but they do not have delusions or auditory hallucinations. *(1:530–1; 2:631–2)*

63. **(C)** The appropriate drug treatment for acute paranoid schizophrenia is *haloperidol.* (1:340–1; 2:386–8)

Chronic amphetamine use can lead to a psychosis very similar to a paranoid schizophrenia. *(1:305–6; 2:342–3)*

64. **(D)** Persons with *passive–aggressive personality disorder* are characteristically demanding and manipulatively dependent and yet act in such a way as to ensure that the help and support they are given is rendered ineffective. They want, they need, and they should be given care and attention but they cannot allow themselves to receive constructively and trustingly.

The young man described in this question manifests some of these symptoms and personality characteristics. *(1:538; 2:641–2)*

65. **(B)** In *syphilitic meningoencephalitis, general paresis (paralysis),* there is inflammation and degeneration initially involving the frontoparietal cortex but later the other cortical areas. Macroscopically the *frontoparietal cortical areas* show atrophy. *(1:269)*

66. **(D)** *Wilson's disease, hepatolenticular degeneration,* is characterized pathologically by degeneration in the brain lenticular nuclei, especially in the putamen and the caudate nuclei, leading to cavity formation in the *basal ganglia.* The patient may show corneal Kayser–Fleischer rings, blue half moons of the fingernails and dementia. *(1:73; 2:290)*

67. **(C)** *Wernicke's encephalopathy or syndrome* occurs most commonly in chronic alcoholism and severe nutritional deficiencies. This rare syndrome is manifested pathologically by congestion, hemorrhages, and necrosis in the areas around the third ventricle and aqueduct and in the mammillary bodies. *(1:290; 2:323)*

68. **(A)** The most common form of infantile cerebral lipoidosis is *Tay-Sach's disease,* where there is loss of cortical architecture due to general neuron lipoid deposition. *(1:693)*

Answers 69 through 73 deal with the schizophrenic syndromes.

69. **(B)** *Residual schizophrenia.* After at least one episode of overt psychosis there are still symptoms of continued illness—blunted or unusual affect, lack of motivation or interest, eccentricities, social withdrawal and mild looseness of thinking—now no longer florid. *(1:217; 2:373)*

70. **(D)** The *disorganized schizophrenic* appears typically "crazy" in the popular sense of the term. These patients are frequently silly, giggling, grimacing, and inappropriate. They show bizarre delusions and hallucinations and their behavior is often markedly regressed. *(1:332–4; 2:371)*

71. **(C)** *Paranoid schizophrenia* tends to occur at a later age, often in the 30s, and there is less overt personality disorganization. Characteristically these patients are suspicious, distrustful, and aloof. They have delusions of grandeur and persecution. These persecutory delusions may provoke them into aggressive or assaultive behavior. *(1:334–5; 2:371)*

72. **(A)** In *catatonic schizophrenia,* there may be episodes of stupor, excitement, or both alternately. Automatisms and negativism may lead to grotesque posturing and bizarre behavior. *(1:334; 2:371–2)*

73. **(E)** *Schizoaffective disorder* presents with schizophrenic personality disorganization plus strong affective symptoms. The affective disorder may be prominent but the personality decompensation denotes a schizophrenia. These patients show depression and elation, often with marked anxiety, together with generally bizarre thought processes. *(1:339; 2:415–6)*

Answers 74 through 83 deal with electroencephalogram recordings. (1:76–82; 2:256–7)

74. **(E)** *Following withdrawal of alcohol* (or barbiturates) in chronic users, there is a *rebound increase in REM sleep,* often with disturbing *nightmares.* *(1:288–9, 472; 2:322–3)*

75. **(B)** *Three-per-second spike and wave* patterns on the electroencephalogram are characteristic of *absence seizures, petit mal.* *(1:263)*

76. **(D)** In *psychomotor epilepsy* usually four- to eight-per-second *temporal lobe* discharge foci can be noted on the electroencephalogram. *(1:263–6)*

77. **(A)** Episodes of *REM sleep activity* on the electroencephalogram are associated with *narcolepsy* attacks. *(1:475; 2:747–8)*

78. **(C)** In delirium, commonly there is an increase in *diffuse slow-wave* activity on the electroencephalogram as the subject becomes more clouded intellectually. *(1:243)*

79. **(C)** After *barbiturate withdrawal,* in chronic users, there is a "rebound" increase in total REM sleep, often with frightening nightmares. *(1:294–5, 472; 2:328–30)*

80. **(A)** In the *newborn,* up to 50% of the sleep cycle is taken up with REM sleep. *(1:468; 2:103)*

81. **(E)** During *sensory deprivation,* the alpha rhythm of the electroencephalogram decreases and there is increasing slow-wave activity. *(1:126–7)*

82. **(B)** *Amphetamines* suppress or block *REM sleep.* Since *narcolepsy* is associated with REM sleep patterns, amphetamines are specifically used in the treatment of this disorder. *(1:306–7,658–60; 2:747–8)*

83. **(D)** Sleepwalking usually occurs in the course of deep sleep, during stage 3 or 4 *non-REM sleep.* *(1:477; 2:749–50)*

84. **(C)** In *acute intermittent porphyria*, there are excreted in the urine large amounts of uroporphyrin and porphobilinogen, which give the classical "port-wine" reddish-brown urine. *(1:212; 2:283)*

85. **(D)** A *lowered serum ceruloplasmin* level, with increased copper deposition especially in the liver and brain, is found in *Wilson's disease, hepatolenticular degeneration. (1:73; 2:290)*

86. **(A)** *Basophilic stippling* of the red cells on the peripheral blood film is a readily available sign of chronic lead poisoning. Usually there is a co-existent hypochromic anemia. *(1:692,740; 2:680–1)*

87. **(E)** There is a reduction of *dopamine* levels in the basal ganglia in *parkinsonism*. Levodopa is used specifically to treat the parkinson syndrome. *(1:72–3; 2:18–9)*

88. **(B)** Pathologically, *neurofibrillary tangles* and *senile plaques* are typically found in the frontal cortex and the hippocampal region in *Alzheimer's disease,* a form of senile dementia. *(1:810–1; 2:285–7)*

Answers 89 through 93 deal with the symptoms typically seen in the schizophrenic syndromes. (1:332–7; 2:371–4)

89. **(B)** The patient with *residual schizophrenia* is lacking in energy, apathetic and aimless, and withdrawn, with illogical thinking and loose associations. *(1:336; 2:373)*

90. **(D)** The patient suffering with *disorganized schizophrenia* usually is socially *silly*. Frequently the patient shows inappropriate *grinning, grimacing*, and *regressed behavior*. Bizarre *hallucinations* are common. *(1:332–4; 2:371)*

91. **(A)** The *paranoid schizophrenic* usually shows less personality disorganization. The psychotic process is often not diagnosed until the third or fourth decade of life. In this illness, the patient presents with *organized delusions of persecution or grandiosity. (1:334–5; 2:376–371)*

92. **(E)** The *catatonic schizophrenic* may show stupor or excitement. In both catatonic syndromes, negativism is often marked. The stuporous catatonic is mute and frequently posturally rigid. Bizarre posturing is a common symptom. *(1:334; 2:371–2)*

93. **(C)** In *schizoaffective schizophrenia*, the patient shows symptoms both of a thought disorder (schizophrenia) and a mood disorder (depression or mania). These patients show periods of at least two weeks when they have disturbances of thinking without affective symptoms. Schizoaffective disorder patients tend to show less deterioration than patients with other schizophrenic syndromes. *(1:351–3; 2:415–6)*

94. **(B)** *Confabulation,* the falsification of memory to fill gaps in recall ability, is most often seen in *Korsakoff's syndrome* and associated organic brain disorders. *(1:255, 290; 2:323)*

95. **(E)** *Transvestic fetishism* is a paraphilia, starting most frequently in adolescence and occurring usually in males, where the subject obtains sexual pleasure by dressing in clothing of the opposite sex. *(1:446; 2:592)*

96. **(A)** *La belle indifference,* an unusual equanimity in the face of usually distressing physical or psychological symptoms, is typically manifested by patients showing a *conversion disorder*. However, this symptom occurs in other syndromes and in normal people. *(1:419; 2:539)*

97. **(D)** In the *Ganser syndrome,* sometimes called the "prison psychosis," the subject gives an approximate answer to even simple basic questions.
   "What is two plus two?"
   "Five."
   "How old are you?" (correct answer 36)
   "Thirty seven."
   "How many brothers have you?" (correct answer two)
   "One brother." *(1:435–6; 2:582)*

98. **(C)** When the flow of thought is excessively rapid and there is said to be a *flight of ideas,* the subject is usually manifesting symptoms of a bipolar disorder, manic type. *(1:219,371; 2:189,405)*

Answers 99 through 103 deal with the definitions of diagnostic terms.

99. **(A)** A *psychosis* is an emotional illness where the subject shows a *marked impairment of reality contact,* often with *severe personality disorganization.* *(1:227; 2:1264)*

100. **(D)** In *anxiety disorders,* there is a *maladaptive reaction to anxiety* without, however, severe reality distortion or personality disorganization. In the anxiety syndrome, the subject is constantly attempting to cope with inner anxiety. *(1:227; 2:1259)*

101. **(B)** A *conduct disorder* is a *stable maladaptive behavior pattern* seen in the *developmental years.* This is a relatively fixed but unproductive way of coping where, however, the personality is not yet finalized. There is always the hope with these children and adolescents that they will grow out of it. Many do not. *(1:722; 2:664)*

102. **(C)** An *adjustment disorder* at any age is a *temporary acute reaction* to *stress*. When the stress is removed or reduced or the subject learns to cope more effectively, the individual returns to the pre-existing level of adaptation. *(1:494; 2:606–7)*

103. **(E)** A *personality disorder* is characterized by chronic fixed maladaptive behavior patterns that are usually recognizable by the teenage years. People with personality disorders typically feel little anxiety themselves about their behavior that, however, makes other people anxious. *(1:525; 2:621)*

Answers 104 through 108 deal with disorders presenting with sexual symptoms, paraphilias. (1:443–8; 2:587–95)

104. **(C)** The *pedophile* achieves sexual *gratification* through contact with *children thirteen years or younger*. This diagnosis usually implies adult sexual interest in an immature child. Sexual play between children would not be included in deviant sexuality. *(1:444–5; 2:592–5)*

105. **(D)** In *transvestic fetishism,* the subject is satisfied with his or her own gender but gains erotic pleasure through dressing in the *clothing of the opposite sex*. Usually the transvestite is a heterosexual male who dresses in female clothing; a heterosexual female who dresses in male clothing is less likely to be labelled as transvestite by present day society. *(1:446; 2:592–5)*

106. **(A)** In *fetishism,* the *fetishist* gains sexual gratification through contact with an inanimate object, such as a shoe or a piece of clothing (the *fetish*). *(1:446; 2:592–5)*

Pedophilia, transvestism, fetishism, and exhibitionism are paraphilias, sexual disorders where the individual is sexually aroused and gratified by sexual objects or situations that are not part of the normal sexual bonding, caring, and procreative patterns.

107. **(B)** The *transsexual* does not accept his or her anatomic sex and has a need to be changed to the opposite sex, usually by surgical means. Transsexualism is a *gender identity disorder*. *(1:752–3; 2:588–91)*

108. **(E)** The *exhibitionist,* usually a male, gains sexual gratification by *genital self-exposure,* usually to members of the opposite sex. *(1:449–450; 2:592–5)*

109. **(B)** In a *conversion disorder,* unacceptable feelings are repressed but are manifested outwardly in *symbolic* fashion by a *physical symptom* involving the voluntary musculature or the special senses. The term *conversion* implies a process that has not been proven to occur. *(1:418–20; 2:535–40)*

110. **(E)** When the subject has a *déjà vu* reaction, he has the *illusion* of having experienced his present reality at some time past. This sensation occurs with normal people especially during the teenage years but may also indicate a developing emotional illness. *(1:221; 2:1248)*

111. **(A)** A *catastrophic reaction* is manifested by acute disruptive agitation that develops when a brain-injured person cannot solve a problem and is faced suddenly with the reality of his intellectual handicap. *(1:246; 2:285)*

112. **(D)** *Bruxism* is the symptom of *compulsive chewing* and *teeth grinding*. Chronic bruxism can wear down the teeth. Bed partners may be awakened by sleep-related bruxism in a fellow sleeper. *(1:478; 2:1244)*

113. **(C)** *Bulimia* is obsessive overeating and food gorging that sometimes alternates with bouts of dieting and self-starvation. *(1:746–8; 2:760–3)*

114. **(C)** *Multiple personality disorder* is a dissociative disorder in which the subject develops two or more distinct personalities. There is much discussion as to how common this syndrome actually is and what are the causative factors. Studies have indicated that many of these patients have a history of sexual abuse but these findings also have been questioned. *(1:431–3; 2:569–79)*

115. **(F)** In a *conversion disorder*, intolerable or unacceptable feelings are repressed, unconsciously and automatically removed from awareness, and then dealt with through a loss or change in function of a bodily function under control of the voluntary muscles or special senses. Conversion disorder is more common in women, in certain cultures, and in lower socioeconomic groups.

In this clinical situation, this married woman dealt with very rageful feelings towards her husband by repressing the rage and by losing her voice that might otherwise have shrieked rage at him. Often the repressed feeling is acted out in the symptom—the woman's anger at her husband is being expressed by forcing him now to attend to her and take over some of her duties. The lady's lack of concern is *la belle indifference*, a lack of anxiety about a situation that normally would be anxiety arousing. The subject also is having much secondary gain in all the attention she is now getting from family members. The *primary gain* is the emotional relief produced by the conflict repression and the symptom development. *(1:418–20; 2:535–40)*

116. **(D)** Chronic cocaine abusers are likely to develop a *cocaine delusional disorder*, a delusional state in which the patient may show symptoms similar to paranoid schizophrenia. Tactile hallucinations *(formication)* of insects crawling in or under the skin may be present—*cocaine bugs*. Abuse of other stimulants such as amphetamines may produce a similar psychotic disorder. *(1:304; 2:337–42)*

117. **(A)** *Agoraphobia* is the fear of social situations from which escape would be difficult or where help would be difficult to obtain in the event the subject begins to lose control or be overwhelmed in some way. A *phobia* is a persistent irrational fear of a specific object, place, or situation. Agoraphobia is a phobia of the marketplace, from the Greek word *agora*. Agoraphobia can be socially and emotionally very incapacitating. *(1:397–400; 2:458–72)*

Somatic Treatments
Questions

INTRODUCTION

For examination purposes and, more important, for general clinical practice, the standard psychiatry texts give too generalized a discussion of the somatic therapies. The student and the practitioner should supplement their understanding of these most important procedures from more specialized books.

REFERENCES

1. Chapter 30,   The Biological Therapies, pp 606–77
2. Chapter 24,   Psychopharmacology and Electroconvulsive Therapy, pp 767–853

    Chapter 30,   Treatment of Children and Adolescents: Somatic Treatments, pp 986–1002

DIRECTIONS (Questions 1 through 20): Each of the numbered items or incomplete statements in this section is followed by answers or by completions of the statement. Select the ONE lettered answer or completion that is BEST in each case.

1. Before therapeutic response is evident, amitriptyline will usually have to be given for a period of

    (A) 3–4 days
    (B) 10–14 days
    (C) 3–4 weeks
    (D) 3–6 months
    (E) 6–8 months

2. All of the following statements are true about treatment with lithium carbonate *except*

    (A) therapeutic serum level 0. 8–1. 2 mEq/L
    (B) may produce goiter
    (C) slurred speech may indicate toxic levels
    (D) additive therapeutic effect with amphetamines
    (E) causes worsening of psoriasis

3. Side effects of chlorpromazine include

    (A) photosensitivity
    (B) gynecomastia
    (C) urinary retention
    (D) pigmentary retinopathy
    (E) false pregnancy test

4. Before giving patients a course of modified electroconvulsive therapy, they should be warned of side effects, which include all of the following *except*

    (A) amenorrhea in women for 2 to 3 months
    (B) headaches
    (C) loss of memory for recent events
    (D) increase in weight
    (E) sleeplessness for 1 to 2 weeks

5. Convulsions may develop on drug withdrawal after chronic use of

    (A) chlorpromazine
    (B) reserpine
    (C) lithium
    (D) meprobamate
    (E) imipramine

6. For the effective treatment of bipolar disorder, depressive type, the number of electroconvulsive therapy treatments necessary for full benefit is likely to be

    (A) 1–3
    (B) 5–10
    (C) 15–25
    (D) 25–50
    (E) over 50

7. A 21-year-old student is brought to the student clinic by his roommate. The young man is anxious, restless, and confused. The roommate reports that the patient has been taking large amounts of a popular over-the-counter sleeping preparation. In treating this patient, you may want to use intramuscular injections of

    (A) scopolamine
    (B) amphetamine
    (C) ergotamine
    (D) diphenhydramine
    (E) physostigmine

8. Electroconvulsive therapy is often very effective in

    (A) opioid abuse
    (B) ulcerative colitis
    (C) conversion disorder
    (D) schizophrenia, catatonic type
    (E) phobic disorder

9. Pigmentary retinopathy is seen in patients receiving high doses of which drug?

    (A) propanolol
    (B) lithium carbonate
    (C) fluoxetine
    (D) methylphenidate
    (E) thioridazine

10. All of the following statements about bupropion are correct *except*

    (A) does not have anticholinergic side effects
    (B) increased risk of seizures with higher doses
    (C) fewer adverse cardiac effects than tricyclic antidepressants
    (D) effective in treatment of patients with major depression
    (E) related to tetracyclic antidepressants

11. You have maintained a 55-year-old depressed man on tranylcypromine for 8 weeks with only moderate symptomatic relief, so you decide to change his medication to amitriptyline. Accordingly, you should plan to

    (A) gradually decrease the tranylcypromine as you give increasing dosages of amitriptyline
    (B) stop the tranylcypromine; after 14 days, start amitriptyline in increasing doses
    (C) stop the tranylcypromine and immediately begin amitriptyline

(D) continue tranylcypromine at present levels as you give amitriptyline in increasing doses to a therapeutically effective level

(E) check thyroid and kidney functions

12. A dangerous effect of reserpine is

(A) bilateral nerve deafness

(B) acute manic state

(C) aggressive hypersexuality

(D) acute schizophrenic reaction

(E) suicidal depression

13. Electroconvulsive therapy has its therapeutic effect due to

(A) increase in total REM sleep

(B) elevation of serum catecholamines

(C) behavior modification

(D) dopamine receptor blockage

(E) none of the above

14. All of the following statements about *clozapine* are correct *except*

(A) used to treat patients who have disabling side effects with traditional antipsychotic medication

(B) does not produce parkinsonian symptoms

(C) seizures tend to occur with high doses

(D) chemically is a piperazine

(E) withdrawal may cause sweating, diarrhea, and restlessness

15. Common benzodiazepine withdrawal symptoms include all of the following *except*

(A) insomnia

(B) heart block

(C) seizures

(D) depression

(E) sweating

16. Electroconvulsive therapy is usually contraindicated by

(A) pregnancy

(B) age over 65

(C) brain tumor

(D) hypotension

(E) angina pectoris

17. All the following statements are true about tardive dyskinesia *except*

(A) may appear or worsen after phenothiazine is stopped

(B) lip sucking and smacking, choreiform arm movements

(C) does not occur in preadolescent children

(D) antiparkinsonian drugs do not help and may worsen symptoms

(E) may be caused by amoxapine

18. Akathisia is

(A) a form of mutism seen in profound barbiturate overdose

(B) an extrapyramidal symptom most commonly associated with piperazines

(C) the type of bluish-gray skin coloration in exposed areas, occurring with prolonged high dosage of chlorpromazine

(D) form of sudden death, possibly due to ventricular fibrillation, in cases with long-term phenothiazine intake

(E) cholestatic jaundice possibly due to individual sensitivity to chlorpromazine

19. When a tricyclic antidepressant is therapeutically effective in treating the depression of a bipolar disorder, the drug should be maintained

(A) 3 weeks from starting the drug

(B) 3 to 6 months after good therapeutic response is noted

(C) 1 to 2 years after depression is cleared

(D) until hypomanic state occurs

(E) 3 weeks from time of beneficial response

20. Which antidepressant is most likely to cause akathisia, parkinsonism, and tardive dyskinesia?

(A) fluoxetine

(B) nortriptyline

(C) tranylcypromine

(D) amoxapine

(E) doxepin

DIRECTIONS (Questions 21 through 50): Each set of matching questions in this section consists of a list of four to eight lettered options followed by a set of numbered words or phrases. For each numbered word or phrase, select the ONE lettered option that is most closely associated with it. Each lettered option may be selected once, more than once, or not at all.

Questions 21 through 28

(A) chlorpromazine

(B) barbiturates

(C) monoamine oxidase inhibitors

(D) amphetamines

(E) lithium

(F) trazodone

(G) valproic acid

For each of the side effects listed below, select the most likely causative medication.

21. Paranoid psychotic reactions

22. Hypertensive crisis precipitated by bee sting

23. Acute confusional state in elderly

24. Exacerbation of acute intermittent porphyria

25. Purplish-gray suntan reaction

26. Priapism

27. Ebstein's anomaly of the tricuspid valve

28. Pancreatitis

Questions 29 through 34

(A) disulfiram
(B) lithium carbonate
(C) chlordiazepoxide
(D) penicillamine
(E) ammonium chloride
(F) clonidine

For each syndrome listed below, select the most appropriate treatment.

29. Delirium tremens

30. Chronic alcoholism

31. Chronic bromism

32. Bipolar disorder, manic type

33. Tourette's Disorder

34. Wilson's disease

Questions 35 through 40

(A) electroconvulsive therapy
(B) physostigmine salicylate
(C) amantadine
(D) dantrolene
(E) ergotamine tartrate
(F) pimozide

For each syndrome, select the most appropriate treatment.

35. Toxic psychosis due to scopolamine-containing sleeping preparations

36. Tourette's Disorder

37. Akathisia

38. Migraine

39. Acute mania

40. Neuroleptic malignant syndrome

Questions 41 through 45

(A) chlorpromazine
(B) amphetamines
(C) benztropine
(D) bromocriptine
(E) calcium disodium versenate (EDTA)

For each syndrome listed below, select the correct treatment.

41. Narcolepsy

42. Neuroleptic malignant syndrome

43. Rabbit syndrome

44. Mania

45. Lead poisoning

Questions 46 through 50

(A) haloperidol
(B) methylphenidate
(C) dimercaprol
(D) methadone
(E) imipramine

For each disorder, select the correct treatment.

46. Attention deficit hyperactivity disorder

47. Functional enuresis, enuresis

48. Tourette's Disorder

49. Chronic mercury poisoning

50. Heroin addiction

Answers and Explanations

1. **(C)** Though *amitriptyline* may produce improvement in appetite, sleeping and energy level within 5 to 15 days, with many patients a significant improvement in mood is not noted until the medication has been given for at least *3 to 4 weeks*. When the antidepressant is being given at an effective level, the medication should be maintained for 3 to 6 months at this dose.

   In the management of depressed patients, it should be noted that the patient is likely to have increased energy before feeling relief from the depression and so is at increased risk for suicide at the early stage of antidepressant treatment. Very often one week's supply of a tricyclic antidepressant would be a lethal dose if taken in a suicide attempt. *(1:664–5; 2:396–7)*

2. **(D)** *Lithium* has no symptomatic additive effect with amphetamines. The therapeutic blood serum level for lithium is 0.8–1.2 mEq/L, though some clinicians suggest a safer therapeutic level is 0.7–1.0 mEq/L, especially in the elderly. Patients on lithium may complain of dry skin, dry hair and hair loss especially in women, acne and a worsening of psoriasis. Speech slurring is more common at higher dose levels. Goiter may also be a side effect of lithium treatment. *(1:652–5; 2:822–6)*

3. **(D)** In patients taking *chlorpromazine*, excessive photosensitivity can occur, leading to disabling sunburn. Sometimes these patients develop a metallic or purplish skin color after exposure to sunlight. Like many anticholinergic neuroleptics, chlorpromazine may produce constipation and *urinary retention*. The drug should be used with caution where there are preexisting micturition difficulties. Women can have false positive pregnancy tests. Male patients, especially adolescents and young adults, may become very disturbed at the *gynecomastia* that is sometimes produced by the neuroleptic induced hormonal changes. Pigmentary retinopathy is not caused by chlorpromazine. *(1:642–6; 2:779–88)*

4. **(E)** *Sleeplessness* is not a major side effect of electroconvulsive therapy.

   Amenorrhea is likely to be present in women patients for 2 to 3 months after a course of convulsive therapy. Headache is a frequent complaint after the treatments and usually responds readily to symptomatic treatment.

   After several treatments, the patient usually develops moderate memory loss for more recent events. The amnesia should clear gradually within 2 to 4 weeks of cessation of treatment. *(1:672–3; 2:840–1)*

5. **(D)** *Convulsions* may occur when *meprobamate* is withdrawn after a period of chronic use. Convulsions can also occur on withdrawal of *barbiturates, benzodiazepines*, or *alcohol* in chronic users. *(1:621–2; 2:818)*

6. **(B)** Usually 5 to 10, with an average of 9 or 10, *electroconvulsive treatments* are necessary to treat and maintain therapeutic benefits in bipolar disorder, depressive type. Symptomatically the painful depression is often relieved by 3 or 4 treatments, but further treatments are necessary to prevent early relapse. *(1:672; 2:839–40)*

7. **(E)** A *toxic psychosis* due to the chronic ingestion of over-the-counter sleeping medication is often caused by the scopolamine or belladonna-related compounds in the preparation. Intramuscular injection of physostigmine salicylate 1 mg repeated after 15 to 20 minutes is the treatment of choice. Patients may develop serious hypotension when given phenothiazines. *(1:281; 2:784–5)*

8. **(D)** *Catatonic schizophrenia,* especially the excited type, often responds very well to a course of electroconvulsive therapy. Apathetic or stuporous catatonia may show symptomatic improvement, but relapse is common. Convulsive therapy would not be indicated for ulcerative colitis, conversion or phobic disorders, or opioid abuse. *(1:671; 2:838)*

9. **(E)** *Pigmentary retinopathy* has been reported in patients receiving 800 mg or more of *thioridazine* over several weeks or months and can occur at lower dose levels. The retinary pigmentation is

permanent and can progress to blindness. This side effect is also reported with mesoridazine. *(1:642–3; 2:786)*

10. **(E)** *Buproprion* is effective in treating major depression. It is not related to either the tricyclic or the tetracyclic antidepressants. Buproprion does not have anticholinergic side effects or the quinidine effect of the tricyclic antidepressants on the heart. Especially with higher doses, over 450 mg per day, there is a significant risk of seizures with buproprion. *(1:628–30; 2:803–4)*

11. **(B)** Stop the tranylcypromine and only after 14 days start amitriptyline in increasing doses.

When a monoamine oxidase inhibitor is given in combination with a tricyclic antidepressant, the patient may develop potentially fatal restlessness, twitching, hyperpyrexia, and convulsions. If the patient has been taking monoamine oxidase inhibitors, a minimum 10 to 14 day washout period is recommended before a tricyclic is started. Some clinicians prefer to wait 14 days to insure the patient is free from this cross-reaction. Monoamine oxidase inhibitors irreversibly inhibit monoamine oxidases; these monoamine oxidases take about 14 days to reach previous baseline level after the MAOI inhibitors are stopped. Under very carefully controlled clinical conditions, these drugs may be used in combination and may prove effective in previously refractory depressive states. *(1:656–7; 2:802)*

12. **(E)** The most dangerous side effect of *reserpine* is the production of depression or the increase of existing *depression* in patients taking the drug. These depressive states may result in *suicide* or may require intensive antidepressant treatment.

Reserpine is rarely used now for its tranquilizing effect. *(1:569; 2:416–7)*

13. **(E)** *None* of the suggested theories about the effect of *electroconvulsive therapy* has been *validated*—and there are now hundreds of proposed theories. The use of this treatment procedure is solely based on its demonstrated efficacy in certain psychiatric states. *(1:670; 2:837)*

14. **(D)** *Clozapine* is a dibenzodiazepine antipsychotic; it is not a benzodiazepine. Clozapine has no extrapyramidal or parkinsonian side effects but with increasing doses there is a rapidly increasing risk of seizures. Drug treatment should be discontinued by tapering the dosage to avoid a cholinergic rebound syndrome with sweating, diarrhea, flushing and restlessness.

Clozapine is used with psychotic patients who have not responded to usually adequate treatment with at least three different types of antipsychotic

drugs or who have intolerable and incapacitating side effects with the traditional neuroleptics. *(1:647–9; 2:773)*

15. **(B)** The symptoms seen with *benzodiazepine withdrawal* depend on how long the drug has been taken, the dosage level, the half life of the benzodiazepine and the speed with which the drug is being tapered. Withdrawal symptoms typically include anxiety, insomnia, restlessness and irritability, sweating and headache. Seizures may occur during withdrawal. Heart block is not a symptom of benzodiazepine withdrawal. Severe depression with suicidal feelings and impulses can occur as part of a withdrawal syndrome. *(1:622–6; 2:328–9, 815–6)*

16. **(C)** With full treatment and support facilities, there are probably very few absolute *contraindications* to the use of *electroconvulsive therapy* in a psychiatric emergency. However, a *brain tumor* is usually considered a specific contraindication. The rise in intracranial pressure during an induced convulsion can prove fatal in patients with brain neoplasm. *(1:672–3; 2:838)*

17. **(C)** *Tardive dyskinesia* is increasingly being diagnosed in children and adolescents.

Tardive dyskinesia may occur at any time during phenothiazine treatment and can appear or worsen when the drug treatment is stopped. Amoxapine may produce tardive dyskinesia. Symptoms of the syndrome include lip sucking and smacking, tongue protrusion, choreiform arm movements, and tonic spasms of the neck and back muscles.

Antiparkinsonian drugs do not relieve the symptoms and may indeed cause them to worsen. *(1:644–6; 2:781–3,998–9)*

18. **(B)** *Akathisia* is an *extrapyramidal* symptom, most often associated with the *piperazine* group of tranquilizers. With this side effect, patients feel restless, cannot sit still, pace about, and tend to complain that their feet or legs are "restless." *(1:644; 2:823; 3:118)*

19. **(B)** A *tricyclic antidepressant,* given in adequate dosage, may take 3 to 4 weeks to achieve full therapeutic effect in the treatment of *depression* and should then be continued for 3 to 6 months to maintain the improvement and to prevent relapse. *(1:665; 2:796–7)*

20. **(D)** *Amoxapine,* a dibenzoxazepine antidepressant, derived from the antipsychotic loxapine has dopamine receptor blocking effects and can cause akathisia, parkinsonism, and tardive dyskinesia. *(1:662,666; 2:801)*

21. **(D)** *Amphetamines* typically produce *paranoid psychotic reactions*, especially with chronic use. *(1:307; 2:342–3)*

22. **(C)** Patients taking *monoamine oxidase inhibitors* must be warned against ingesting aged cheese, beer, wines, chicken liver, pickled herring, and other foods rich in tyramine. The hypertensive effect of the dietary tyramine is potentiated by the monoamine oxidase inhibitor, and *severe hypertensive crisis* may occur. Bee stings may cause a hypertensive crisis. *(1:657–8; 2:802–5)*

23. **(B)** *Barbiturates* should not be used for sedation in the *elderly* because they are liable to precipitate *acute confusional states*. *(1:817; 2:1135)*

24. **(B)** *Barbiturates* are absolutely contraindicated in patients with *acute intermittent porphyria* because the drug can precipitate an acute attack.

    Chlorpromazine is useful in the symptomatic treatment of an acute episode of porphyria. *(1:267)*

25. **(A)** Chronic users of *chlorpromazine* are liable to develop a *purplish-gray suntan* reaction due to the development of skin pigmentation. Penicillamine has been used with benefit to treat the pigmentation. *(1:649; 2:786)*

26. **(F)** *Trazodone* may produce *priapism* which can be painful, irreversible and lead to impotence. Persistent priapism will require surgical treatment. *(1:661; 2:800)*

27. **(E)** *Lithium* is contraindicated during pregnancy. When lithium is given during the first trimester of pregnancy, Ebstein's anomaly of the tricuspid valve is likely to occur. Lithium given late in pregnancy can cause lithium toxicity in the newborn. Lithium is excreted in part in the breast milk and so can affect the nursing infant. *(1:651–5; 2:821)*

28. **(G)** *Valproic acid*, an anticonvulsant used in the treatment of bipolar disorder, may cause serious and sometimes fatal pancreatitis, especially in the first six months of treatment. *(1:668–9; 2:819,829)*

29. **(C)** *Delirium tremens, alcohol withdrawal delirium*, an acute delirious state, is best treated by *benzodiazepines;* chlordiazepoxide and diazepam are the most often used. Nutritional deficiencies need to be corrected and the fluid balance carefully monitored. *(1:288–9; 2:324–4)*

30. **(A)** In treating the *chronic alcoholic* who wishes to give up drinking, *disulfiram* (Antabuse) can be used to help make alcohol intake disagreeable. *(1:291–2; 2:326)*

31. **(E)** *Chronic bromide intoxication, chronic bromism*, is treated by discontinuing all bromide ingestion and eliminating bromide from the body.

    Clearing of bromide is accelerated by taking extra salt and fluids to flush out the bromide. Bromide excretion is hastened by the use of *ammonium chloride* rather than *sodium chloride*. The ammonium salt itself has a diuretic action. *(1:565)*

32. **(B)** *Lithium carbonate* is used in the treatment of *bipolar disorder, manic type*, especially in the treatment of moderate manic states and in the prevention of manic recurrences. In acute manic states, lithium carbonate is usually too slow-acting to be useful, and one of the antipsychotics is used. *(1:651; 2:820)*

33. **(F)** *Clonidine* is used in the treatment of patients with Tourette's Disorder especially where the patient has attention disorder, hyperactivity disorder, or where haloperidol and pimozide cause distressing side effects. *(1:762; 2:688)*

34. **(D)** *Penicillamine* is used to increase copper excretion and to prevent or minimize symptoms in *hepatolenticular degeneration, Wilson's disease*, where there is increased deposition of copper in the tissues, especially of the basal ganglia and the liver. *(1:73,758; 2:290)*

35. **(B)** *Toxic psychoses* may occur due to chronic use of nonprescription *scopolamine-containing sleeping preparations*. Intramuscular *physostigmine salicylate* is the specific antidote. *(1:619,666; 2:785)*

36. **(F)** *Pimozide*, an antipsychotic, is used to treat patients with *Tourette's Disorder*. It may cause less cognitive dulling than haloperidol but is more cardiotoxic, especially at higher doses. *(1:762; 2:688)*

37. **(C)** *Akathisia*, the restless leg syndrome, is an extrapyramidal side effect of dopamine receptor-blocking antipsychotic medications. Many akathisia patients may look anxious because they are motorically restless but will state that emotionally they do not feel anxious, even though the akathisia can feel unpleasant. *Amantadine* or *propanolol* can be used to treat this side effect without having any additive anticholinergic side effects. *(1:617–8; 2:780)*

38. **(E)** The treatment for *migraine acute attacks* is *ergotamine tartrate* by mouth or subcutaneous injection. Ergotamine may be combined with caffeine, antispasmodics, or sedatives. *(1:507; 2:900, 921)*

39. **(A)** Electroconvulsive therapy will quickly bring manic symptoms under control. *(1:670; 2:838)*

40. **(D)** *Neuroleptic malignant syndrome,* a most serious neuroleptic side effect that can be rapidly fatal, is treated by immediately stopping the neuroleptic, very active symptomatic treatment, and the use of *dantrolene* and *bromocriptine.* (1:646; 2:783–4)

41. **(B)** *Amphetamines* are the drugs specifically used for *narcolepsy.* Many narcoleptic patients show REM sleep patterns on their electroencephalograms during attacks; amphetamines inhibit REM sleep. (1:475; 2:747–8)

42. **(D)** *Bromocriptine,* a dopamine agonist, is frequently used in the treatment of the *neuroleptic malignant syndrome.* (1:646; 2:291)

43. **(C)** The *rabbit syndrome,* manifested by rabbit-like perioral movements, is a relatively late onset parkinsonian side effect of the neuroleptics that is a common examination topic. The syndrome usually responds to benztropine and other anticholinergic medications. (1:644; 2:780–1)

44. **(A)** Chlorpromazine in high dosages is very effective in treating mania. (1:639–40; 2:774)

45. **(E)** For *lead poisoning,* a treatment program of *calcium disodium versenate (EDTA)* should be instituted after the source of the lead intake has been blocked. (1:692,740; 2:680–1)

46. **(B)** *Methylphenidate* is the medication presently most often used for patients with *attention deficit hyperactivity disorder.* This medication produces symptomatic improvement in about 70% of cases. Growth stunting with chronic use has been reported but with adequate monitoring and drug-free periods at weekends and holidays, when therapeutically reasonable, growth retardation is not a major problem. (1:729; 2:660–3)

47. **(E)** With *enuresis,* many different treatments work with different clinicians and different children.

Imipramine will often produce symptomatic benefit but the improvement may not continue after the medication is stopped. Because tolerance to the drug can occur within several weeks, the symptoms are likely to recur even when the treatment is continued. (1:767; 2:994–5)

48. **(A)** *Haloperidol,* one of the butyrophenones, is often effective in producing symptomatic improvement in patients with *Tourette's Disorder.* Even though the multiple tics, coprolalia, and echolalia shown by these subjects are often totally incapacitating without effective treatment, many patients stop the haloperidol due to the side effects of the antipsychotic. While patients with Tourette's Disorder usually show symptomatic improvement at a lower dose level of haloperidol than is used in treating psychosis, tardive dyskinesia is noted as an antipsychotic-induced side effect in these patients. (1:762; 2:688)

49. **(C)** In the treatment of *mercury poisoning,* the patient should be removed from the source of the mercury. Usually mercury poisoning is an occupational hazard. The Mad Hatter in "Alice in Wonderland" was mad because mercury poisoning was an occupational hazard of hatters in Victorian England.

    Dimercaprol (BAL) is used to increase mercury excretion. (1:212; 2:254)

50. **(D)** *Methadone* is used to withdraw a patient from heroin or to substitute as a maintenance drug instead of heroin in patients with *heroin addiction.* Methadone is an addicting narcotic itself but it can be given orally once daily, and causes less euphoria and drowsiness than heroin.

    L-alpha acetyl methadol (LAMM) can suppress opioid withdrawal symptoms for three to four days so can be given three times a week instead of methadone. (1:301; 2:334–5)

CHAPTER 6

Psychological Treatment and Management
Questions

INTRODUCTION

Examination candidates will be expected to know in general about different types of psychological treatment but should anticipate more detailed questions on two very different aspects of clinical practice—the management of the difficult patient and the process and planning of psychoanalytic psychotherapy.

The trainee will face questions about difficult patients, such as those who are seductive, manipulative, aggressive, or otherwise disturbing. The questions will be phrased in such a way that the student is expected to recognize the problem posed by these patients, to be aware of the doctor's natural human reaction to such a patient, and yet to be able to plan the necessary examination, management, and treatment that these people, like any other patients, should have.

Frequently in clinical psychiatry examinations, there are questions about the theoretical aspects of psychotherapy, usually from the psychoanalytic standpoint. These questions test the student's understanding of the way the psychotherapy process can be developed and strengthened in a treatment situation where the purpose is to help patients understand what they are feeling, thinking, saying, and doing. In order to make these questions about psychotherapy sufficiently specific, the questions posed and the answers required may sometimes seem rather unrealistic.

REFERENCES

1. Chapter 7.1, Clinical Examination of the Psychiatric Patient.

   Psychiatric Interview, History and Mental Status Examination, pp 193–205

   Chapter 29, Psychotherapies, pp 571–605

   Chapter 44, Psychiatric Treatment of Children and Adolescents, pp 787–806

2. Chapter 6, Psychiatric Interview, Psychiatric History and Mental Status, pp 163–199

   Chapter 25, Individual Psychotherapies, pp 855–889

   Chapter 26, Behavior Therapy, pp 891–928

   Chapter 28, Family Therapy, pp 929–949

   Chapter 29, Group Therapies, pp 951–984

   Chapter 30, Treatment of Children and Adolescents, pp 985–1020

DIRECTIONS (Questions 1 through 18): Each of the numbered items or incomplete statements in this section is followed by answers or by completions of the statement. Select the ONE lettered answer or completion that is BEST in each case.

1. All of the following statements about behavior therapy are correct *except*

   (A) deals with observable behavior
   (B) attempts to uncover underlying dynamics
   (C) is based on learning theory
   (D) problems should be clearly outlined
   (E) goals should be definitely established

2. All of the following statements about behavior modification are correct *except*

   (A) helpful in teaching communicative language to autistic children
   (B) medications are unhelpful in behavior modification treatment
   (C) phobic adults may be treated by flooding
   (D) electric shock has been used to treat sexual deviates
   (E) effective in treating infant rumination disorder

3. Behavior modification is based on

   (A) transference
   (B) reinforcement
   (C) counseling
   (D) hypnosis
   (E) group interaction

4. Psychoanalysis is of greatest value in treating

   (A) schizophrenia
   (B) borderline retardation
   (C) adolescent identity crises
   (D) major depression
   (E) obsessive–compulsive disorder

5. Transference is the

   (A) manifestation of the psychotherapist's feelings toward the patient
   (B) development of warm feelings between patient and psychotherapist
   (C) carryover of patient's feelings from an earlier relationship onto the psychotherapist
   (D) ability to feel with the other person and to understand his feelings
   (E) splitting of an idea from its accompanying emotion

6. You are seeing a 24-year-old woman in psychotherapy. During the third session, she begins to cry loudly as she talks about her marriage. To enhance the treatment process, you should

   (A) encourage her to continue crying, to let out her feelings
   (B) point out that she is trying to share information and crying may be her way of not sharing
   (C) acknowledge her crying and continue to discuss this topic with her
   (D) bring the session to an end so that the patient does not become too upset
   (E) change the subject and deal with something less tension provoking

7. A 35-year-old unmarried schoolteacher is too fearful to go to work. She begins psychotherapy. In her third interview, she admits she is afraid she will be attacked by some of her older students and adds, "All the other women teachers are scared too. Several have been assaulted." To facilitate her treatment, you should say

   (A) "Well, it is reassuring to know you have the same anxieties that the other teachers have."
   (B) "But they have been able to continue working in school."
   (C) "When you say 'assaulted,' perhaps you are worried about a sexual attack."
   (D) "First let us try to understand your feelings and what these feelings do to you."
   (E) "Working in our schools is certainly difficult nowadays."

8. During her fourth psychotherapy session, a 26-year-old married woman asks, "Do you like my new hairstyle?" She really looks dreadful. Your response should be

   (A) "No, you look dreadful."
   (B) "Yes. You look very attractive."
   (C) "Why do you ask?"
   (D) "Are you testing me?"
   (E) "You should not ask personal questions in therapy."

9. You are a male psychotherapist and have just started to see a 44-year-old man in psychotherapy. At the start of the second interview, he gives you a most attractive tie. You should say something like

   (A) "Why do you want to give me this gift?"
   (B) "Are you are trying to buy my approval?"
   (C) "Thank you very much."
   (D) "A tie has male sexual symbolism."
   (E) "I never accept personal gifts."

10. For 2 weeks a paranoid schizophrenic man has been under your care in a general hospital psychiatric unit. During an interview, he shows you a switchblade he carries around for protection. You should

   (A) ask the patient for the knife. If he refuses, you are required to keep the matter confidential

   (B) ask the patient for the knife. If he refuses, call in the security personnel to take the knife from him

   (C) ask the patient for the knife. If he refuses, catch hold of him, refusing to let go until he gives you the knife

   (D) tell the patient that knives are totally forbidden on the unit. Insist that he get rid of the switchblade

   (E) increase the frequency of his appointments so you can work through his insecurity and need to carry a weapon

11. An 18-year-old college student has been hospitalized for recurrent hyperventilation attacks. When you are called in consultation by his physician, you should

   (A) reassure the patient that he is physically well

   (B) explain the purpose and nature of the interview

   (C) try to look the patient directly in the eye

   (D) first discuss the situation with the Dean of Students

   (E) recommend that the patient be discharged from the hospital

12. While the local family doctor is on vacation, you are looking after his practice for him. For the third time this week, you have been interrupted after office hours by a 45-year-old married woman coming to see "her doctor." She has been complaining of recurrent low back pain but, in brief examinations, you have found nothing wrong. Your office nurse has just left for home when you hear this woman patient rapping impatiently on the office door. You should

   (A) ignore her knocking and leave by the back door

   (B) point out that her aches are purely functional and she should pull herself together

   (C) tell her that she requires careful, thorough evaluation. Give her the next available appointment during office hours

   (D) bring her in and give her the most thorough physical examination. Then point out her seductive behavior

   (E) call her husband and point out that she obviously wants companionship and understanding

Question 13

You are starting psychotherapeutic treatment with a 23-year-old man. In his second interview he asks, "What should I do to get well?"

13. To facilitate the treatment process you should answer

   (A) "Just trust in me and be sure to share your true feelings."

   (B) "That is not up to me to tell you."

   (C) "How do you feel about that yourself?"

   (D) "It is too early in the treatment to tell you yet."

   (E) "Try to avoid being bothered by specific details at this time."

Question 14

The wife of a 45-year-old man is very concerned about her husband's increasing alcoholism. She wants you to prescribe something for him that "will settle his nerves." He does not have the time to come to see you himself.

14. You should

   (A) prescribe a mid-potency tranquilizer such as chlordiazepoxide

   (B) insist on seeing the husband before you prescribe any treatment

   (C) suggest that he would be better with Antabuse

   (D) point out that his inability to come to see you is a sign of his resistance to treatment

   (E) give the wife some sedation to help her relax

Question 15

One Sunday afternoon you are asked to see a 19-year-old male college student as an emergency consultation. His parents, who bring him to your office, complain that he is "totally out of control," "weird," and "unable to look after himself." The young man looks unkempt and rather dirty but steadfastly refuses to talk with you; he states he is not sick and "it is none of your business."

15. The only correct statement that follows is

   (A) he should be hospitalized for further evaluation and treatment
   (B) you have insufficient information to take any definite action
   (C) he is most likely an early schizophrenic and should respond to a neuroleptic
   (D) he is probably emotionally normal and you are being pulled into a family conflict
   (E) the parents may well be too authoritarian and intrusive themselves and need counseling

Question 16

A 43-year-old married woman comes to see you about her 75-year-old mother. The mother lives by herself in a big old house, her home for the past 40 years. Her memory is not as good as it used to be. She leaves lights on, doors unlocked, and water faucets running. The daughter wants her mother to have the security and care of the local state hospital.

16. You should

   (A) prepare a commitment certificate for the mother
   (B) point out to the daughter that she appears to be trying to get her mother's possessions
   (C) agree to interview and examine the elderly woman if she is willing to be examined
   (D) refer the case to the local Adult Protection agency
   (E) suggest that the daughter herself may be undergoing emotional difficulties common at menopause

17. A young woman physician refuses to work with alcoholic patients. She states that these patients do not want to change, have learned to manipulate the system and are unnecessarily dependent. The doctor's attitude is a manifestation of

   (A) reaction formation
   (B) countertransference
   (C) rationalization
   (D) paranoid delusion
   (E) inappropriate affect

18. In the course of psychotherapy, all of the following are likely to indicate therapist countertransference *except*

   (A) allowing the patient to stay longer than the scheduled time
   (B) terminating the session when the patient threatens violence
   (C) becoming drowsy during the sessions
   (D) arriving late for the appointments
   (E) forgetting the patient's name

DIRECTIONS (Questions 19 through 30): Each group of items in this section consists of lettered options followed by a set of numbered words or phrases. For each numbered word or phrase, select the ONE lettered option that is most closely associated with it. Each lettered heading may be selected once, more than once, or not at all.

Questions 19 through 24

   (A) patient's emotional reaction to the therapist as if he or she were another significant person
   (B) conscious or unconscious emotional reaction of the psychotherapist to the patient
   (C) the planned giving of insight into the dynamics of feelings and behavior
   (D) requirement that patient delay gratification and discuss in therapy sessions
   (E) uncensored verbalization of thoughts and feelings
   (F) committment of therapist and patient to bring about reasonable improvement or cure
   (G) opposition to revealing unconscious material

Match the numbered psychoanalytic term with the appropriate lettered definition.

19. Resistance

20. Countertransference

21. Free association

22. Transference

23. Interpretation

24. Therapeutic alliance

Questions 25 through 30

   (A) unpleasant stimulus paired with stimulus that causes maladaptive behavior
   (B) rewards for desired behavior
   (C) remove reward for inappropriate behavior so maladaptive response decreases

(D) produce paired response antagonistic to undesired behavior

(E) gradually increased exposure to stimulus, so
even high intensity no longer produces maladaptive behavior

(F) patients directly confronted with feared situation

Match the numbered behavior therapy term with the appropriate lettered definition.

25. Positive reinforcement

26. Conditioned avoidance

27. Flooding

28. Reciprocal inhibition

29. Desensitization

30. Extinction

Answers and Explanations

1. **(B)** *Behavior therapy* deals with *clearly observable behavior* of the subject. This treatment approach is based on learning theory and does not attempt to uncover underlying *dynamics* for the maladaptive behavior. For most efficient treatment, the problems should be clearly defined and the goals definitely established. When the desired behavior occurs, it is strongly *reinforced positively* while the unwanted or unacceptable behaviors are *negatively reinforced* or the undesired behavior meets with no results, leading to *extinction* of this behavior. *(1:595–9; 2:891–905)*

2. **(B)** Medication is often very useful in facilitating *behavior modification* treatment. Behavior modification has been successfully used to teach communicative language skills to *autistic children.* Infants with *rumination disorder* often respond swiftly to mildly adversive stimuli (such as putting a few drops of lemon juice on the child's tongue to dissuade rumination). *Phobic adults* can be treated by *flooding*—by direct confrontation with the feared situation. Patients with *paraphilias* are treated with various adversive conditioning procedures including electric shocks; such techniques require careful monitoring of the use of these potentially painful stimuli. *(1:595–9; 2:891–905)*

3. **(B)** *Behavior modification* is based on *reinforcement* where desired behavior is rewarded and sometimes undesired behavior brings an unpleasant result. *(1:597; 2:892)*

4. **(E)** Psychoanalysis is of greatest value in treating *anxiety disorders, obsessive–compulsive disorder, phobias, dysthymia,* and selected *personality disorders.*

   Psychoanalytic techniques can be used or modified in the treatment of patients with schizophrenia, borderline retardation, adolescent identity crises, and even major depression. In these syndromes, usually the analytic approach must be adapted and combined with other treatment procedures including environmental manipulations, family counseling, and pharmacotherapy. *(1:574; 2:859)*

5. **(C)** *Transference* is the carryover of the patient's feelings from an earlier significant relationship onto the psychotherapist. *(1:573; 2:857)*
   A. *Countertransference* is the manifestation of the therapist's conscious and unconscious feelings toward the patient. *(1:573; 2:857)*
   B,D. The development of warm feelings between patient and psychotherapist would be the development of *empathy* where these feelings were objective, or of *sympathy* where the feelings were subjective. *(1:586; 2:1251)*
   E. *Isolation* is the defense mechanism whereby an idea is split off or separated from the normal feelings that would accompany the idea but are repressed. *(1:184; 2:1256)*

6. **(C)** Whenever the patient manifests a disturbing symptom in the course of psychotherapy, the symptom generally should be openly recognized and the patient gently helped to discover how the symptom arose.
   A. The psychotherapist needs to understand, if possible, why the patient is crying so he can help her. Mere pouring out of feeling without sharing will not necessarily promote therapeutic movement.
   B. Some patients do indeed cry or show emotion, not to communicate but to block more meaningful sharing. This interpretation may be correct but the psychotherapist probably needs more information before making such a comment. If the statement is not valid, the patient is liable to feel attacked or reprimanded.
   D. Because the patient is distressed, there is no reason to bring the session to an end. The patient might feel the therapist was scared of her feelings.
   E. If the psychotherapist changes the topic of the discussion away from a distressing subject, the patient may believe with good reason that the therapist is feeling anxious about this subject. *(1:7–9; 2:174–83,880–2)*

7. **(D)** This would be the most appropriate comment, planned to facilitate further communication without judgments and without presuppositions.
A. At the initial stages of psychotherapy, it is more important to gain understanding than it is to reassure the patient. Premature reassurance may tend to block communication.
B. This statement may be correct but may be directly challenging. At this third session, such a comment could provoke more anger or anxiety than the patient can tolerate and lead her to discontinue therapy. The same interpretation could be made in a more supportive fashion, leading the patient to share and understand her feelings more.
C. This is again a valid comment but a statement that may be out of place. When the psychotherapist raises potentially distressing concepts, he or she should be sure that the psychotherapy bond can tolerate the stress. Also the therapist should beware of raising provoking subjects before having a thorough understanding of the patient, which he may not have by the third interview.
E. Reassurance may be comforting to the patient and to the psychotherapist, but reassurance does tend to block rather than facilitate communication. *(1:5–9; 2:171–83)*

8. **(C)** While patients need good reality reinforcement, in psychotherapy it is more important for patient and psychotherapist to know why a question was asked than to have an answer.
"Why do you ask?" is the correct answer. The therapist and patient need to know what exactly the patient is asking for and why.
A. Later in the psychotherapy process this might be an appropriate answer when said in a supportive fashion to a patient who needs to know reality. At this stage in treatment, such an answer is likely to bring an end to that communication.
B. Not only does this response block communication, it is also untrue and deceitful. The therapist must never base the treatment on deception, however kindly meant. His task is to help the patient adapt to generally accepted reality.
D. The psychotherapist should avoid personalizing any issue in psychotherapy. This is a manifestation of acted out countertransference.
E. This is a direct block to communication. *(1:5–9; 2:171–83)*

9. **(A)** It is more important to gain understanding in the psychotherapy process.
Sometimes patient and psychotherapist will find themselves acting together in a way that delays or minimizes communication.
By bringing a gift the patient is tuning in to the psychotherapist's personality and the therapist must handle the situation with full objectivity.
"Why do you want to give me this gift?" would

tend to support increased communication. The psychotherapist is not seduced, threatened, or judgmental. His role is to help the patient and he will not be deflected by a gift.
A. At only the second interview, this is a presumptuous comment by the psychotherapist, who cannot yet know the many reasons for such a gift.
C. To accept any gift without understanding the underlying communication bodes ill for the development of the psychotherapy process. The therapist needs to know much more.
D. This comment is liable to be unnecessarily anxiety arousing. To make or to suggest an individual interpretation based on a theoretical concept is unlikely to be useful at this early stage in therapy.
E. The therapist should not make such a comment. He does not know if the tie is a gift, a bribe, a threat—or what.
Again, the therapist and patient must understand what is happening before they feel any need to respond. *(1:5–9; 2:171–83)*

10. **(B)** The difficult problem of managing the dangerous patient is inadequately discussed in standard textbooks. The cardinal rule is that the clinician cannot allow the patient to hurt himself or those around him in any lasting fashion. This responsibility to the individual patient and to society far outweighs any limitations imposed by rules or requirements of confidentiality.
The therapist must attempt to ally himself or herself with that part of the patient's personality that is willing to relinquish this potentially lethal weapon. The physician should emphasize that he is not willing to allow the patient to run the risk of hurting himself by using the knife in any fashion. For the patient's sake, he must be relieved of the knife. If the patient refuses to give up the knife, the doctor should call in police or security personnel to relieve the patient of the knife. The patient will almost surely need hospitalization for his protection and the protection of others until his paranoid symptoms are brought under control.
A. A patient carrying a knife or any other dangerous instrument or weapon is not tolerable in any hospital unit. If the therapist hides behind the barrier of confidentiality, he is leaving his patient, this paranoid schizophrenic man, and the staff and patients of the unit, liable to be severely hurt.
C. There is no point in appearing to threaten the patient in any way that may provoke a sudden attack. There is no benefit in becoming a dead hero. In society there are people trained to disarm potentially dangerous people. If the paranoid schizophrenic patient seems unlikely to surrender his switchblade to the psychotherapist or to the unit staff, the physician in charge should not hesitate to call on the assistance of the appropriate legal authorities.

D. If the psychotherapist insists that the patient accept the full responsibility of getting rid of the switchblade, the therapist is avoiding his clinical responsibility. The physician must make sure that the knife is placed in safe custody or destroyed. If the patient is required only to put it away, he can get it back with equal ease. If he hides it, someone else can find it. The possibilities for acting out are endless.

E. As long as this psychotic patient has possession of a potentially lethal weapon, he is a danger to himself and to society and no number of appointments can get around this reality. Psychotherapy cannot dissolve a weapon. This is one example of a reality where the therapist must act first and then work through the feelings later. *(1:560–3; 2:182–3)*

11. **(B)** As in any consultation, a good introductory move is always to introduce yourself and explain the nature and purpose of the visit.

A. Premature reassurance blocks communication that may be vital. Until the consultant has thoroughly evaluated the patient, reassurance is out of place.

C. Too much nonsense is written about looking patients "in the eye." In any evaluation procedure, the consultant notes and considers every communication including the reality of whether there was eye contact or not. Each patient, like each individual, has his or her own way of communicating, and the consultant should not try to impose an unacceptable or uncomfortable communication. In some cultural groups, it is rude to look another person directly in the eye.

D. The consultant must be careful to maintain routine confidentiality. Unless the patient gives written permission to discuss his situation with the Dean of Students, even acknowledging the fact of his hospitalization is a breach of professional confidentiality. (Even though colleges and universities maintain that a history of emotional illness does not hinder a student's chance of acceptance, it is understandable that Admission Committees prefer to accept students with no risk of psychiatric difficulty.)

E. Hospitalization can serve many therapeutic functions for the patient, his family, his culture, and his physician. The consultant must thoroughly evaluate all factors before recommending discharge; the consultant should propose alternative treatment or support if such is required. *(1:7–9,567; 2:182,502–3)*

12. **(C)** The seductive patient is a favorite examination subject. Often these questions seem contrived, but they serve to point out several things. The physician must be able to recognize a seductive patient, male or female. The clinician must be sensitive to his own reactions to such a patient. The

doctor must continue to evaluate and treat the patient in the most supportive professional way.

Each patient, even a seemingly neurotic patient, needs to be treated with respect as a first step to maintain or build self-respect. Any patient is entitled to a thorough medical and psychological evaluation. With the office nurse present, the patient may communicate in other more direct and appropriate ways.

A. The physician cannot avoid professional responsibilities by rejecting or avoiding the patient. This patient, in her own way, is asking for help.

B. It would be wonderful if we could all "pull ourselves together" on the basis of our own inner strengths. Before the physician makes such a demand, the clinician needs to know why the patient should be expected to "pull himself together." How will this benefit the patient? Or will it? The physician should know whether the patient has the emotional capacity to pull together and stay together. The doctor has to recognize that these aches and pains are a communication about something. As the physician, you should know what this message is before you insist that the communication stop.

D. The doctor should hesitate acting out any patient's wish for private closeness even in order to point out seductiveness. Such an interaction is open to misinterpretation and can easily get out of control.

E. Until the doctor has evaluated the patient thoroughly, medically and psychiatrically, the doctor does not know whether or not the patient needs companionship. If it becomes obvious that this is indeed the situation, it is better to invite the spouse to meet the doctor at the office and discuss the situation. A telephone call can be too abrupt, open to misinterpretation, and too brief for resolution of feelings. *(1:3–4; 2:171–83)*

13. (C) "What should I do to get well?" is a common question asked by patients and an easy way to pass the responsibility totally over to the psychotherapist. No matter how directly the therapist tries to answer this question, any specific response he or she gives will be wrong in some way. The therapist will better help the patient get well by allying himself with the healthy aspects of the patient's personality.

This is an awkward but correct response. The therapist wants to say to the patient that he will join with the patient in considering everything together. The psychotherapist's task is to help develop the patient's own individual strengths.

A. By saying "Trust in me," the therapist has told the patient that the doctor will carry the total burden. If the patient is to grow emotionally, he must learn to carry his own emotional responsibilities more capably. This response can be felt by the patient as an invitation to regression and dependency.

B. "That is not up to me to tell you" is the opposite quality of response where the psychotherapist refuses to accept any responsibility in what should be a shared therapeutic alliance. Many patients do need guidance, prompting, suggestions, and models.

D. This response blocks communication. The therapist does not know why the patient was asking or what specifically the patient was requesting; so it was bad technique to shut off the communication by this response.

E. Here the therapist is trying to give a specific answer that any patient can quickly make appear ridiculous. (1:7–9; 2:174–80)

14. (B) You must see the husband to evaluate him before deciding on any treatment.

A,C. Never diagnose or treat a patient by proxy or in abstentia. You do not know what this man's alcoholic intake signifies—normality, depression, psychosis, early senility, marital difficulties—the possibilities are endless. You should not treat what you do not know or understand.

D. You do not know whether his inability to come to see you is a sign of resistance. He may work an inflexible schedule, so you may need to make your schedule more flexible. His wife may have asked him to come to see you in a way that persuaded him not to come.

E. If the wife is given sedation to block out reality, you are trying to build a barrier of denial. Denial takes a great deal of psychic energy and tends to distort reality. It would be more productive to help the wife cope with the situation with less denial and more productive personal adaptation. (1:589; 2:931–5)

15. (B) The doctor who is asked to bring children "under control" is faced with a common problem. It is not the task of clinicians to provide control or to ensure that some individuals, even parents, maintain dominance over other people.

The physician has the responsibility of examining whether the conflict is a manifestation of emotional maladaption or illness. He can only evaluate where the patient wishes to be evaluated or where the legally responsible people can insist on maintaining an evaluation.

This 19-year-old man is past the age of full legal responsibility. He states directly that his life is not the physician's concern. Unless the doctor has clear evidence of markedly inappropriate behavior, he cannot interfere in this young man's life.

You do not have sufficient information to take any action and you should so inform the parents and the son. However, you can continue to offer to work with them as parents, as a family, or as individuals because their present interaction is mutually unproductive.

A. With no other signs of disturbed behavior, forced hospitalization would grossly infringe on the young man's legal rights and leave everyone involved open to legal suit.

C. The fact that the young man is unkempt, dirty, and refuses to cooperate does not in any way suggest that he is an early schizophrenic. For such a diagnosis, much more information about his personality and relationship ability is needed. The doctor must not confuse a personal dislike for the patient's style of life with evidence of emotional illness.

D. Equally there is insufficient evidence for a diagnosis of normality.

E. The parents may or may not be disturbed or disturbing. You have insufficient information.

Here is a family in pain. It is unclear from where the pain is originating. You should not act out family anxieties or psychopathology but you must be supportive to all family members. (1:679, 803; 2:115–20,935–42)

16. (C) Unless this elderly woman is grossly incompetent socially or a danger to herself or to society, she cannot be obliged to be examined psychiatrically. At the same time you cannot and must not attempt to diagnose her without seeing her.

A. Commitment necessitates direct examination of the patient.

B. Even if this statement were true, the physician serves little therapeutic purpose by merely antagonizing a patient or a patient's relatives.

D. When a doctor is asked for help, he is being requested to respond to some pain, anxiety, or maladjustment in the family. He may not like the message or the manner of the request for assistance, but he cannot refuse to help or attempt to help this woman and her family.

E. Menopause tensions do indeed lead to many psychological problems, but too often this reason is used to explain away many unrelated physical and emotional difficulties. Before such a diagnostic comment is made, the daughter should be evaluated thoroughly. (1:807–9,818; 2:251–2)

17. (B) Rather than allowing herself to evaluate and manage each patient based on the way the patient presents, this physician is responding to her own *countertransference*. She is projecting onto these patients her own feelings, based on her previous relationships, and is then reacting to these projections, these emotions and qualities, as if they belonged to the patients. (1:3–4; 2:172)

18. (B) The violent patient has to be given the controls and the protection that the patient and the community needs. It is not the role of the therapist to provide these controls. If a patient threatens violence or becomes violent, it is both therapeutic and appropriate to stop the session and call for the

needed security or legal personnel to provide the patient with the controls he needs at that moment. Not to stop the session or to call for outside controls is most likely to be a manifestation of therapist countertransference.

Answers 19 through 24 deal with psychoanalytic technique. (1:571–4; 2:171–4,857–60)

19. **(G)** *Resistance* is the conscious and unconscious opposition to the revealing of unconscious material, usually by a patient in treatment. *(1:573–4; 2:173)*

20. **(B)** *Countertransference* is the conscious and unconscious emotional reaction of the psychotherapist to the patient.
    Many psychotherapists use their countertransference as a useful diagnostic and therapeutic tool. *(1:573; 2:172,857)*

21. **(E)** *Free association,* a prerequisite for analytic treatment, is the uncensored verbalization of all thoughts and feelings. *(1:573; 2:858)*

22. **(A)** *Transference* is the patient's emotional reaction to the therapist as if the psychotherapist were another significant person. Feelings from an early nuclear relationship are transferred to the therapist in the therapeutic interaction. *(1:573; 2:171–2,857)*

23. **(C)** In psychotherapy, *interpretation* is the psychotherapist's method of giving the patient planned insight into the dynamics of the patient's feelings and behavior. Sometimes this insight leads to the release of unconscious emotions with the outward release of feelings (catharsis). *(1:573; 2:176,857–9)*

24. **(F)** The *therapeutic alliance* is the reality-based commitment of both therapist and patient to work together to bring about a cure or a reasonable improvement in the patient's situation. *(1:573; 2:172–3,858)*

Answers 25 through 30 deal with Behavior Therapy. (1:109–12,595–9; 2:891–905)

25. **(B)** *Positive reinforcement* rewards the subject for producing or manifesting the desired behavior. *(1:111,598; 2:891,1005)*

26. **(A)** When an unpleasant stimulus is paired with the stimulus that usually causes the maladaptive behavior, this is termed *conditioned avoidance.* The alcoholic taking disulfiram (Antabuse) feels physically uncomfortable when he tries to enjoy alcohol. *(1:110–1,597–8; 2:891–2)*

27. **(F)** In *flooding,* the patient is confronted with the feared situation and prevented from escaping. The patient's anxiety gradually becomes less and more tolerable and the patient finds that he can survive the anxiety-arousing experience. Escaping the feared situation tends to reinforce the anxiety-causing effect of the situation. However, many patients refuse to undergo a flooding experience because it may be so stressful. *(9:597; 2:1253)*

28. **(D)** *Reciprocal inhibition* works by pairing a response antagonistic to the undesired behavior with this behavioral response. Wolpe has emphasized the technique of developing progressive relaxation simultaneously with the anxiety-arousing stimulus. *(1:112,596; 2:892–4,1265)*

29. **(E)** In *desensitization,* the patient is given gradually increased exposure to the anxiety-provoking stimulus, starting from a low intensity, so that eventually even a high-intensity stimulus no longer produces the maladaptive behavior.
    The patient who is phobic for white rabbits could be progressively desensitized to white wool, a white rabbit toy, and then a live white rabbit. *(1:110,459–60,597; 2:893)*

30. **(C)** *Extinction* involves removing the reward for the inappropriate behavior so that the maladaptive behavior gradually decreases.
    Often a child's "bad" behavior is perpetuated by all the attention this behavior brings. When this behavior is ignored, the youngster may gradually cease to act in this fashion and extinction has occurred. *(1:110; 2:892–4,1005)*

CHAPTER 7

Social Psychiatry and Forensic Psychiatry
Questions

INTRODUCTION

In this era of social awareness, much attention is given to the concept of community psychiatry. Unfortunately, basic principles and goals have yet to be defined and tested. Each standard textbook deals with some aspects of community work, but as yet there is no clear agreement as to what is required from the examination candidate. Most examinations have specific questions dealing with community psychiatry as one facet of social psychiatry.

Forensic psychiatry is included in this brief chapter as an increasingly important part of the clinician's work. For clinical work and for examinations, the student and physician must know certain basic principles of legal psychiatry, which are asked about in most examinations, often in several different ways.

REFERENCES

Social Psychiatry

1. Chapter 4,   Contributions of the Psychosocial Sciences to Human Behavior, pp 104–154
2. Chapter 37,   Community Psychiatry and Prevention, pp 1141–60
    Chapter 38,   Administration in Psychiatry, pp 1161–78

Forensic Psychiatry

1. Chapter 41,   Forensic Psychiatry, pp 820–31
2. Chapter 33,   Psychiatry and the Law, pp 1059–84

DIRECTIONS (Questions 1 through 18): Each of the numbered items or incomplete statements in this section is followed by answers or by completions of the statement. Select the ONE lettered answer or completion that is BEST in each case.

1. The fourth pregnancy of a 42-year-old mother has resulted in a child with Down's syndrome. You begin a program of counseling with the parents and encourage them to join the local association of parents of retarded children. Your work with the parents in dealing with their new child could be classified as

   (A) primary prevention
   (B) genetic counseling
   (C) secondary prevention
   (D) tertiary prevention
   (E) suppression

2. Primary prevention programs

   (A) are planned for early identification and treatment of an illness
   (B) minimize the handicapping effect of any illness
   (C) work to lower the incidence of a disease
   (D) deal with the initial symptoms of a disorder
   (E) focus on the outward manifestations of an illness rather than the underlying causes

3. A community is likely to define a substance as a "drug of abuse" when

   (A) the drug is shown to cause liver or brain damage
   (B) the substance is used by a small segment of the population
   (C) the use of the drug conflicts with community standards
   (D) prolonged use leads to physical dependence
   (E) the drug is liable to be impure or diluted with toxic substances

4. In planning a primary prevention program for the management of mental retardation, you would want to establish all of the following *except*

   (A) genetic counseling for parents
   (B) antenatal care programs
   (C) physical rehabilitation services for the retarded
   (D) public education campaigns
   (E) easily accessible pediatric services

5. A 76-year-old woman lives by herself in a small apartment. Her married daughter would like to move her mother to a comfortable rest home. You advise the daughter that

   (A) the move would help encourage her mother to be more socially outgoing
   (B) the move is liable to precipitate physical and psychological deterioration
   (C) the move would lessen her mother's workload and lengthen her life
   (D) the move to a country environment would act as a physical tonic

6. You have just been appointed director of a community health center. Your main professional role should be

   (A) direct care for patients
   (B) clinical supervision of the social workers, psychologists, and paraprofessionals
   (C) consultation with the other agency psychiatrists
   (D) public relations work for the agency
   (E) supervision and coordination of all the agency staff

7. By diagnosis, the largest group of patients in state mental hospitals are

   (A) alcoholic
   (B) senile
   (C) depressed
   (D) schizophrenic
   (E) affected by personality disorders

8. Tertiary prevention

   (A) reduces the residual handicapping of an illness
   (B) provides the earliest possible treatment of a disease
   (C) works for the earliest identification of an illness
   (D) necessitates easily available genetic counseling
   (E) aims to reduce the occurrence of a disorder

9. In a hotly contested political election, you are working actively for one of the candidates. You sincerely believe that the other candidate is unsuited for office. On a radio interview show, you are asked for your clinical opinion of the opposition candidate's mental condition. In response, you should

   (A) give a clear, concise evaluation of the opposition politician but point out that your opinions are not based on direct examination
   (B) give a thoughtful in-depth opinion based on everything you know about the subject
   (C) refuse to give any clinical opinion

(D) take the opportunity to make known your professional doubts about the opposition candidate's psychological competence

(E) respond with a joking comment if possible

10. According to recent epidemiological studies, the mental disorder with the highest prevalence rate is

(A) panic

(B) schizophrenia

(C) antisocial personality

(D) dysthymia

(E) phobia

11. To be competent to stand trial, the accused must have the ability for all of the following *except*

(A) understanding questions

(B) remembering

(C) distinguishing fantasy from reality

(D) reading and writing

(E) cooperating in his own defense

12. To make a legally acceptable will, the person making the will must fulfill all of the following criteria *except*

(A) understand that he is making a will

(B) be able to read and write

(C) know the nature and extent of his property

(D) be aware of the "natural objects of his bounty"

(E) be able to understand the interrelationship of these factors

13. All of the following statements about confidentiality are correct *except*

(A) confidentiality is waived when a patient is suing the doctor

(B) patients can waive confidentiality when they so decide

(C) the doctor can maintain confidentiality whenever he considers it in the patient's best interests

(D) confidentiality does not exist in military courts

(E) confidentiality is waived in cases of alleged child abuse

14. The M'Naghten rule

(A) is a test of sanity

(B) provides guidelines for commitment

(C) defines criminal responsibility

(D) indicates criteria for testamentary capacity

(E) outlines the grounds for divorce on the basis of insanity

15. As a result of the Tarasoff rulings of the California courts, many states have now changed their laws regarding the clinician and

(A) involuntary commitment

(B) threats against a third party

(C) alleged child abuse

(D) criminal responsibility

(E) informed consent

16. Your patient wishes to make a will. To minimize the risk that this will be challenged on grounds of mental incompetency, you should

(A) take a very thorough history from the patient

(B) examine the patient carefully at the time the will is made and record all your findings

(C) make a careful note of your diagnosis at the time the will is being written

(D) discharge the patient temporarily from psychiatric treatment until the will has been written and filed

(E) meet with the family members and do a thorough family evaluation

17. The M'Naghten rule in determining responsibility is concerned with

(A) irresistible impulse

(B) whether the criminal act was a product of mental illness

(C) competence to stand trial

(D) understanding of right and wrong

(E) ability to act as a witness

18. To practice psychiatry in a state requires

(A) specialist board certification

(B) a state medical license

(C) an acceptable residency training

(D) a personal psychoanalysis

(E) none of the above

19. Testamentary capacity is

(A) competency to act as a witness

(B) ability to handle one's own affairs

(C) competency to make a will

(D) ability to take part in one's own legal defense

(E) the knowledge of right and wrong

20. For a patient to give informed consent regarding a proposed treatment, all of the following are applicable *except*
    (A) the patient is not psychotic
    (B) the patient understands the benefits and the risks of the treatment
    (C) the patient knows the alternate treatments possible
    (D) the patient gives consent voluntarily
    (E) the patient appreciates the risk of no treatment

21. Which of the following statements about the physician as an expert witness is correct?
    (A) Board certification is required to be recognized as an expert witness
    (B) a resident in training cannot be an expert witness
    (C) the expert witness may testify on hearsay evidence
    (D) the expert witness cannot use notes or records
    (E) an expert witness can only testify regarding direct observations on the case

22. A 13-year-old girl is brought for evaluation because of recent irritability, rebelliousness and failing school grades. In the course of the examination, she mentions that her "Paw-paw," her 74-year-old grandfather, comes into her room almost every night and touches her genitals. Her mother, who is very upset about this information, states firmly that she will deal with this family situation but asks that you say nothing to her father, the patient's grandfather, because "It will kill him." Which action should the physician take first?
    (A) set up an interview with the grandfather
    (B) report the alleged behavior to the child protection agency
    (C) set up regular counseling sessions with the teenage patient
    (D) begin family therapy with the patient, parents, and grandparents
    (E) plan further interviews with the girl to gather more detailed information

Questions 23 through 25

Match the legal reference with the appropriate patient legal concept.
    (A) Wyatt v. Stickney
    (B) Tarasoff v. Regents of University of California
    (C) American Law Institute Model Penal Code

23. criminal responsibility

24. right to treatment

25. duty of physician to warn

Answers and Explanations

1. **(C)** *Secondary prevention* aims to diagnose the illness or malfunctioning early and treat the disease intensively, after it has occurred. In the case described, you cannot prevent the malfunctioning from occurring (which would have been primary prevention), but you can help the parents deal productively with their anxieties and anger and assist them in working to minimize their child's limitations. *(1:144; 2:1155)*

2. **(C)** *Primary prevention* programs work to lower the incidence of a disease—to prevent the disorder, maladaptation or malfunctioning from ever occurring. *(1:144; 2:1155–6)*

   Programs for early identification and treatment that deal with initial symptoms are included in *secondary prevention*. Once a disease has occurred and chronic handicapping has developed, programs to limit or reduce the handicapping would be considered *tertiary prevention*.

3. **(C)** A substance is defined as a "drug of abuse" when its use conflicts with community standards. Across the world, alcohol abuse is a major cause of individual, family, and community problems, yet the sale and distribution of alcohol is socially supported and frequently provides a substantial portion of government revenue. *(1:279; 2:314)*

4. **(C)** This is an artificial question since undoubtedly a community planner would not limit a program solely to primary, secondary, or tertiary prevention. This question is designed merely to test the candidates' understanding of primary prevention as a concept. *Primary prevention* prevents the disease from ever occurring. Thus *genetic counseling, antenatal care, public education,* and *accessible pediatric services* all work to prevent mental retardation from occurring. Physical rehabilitation deals with the retarded after they have appeared; that is, after primary prevention has failed or been unavailable. Physical rehabilitation is a form of tertiary prevention, designed to reduce the long-range disability produced by an illness. *(1:144; 2:1155–6)*

5. **(B)** Most human beings develop a very meaningful sense of belonging—to family and friends and to a place. In the very old and the young, this sense of belonging is a critical and stabilizing part of the individual's adaptation. With the aged, familiar surroundings and faces become even more important and, for many, an integral part of their personality and sense of self. Much more than is often realized, the elderly come to depend on the same accustomed environmental cues and stimuli. When an elderly person is removed from her accustomed home, emotional decompensation and disintegration is liable to occur. The healthy elderly woman will state that she has lost a part of herself with a move, and psychologically she is correct. The elderly woman may give up physical and intellectual ties to the living world when moved away from her familiar home. A move that lessens an elderly person's workload may also reduce her purpose for living. *(1:53–5; 2:1136–7)*

6. **(E)** This question attempts to focus on principles of administrative and community psychiatry. The director or focal administration officer must first fulfill the role of decision maker, integrator, and leader for staff. He cannot spend time on direct patient care when his prime function is to run a mental health center. Clinically oriented professionals find it difficult not to spend their time in direct front-line patient care when, in reality, they can best use their talents in supervising and teaching others to handle a much wider group of patients than they could have seen in direct patient contact. The director of any unit must be director and spokesperson for all the staff, not just any one limited professional group, not even his own profession. Similarly, the supervisory responsibilities as director take in all the staff, not just the other professions or his own profession.

   When a director must do public relations work, he cannot work outside the health center at the expense of work with the staff for whom he is responsible.

   Thus, the director of a community health center has, as his main professional role, the task of supervising and coordinating the work of all the agency staff. *(1:143–4; 2:1153–5,1163–76)*

7. **(D)** By diagnosis, the largest group of patients in state mental hospitals are *schizophrenic*. *(1:324; 2: 378)*

8. **(A)** The aim of *tertiary prevention* programs is to *reduce the residual handicapping* of an illness. *(1: 144; 2:1155)*

Primary prevention would include genetic counseling and would aim to reduce the occurrence of an illness or disability.

Secondary prevention is designed to provide early identification and treatment of a disorder.

Primary, secondary, and tertiary prevention programs are seen in every area of social medicine (and thus in the examination for every specialty).

In considering *rheumatic fever, primary prevention* might include prophylactic antibiotics to prevent the spread of streptococcal infections.

Secondary prevention would offer good pediatric diagnostic and treatment services for children with acute rheumatic fever. The illness cannot now be prevented but heart–valve scarring might be minimized.

Tertiary prevention would offer rehabilitation and treatment programs to children with heart–valve scarring, surgery for mitral stenosis and homebound schooling for the incapacitated.

9. **(C)** No clinician gives a clinical opinion without an adequate examination of the patient. All clinicians are ethically bound to confidentiality about their clinical opinions.

A physician, no matter the circumstances, can never avoid his professional responsibilities when acting in any fashion in a clinical capacity. *(1:10, 821; 2:1087–95)*

10. **(E)** The recent *NIMH Epidemiological Catchment Area Program* studies have shown that *phobic disorders have the highest prevalence rates for emotional disorders as defined by DSM III and DSM IIIR*. *(135–7; 2:81–3*

11. **(D)** There is no need for the accused to be able to read or write. But to be *legally competent to stand trial* he must be able to distinguish fantasy from reality, to answer questions, to cooperate in his own defense, and to remember. Competency to stand trial is quite different from criminal responsibility. *(1:827; 2:1061–3)*

12. **(B)** *Testamentary capacity* is a specialized area of competency—the *competency to make a legally acceptable will*.

To be considered legally competent, the person making the will must, at the time of making the will, be able to understand that he is making a

will, know the nature and extent of his property, know who are the "natural objects of his bounty"—wife or husband, children, close relatives—and be able to understand the interrelationship of these factors. He does not have to be able to read or write in this situation. *(1:825–6; 2:1069– 71)*

13. **(C)** The right to maintain *confidentiality* belongs to the patient. The patient can waive confidentiality whenever he or she so decides. The doctor has no power to maintain confidentiality no matter whether the physician believes that the patient's best interest requires confidentiality. Confidentiality is waived when the patient sues the doctor. Confidentiality does not exist in military courts. *(1:821; 2:173–4)*

14. **(C)** The M'Naghten rule,* established in Victorian Britain, defines *criminal responsibility*.

It is not a test of sanity and does not give guidelines for commitment, testamentary capacity, or grounds for divorce. *(1:827–8; 2:1064)*

15. **(B)** Under the *Tarasoff* rulings in California, the clinician is legally obliged to notify the potential victim when a patient has made clear threats to injure or kill that person. *(1:822; 2:1080–2)*

16. **(B)** To protect your patient or client on any occasion against risk of challenge to his or her *mental competency*, you should examine the patient carefully at the time legal action is taken—in this case when making a will—and record all of your findings at that time.

A thorough history focuses on the past and may not in any way indicate the patient's mental and emotional state at the time in question.

A diagnosis is a subjective opinion, open to later question. You must record observed facts. Even though the patient is not labeled as a psychiatric patient, his or her judgment can always be called into question.

A thorough family evaluation may have nothing to do with the patient's mental status. *(1:825–7; 2:1069–71)*

17. **(D)** The *M'Naghten rule* in defining criminal responsibility is concerned with the accused's understanding of right and wrong—did he know the nature and consequences of the act and, if so, did he understand that this act was wrong. *(1:827–8; 2:1064)*

The *Irresistible Impulse Rule* states that the accused cannot be held responsible for his behavior if he could not have resisted the impulse to

* Daniel M'Naghten, after whom the legal rule is named, is listed as McNaugten, M'Naugten, and McNaghten in different textbooks.

this behavior, even when understanding the likelihood of being caught or punished. *(1:828; 2: 1063–6)*

18. **(B)** *To practice psychiatry* in a state requires at present only a valid state medical license.

19. **(C)** *Testamentary capacity* is the *competency to make one's own will. (1:825–6; 2:1069–71)*

    Testamentary capacity has nothing to do legally with competency to act as a witness or in one's own defense or with general competency, nor has it any bearing on the capacity to understand the difference between right and wrong.

20. **(A)** In order to give *informed consent,* it must be shown that the patient knew the benefits and the risks of the treatment, the risks of no treatment at all, and the alternate treatments available. It should be shown that the patient gave consent (or refusal) willingly and not under duress. Psychosis need not prevent the patient giving informed consent or refusal. However, if the patient's psychosis interfered with his ability to understand the situation and the choices available to him, under these circumstances he could not give informed consent. *(1:824–5; 2:1069–71)*

21. **(C)** An *expert witness* can testify on hearsay evidence. The court decides who is an expert witness. Thus Board certification is not a prerequisite to be an expert witness and a resident-in-training can be approved as an expert witness. An expert witness is not limited to direct observations of the case, a witness of fact, and is free to refer to notes or records in giving evidence. *(1:820–1; 2:1059–84)*

22. **(B)** In any situation where the clinician suspects that child abuse may have occurred, the doctor is obliged by law to report immediately to the appropriate child protection agency. The physician who became aware of the abuse possibility has this obligation to report; this reporting obligation cannot be assigned to another staff member or to a family member. The reporting of suspected abuse should not be delayed on account of any clinical or family circumstances. *(1:822; 2:1080–3)*

23. **(C)** The *American Law Institute Model Penal Code* is the present law in Federal Courts and in several states defining *criminal responsibility.* This code states that persons are not responsible for criminal conduct if, at the time of such conduct, as a result of mental disease or defect, they lacked substantial capacity to appreciate the criminality of their conduct or to conform their conduct to the requirements of the law. *(1:828; 2:1064)*

24. **(A)** In his ruling on the *Wyatt v. Stickney* case, the judge noted that a patient committed to an institution had a right to treatment. *(1:824; 2:1071–3)*

25. **(B)** The 1974 and 1976 California Supreme Court *Tarasoff* rulings requires the therapist *to warn* the intended victim when a patient reveals intent to injure or commit homicide on a clearly designated victim. Many other states have passed laws to incorporate the Tarasoff rulings. *(1:822; 2:1080–2)*

CHAPTER 8

History of Psychiatry
Questions

INTRODUCTION

Many of the national examinations do not have questions on the historical background of the various branches of medicine. However, even in these examinations, allusions to historical aspects may be part of individual questions. Certainly in other examinations the candidate must be prepared for questions on the historical evolution of the specialty.

In the behavioral sciences, certain key scientists and seminal concepts are important in clinical work and in 20th-century culture. These investigators and their ideas are the focus of this chapter.

REFERENCE

1. Chapter 48,   History of Psychiatry, pp 836–51

DIRECTIONS (Questions 1 through 6): Each of the numbered items or incomplete statements in this section is followed by answers or by completions of the statement. Select the ONE lettered answer or completion that is BEST in each case.

1. In everyday discussion you may hear the phrase "identity crisis." This is a concept of

   (A) S. Freud
   (B) E. Bleuler
   (C) B. F. Skinner
   (D) E. Erikson
   (E) F. A. Mesmer

2. "Freudian slip" is a popular term for

   (A) parapraxis
   (B) catharsis
   (C) cathexis
   (D) transference
   (E) countertransference

3. The "Oedipus complex" is a concept introduced by

   (A) C. Jung
   (B) A. Adler
   (C) P. Janet
   (D) S. Freud
   (E) I. Pavlov

4. The term "inferiority complex" refers to a concept described by

   (A) A. Freud
   (B) J. Piaget
   (C) A. Adler
   (D) J. Sartre
   (E) W. Reich

5. Jung introduced all the following concepts *except*

   (A) inferiority complex
   (B) collective unconscious
   (C) persona
   (D) introversion and extroversion
   (E) anima

6. In his structuring of the psychic apparatus, Freud included all of the following *except*

   (A) preconscious
   (B) superego
   (C) alterego
   (D) id
   (E) ego ideal

DIRECTIONS (Questions 7 through 36): Each group of items in this section consists of lettered options followed by a set of numbered items. For each numbered item, select the ONE lettered option that is most closely associated with it. Each lettered option may be selected once, more than once, or not at all.

Questions 7 through 11

   (A) basic trust
   (B) neurasthenia
   (C) psychobiology
   (D) schizophrenia
   (E) inferiority complex

Match the concept or term listed above with the appropriate clinician.

7. E. Bleuler

8. G. Beard

9. E. Erikson

10. A. Adler

11. A. Meyer

Questions 12 through 16

   (A) prefrontal lobotomy
   (B) electroconvulsive therapy
   (C) projective tests
   (D) psychodrama
   (E) therapeutic community

Match the lettered procedure with the appropriate name.

12. Moreno

13. Moniz

14. Maxwell Jones

15. Cerletti

16. Rorschach

Questions 17 through 21

   (A) imprinting
   (B) somatotypes
   (C) schizophrenic twin studies
   (D) primate behavior research
   (E) operant conditioning

Match the area of research with the correct researcher.

17. Sheldon

18. Kallmann

19. Harlow

20. Lorenz

21. Skinner

Questions 22 through 26

    (A) collective unconscious
    (B) infantile autism
    (C) unchaining the mentally ill
    (D) infantile sexuality
    (E) intelligence testing

Match the concept or field of research with the appropriate name.

22. S. Freud

23. Binet

24. Jung

25. Kanner

26. Pinel

Questions 27 through 31

    (A) child development
    (B) phenothiazines
    (C) lithium
    (D) electroencephalogram
    (E) borderline personality disorder

Match the above topics with the correct clinician or investigator.

27. Cade

28. Kernberg

29. Piaget

30. Delay

31. Berger

Questions 32 through 36

    (A) *Declaration of Independence* and the first American psychiatry text
    (B) *The Mind That Found Itself*
    (C) *The Anatomy of Melancholy*
    (D) *The Interpretation of Dreams*
    (E) *Confessions of an Opium Eater*

Match the correct authors with the important publications listed.

32. Clifford Beers

33. Sigmund Freud

34. Benjamin Rush

35. Thomas DeQuincey

36. Robert Burton

Questions 37 through 40

    (A) campaigned for improvement of care of mentally ill
    (B) described multiple personality disorder
    (C) set the standard for the large mental hospitals
    (D) founder of American forensic psychiatry

Match the achievement listed above with the American named below.

37. Isaac Ray

38. Thomas Kirkbride

39. Morton Prince

40. Dorothea Dix

Answers and Explanations

1. **(D)** According to *Erik Erikson, adolescence* is the stage when the growing child establishes his or her individual *identity,* and is the developmental period of the *identity crisis,* of ego identity versus role confusion. *(1:42–3; 2:145–6)*

    S. Freud was the originator and developer of *psychoanalysis.*

    E. Bleuler introduced the concept of *schizophrenia.*

    F. Skinner has developed the concept of *operant conditioning.*

    F. A. Mesmer, an 18th-century German physician, briefly popularized hypnosis—hence our word *mesmerize.*

2. **(A)** A *parapraxis,* or *Freudian slip,* is a slip of the tongue betraying underlying unconscious feelings. *(1:218; 2:126)*

    The other terms also refer to psychoanalytic concepts.

    Catharsis is the release of repressed ideas or feelings with appropriate outward emotional reaction.

    Cathexis is the investment of emotional energy in an object, person, or goal.

    Transference feelings are those emotions, initially linked to a significant life figure, that are transferred onto a person in a present relationship.

    Countertransference is the feelings, logical and illogical, of the psychotherapist toward the patient.

3. **(D)** The *Oedipus complex* is a psychological concept introduced by S. Freud. *(1:181; 2:96–7)*

    C. Jung, a Swiss analyst, focused more on the hereditary aspects of the human personality.

    A. Adler, the founder of Adlerian individual psychology, branched off from traditional psychoanalysis to emphasize more the development of the individual in society.

    P. Janet, a French psychiatrist, wrote extensively on hysteria and obsessive–compulsive neuroses.

    I. Pavlov, a Russian physiologist and Nobel Prize winner, introduced and developed the concept of conditioned reflexes and conditioning.

4. **(C)** *Alfred Adler* emphasized the helplessness of the very young child, a helplessness that leads to a lifelong pervasive feeling of inferiority against which the individual constantly strives.

    The *inferiority complex* was one concept derived from Adlerian principles. *(1:186; 2:154–5)*

    Anna Freud, the daughter of Sigmund Freud, has expanded her father's psychoanalytic theory, especially in the field of child and adolescent psychiatry.

    J Piaget was an influential Swiss psychologist who developed an extensive theory of child development.

    J. Sartre was a 20th-century French writer–philosopher.

    W. Reich developed the process of *character analysis.*

5. **(A)** *Carl Jung* introduced the concepts of *collective unconscious, persona, introversion* and *extroversion,* and *anima. (1:188; 2:153–4)*

    Alfred Adler popularized the idea of the *inferiority complex. (1:186; 2:154–5)*

6. **(C)** *H. Kohut* included the *alterego* in his theory of *self psychology.* The *preconscious,* the *superego,* the *id,* and the *ego ideal* were *Freudian* concepts of psychic apparatus. *(1:180–1; 2:132–5)*

7. **(D)** *Eugen Bleuler* delineated the schizophrenic syndromes and introduced the term *schizophrenia.* *(1:320; 2:258–9)*

8. **(B)** In the period after the Civil War, *George Beard,* an American physician, introduced the concept of *neurasthenia. (1:841)*

9. **(A)** *Erik Erikson,* an Austrian psychoanalyst who emigrated to the United States, suggested that infants develop *basic trust* during a stable mother–infant interaction. *(1:34–5; 2:145)*

10. **(E)** *Alfred Adler* postulated that all humankind struggles against a basic feeling of inferiority from the time of infant helplessness. He introduced the term *inferiority complex. (1:186; 2:154–5)*

11. **(C)** *Adolph Meyer* developed the *psychobiologic* approach, which emphasized the study of the whole person in his environment. *(1:190)*

12. **(D)** *Jacob Moreno* developed *psychodrama,* a form of group psychotherapy where a person's or a group's relationships are acted out. *(1:588)*

13. **(A)** *Egas Moniz* was awarded the Nobel Prize for his pioneering work on *prefrontal lobotomy* in the mid-1930s. Though psychosurgery has been largely superseded by psychopharmacologic treatment, Moniz's work opened up a wide field of continuing research. *(1:675; 2:388)*

14. **(E)** *Maxwell Jones,* a British psychiatrist, popularized the *therapeutic community* where patients largely govern their own institutional management in alliance with the professional staff. *(1:131; 2:1174)*

15. **(B)** *Ugo Cerletti,* in collaboration with his colleague *L. Bini,* pioneered *electroconvulsive therapy,* following the use of pharmacologic convulsive treatments by *Meduna.* *(1:669–70; 2:836)*

16. **(C)** *Herman Rorschach* developed the most widely used *projective test,* using a series of ten inkblots as the standard ambiguous stimulus. *(1:159–60; 2:234–5)*

17. **(B)** *W. H. Sheldon* devised a method of human *somatotyping* and postulated a relationship between personality type and body somatotype.

18. **(C)** *Franz Kallmann,* in the United States, did the first extensive *twin study* on the incidence of *schizophrenia.* *(1:842; 2:47)*

19. **(D)** *Harry Harlow,* at the University of Wisconsin, worked extensively in studies on the effects of *maternal deprivation in primates.* *(1:29,125–6; 2:101)*

20. **(A)** *Konrad Lorenz,* in his studies on newly hatched geese, showed the effects of early *imprinting.* *(1:122–3; 2:101)*

21. **(E)** *B. F. Skinner,* a behavioral psychologist, has written extensively about his research in the area of *operant conditioning.* *(1:110–1; 2:891–2)*

22. **(D)** *Sigmund Freud* first popularized the concept of *infant sexuality* as he was developing his psychoanalytic theory of the instincts. *(1:174; 2:128–9)*

23. **(E)** *Alfred Binet,* in France, formulated the first widely used form of *intelligence testing.* His test was later modified and is still in use as the Stanford–Binet test. *(1:155; 2:98)*

24. **(A)** *Carl Jung,* a Swiss psychoanalyst, developed his own school of analysis and included in his theory of personality growth and structure the concept of the collective unconscious, common to every person. *(1:188; 2:153–4)*

25. **(B)** *Leo Kanner,* in 1943, first delineated the syndrome of *infantile autism,* which has led to extensive research in childhood psychoses and early emotional development. His 1943 paper describing the syndrome clearly delineated most of the cardinal features. *(1:699; 2:712)*

26. **(C)** Periodically there are waves of treatment reform when the management of the emotionally ill becomes less custodial and less repressive. *Philippe Pinel* is famed for *unchaining the mentally ill* in France at the time of the French Revolution. *(1:838; 2:1141)*

27. **(C)** *John Cade,* an Australian psychiatrist, first noted the anti-manic effects of lithium. *(1:606,843; 2:819)*

28. **(E)** *Otto Kernberg* studied the group of patients he described as showing *borderline personality organization.* *(1:188; 2:142,636)*

29. **(A)** Based initially on studies of his own children, *Jean Piaget* developed his theory of cognitive development. *(1:104–6; 2:98–101)*

30. **(B)** *Jean Delay* and *Pierce Deniker* introduced chlorpromazine, the first effective phenothiazine antipsychotic, in 1952. *(1:606)*

31. **(D)** *Hans Berger* developed the technique of recording changes in brain potential in an *electroencephalogram.* *(1:76)*

32. **(B)** *Clifford Beers* wrote *The Mind That Found Itself,* the personal story of his recovery from mental illness. *(1:841; 2:1142,1174)*

33. **(D)** *Sigmund Freud* wrote, as one of his earliest and most influential publications, *The Interpretation of Dreams.* *(1:179–80; 2:125–8)*

34. **(A)** *Benjamin Rush* was one of the signers of the *Declaration of Independence* and wrote the first American psychiatry textbook. *(1:838; 2:1173)*

35. **(E)** From his own experiences, *Thomas DeQuincey* wrote *Confessions of an Opium Eater.*

36. **(C)** *Robert Burton* wrote *The Anatomy of Melancholy.* *(1:837)*

37. **(D)** *Isaac Ray,* one of the founders of the American Psychiatric Association, is also considered to

be the father of American forensic psychiatry. He wrote that nonrestraint would not work with liberty-loving Americans who would assert themselves even in the state of insanity. *(1:839)*

38. **(C)** *Thomas Kirkbride*, believed that "asylums can never be dispensed with" and prophesied the social disasters that would result if hospitals were not maintained. He helped develop the imposing, well organized Victorian mental hospitals that until a generation ago were still the standard for good inpatient care. *(1:840)*

39. **(B)** *Morton Prince*, in his book *The Dissociation of the Personality* (1906), described multiple personality disorder. *(1:841; 2:570)*

40. **(A)** For forty years in the mid-19th century, the most effective campaigner for improved care for the mentally ill was *Dorothea Lynde Dix*, a school teacher who retired after developing tuberculosis—and then went on to found or enlarge more than 30 state institutions for the proper care of the insane. *(2:1142,1174)*

CHAPTER 9

Matching Sets Questions
Questions

INTRODUCTION

In most standard examinations there are many matching sets of questions where there are groups of questions related to a common topic. This chapter is devoted to this type of question.

DIRECTIONS: Each set begins with a list of lettered response options followed by a set of numbered words or phrases. For each numbered word or phrase, select the ONE lettered option that is most closely associated with it. Each lettered option may be selected once, more than once, or not at all.

Questions 1 through 10

At what age should the normal child be expected to achieve the following developmental milestones?

   (A) 4 months
   (B) 10 months
   (C) 15 months
   (D) 2 years

Match the numbered developmental level with the appropriate age of first achievement.

1. Aware of strange or different situations

2. Says three to five words with meaningful significance

3. Says "da-da"

4. Speaks of herself by her name

5. Spontaneous social smile

6. Sits alone without support

7. Coos, gurgles, and laughs

8. Responds to "peek-a-boo" or smiles

9. Builds tower of six or seven blocks

10. Walks alone

Questions 11 through 15

   (A) lithium
   (B) monoamine oxidase inhibitors
   (C) diphenylhydantoin
   (D) amitriptyline
   (E) glutethimide

Match the side effect with the most likely causative medication.

11. Toxicity when barbiturates discontinued

12. Restlessness, dizziness, and convulsions when given with tricyclic antidepressants

13. Thyroid goiter

14. Withdrawal convulsions

15. Urinary retention and paralytic ileus when given with thioridazine and antiparkinsonian drug

Questions 16 through 20

   (A) greenish-yellow ring encircling the cornea
   (B) pigmentary retinopathy
   (C) pupils nonreactive to light
   (D) dilated pupils and vertical nystagmus
   (E) peripheral neuropathy

Match the physical sign with the most likely cause.

16. Neurosyphilis—general paresis

17. Thioridazine in high doses

18. Acute intermittent porphyria

19. Hepatolenticular degeneration

20. Phencyclidine use

Questions 21 through 25

   (A) pseudocyesis
   (B) cri du chat syndrome
   (C) Munchausen syndrome
   (D) cocaine delusional disorder
   (E) Lesch–Nyhan syndrome
   (F) Wernicke's syndrome
   (G) Pickwickian syndrome
   (H) Ganser syndrome

Match the symptom presentation with the most likely diagnosis.

21. Ophthalmoplegia, memory loss and confusion

22. Simulated illnesses with multiple hospitalizations

23. Aggressive retarded boys with hyperuricemia

24. False pregnancy

25. Approximate answers

Questions 26 through 30

   (A) Alzheimer's Disease
   (B) autistic disorder
   (C) male erectile disorder
   (D) amphetamine delusional disorder
   (E) adjustment disorder with depressed mood
   (F) multiple personality disorder

(G) Tourette's Disorder

(H) tardive dyskinesia

Match the clinical symptoms with the most likely diagnosis.

26. An 18-year-old boy with multiple tics, coprolalia, and episodic grunting

27. A 24-year-old truck driver, increasingly irritable for the past three months; moods have become unpredictable; now is accusing wife of infidelity

28. A 32-year-old chronic schizophrenic, maintained as an outpatient with treatment at the local mental health center, develops lip-smacking and sideways jaw movements

29. A 54-year-old surgeon recently has forgotten his operative schedules, written incorrect drug prescriptions, and been very abrupt with patients. He walks stiffly and his operative technique seems much slower

30. A 36-year-old man, two weeks after vasectomy, is noted by his wife to be chronically tired, sleeping poorly, and not eating well

Questions 31 through 33

(A) tricyclic antidepressants

(B) haloperidol

(C) lithium carbonate

(D) monoamine oxidase inhibitors

(E) buspirone

Which of the medications listed would be contraindicated with the numbered situation below?

31. Cardiac irregularities

32. First trimester of pregnancy

33. Wine and cheese party

Questions 34 through 37

(A) subject helped to achieve insight as to dynamic basis for feelings and behavior

(B) subject helped to develop better coping behaviors by new learning experiences and different rewards

(C) subject develops a strong emotional reaction to the psychotherapist as if he were a significant figure in the patient's earlier life

(D) subject is helped to strengthen existing defenses and cope with anxiety

Select the correct definition for each psychotherapy term.

34. Interpretive psychotherapy

35. Supportive psychotherapy

36. Behavior therapy

37. Transference neurosis

Questions 38 through 44

(A) Vineland Social Maturity Scale

(B) Bender–Gestalt Test

(C) Children's Apperception Test

Match each statement with the appropriate psychological test.

38. Ambiguous stimuli

39. Tests visual–motor coordination

40. Geometric designs

41. Based on reports rather than direct observation

42. Useful in evaluating brain damage

43. Reveals private fantasies and motives

Questions 44 through 47

(A) Halstead-Reitan Battery

(B) Rorschach Test

(C) Minnesota Multiphasic Personality Inventory

(D) Thematic Apperception Test

(E) Denver Developmental Scale

Match the descriptive statement with the appropriate psychological test.

44. Ambiguous pictures

45. Color stimuli

46. 550 test questions

47. Can be computer scored

Questions 48 through 50

  (A) autosomal recessive gene; defect in leucine, isoleucine, and valine decarboxylation

  (B) autosomal recessive gene; absence or inactivity of liver phenylalanine hydroxylase

  (C) autosomal recessive gene; deficiency of galactose phosphate uridyl transferase

Match the symptom description with the correct metabolic disorder.

48. Small size, fair complexion, convulsions, dermatitis, and retardation

49. Urine has characteristic smell and turns blue with ferric chloride; infant convulsions, rigidity, hypoglycemia, and retardation

50. Jaundice, vomiting, diarrhea, and failure to thrive in infancy; mental retardation, cataracts, hepatic insufficiency

Questions 51 through 54

  (A) narcolepsy
  (B) amphetamine abuse
  (C) bulimia
  (D) acute intermittent porphyria
  (E) panic disorder
  (F) alcohol withdrawal delirium

Match the clinical symptoms with the most likely diagnosis.

51. Calluses on back of fingers and dental erosion

52. Sleeps during work. When laughing, briefly slumps back in chair and then continues talking

53. Elderly society matron, hospitalized with fractured femur, becomes sweaty, restless, and scared of shapes on the ceiling

54. Thin, pale-faced man, restless, suspicious, grinding his teeth

Questions 55 through 58

  (A) undoing
  (B) somatization
  (C) dissociation
  (D) denial
  (E) idea of reference
  (F) inappropriate affect

Match the clinical description with the appropriate term.

55. "Of course I do not know those people together on the other side of the street, but I know they are talking about me"

56. The nurse has a rapidly enlarging lump in her right breast, but she is not concerned, nor does she think she should consult a physician

57. The psychotic patient giggles and laughs as she tells how she did her supermarket shopping, deposited money in the bank, and washed the windows of her house

58. The teenage girl goes upstairs and vomits when she has been refused permission to go out

Questions 59 through 64

  (A) derealization
  (B) somatic delusion
  (C) neologism
  (D) illusion
  (E) compulsion
  (F) echolalia

Match the clinical description with the correct term.

59. "Everything seems strange. People are so far away"

60. "My insides are rotting away"

61. "What time is it?" "What time is it, time is it." "What is your name?" "Name." "What is the date today?" "Date today"

62. The wind is blowing the tree branches. The old man interprets the moving shadow under the tree as people pointing at him

63. The schizophrenic refers to his wife as "Jinwhanny"

64. On the way home from school, the eight-year-old must walk only on the cracks in the sidewalk. If he steps off a crack he must go back to the beginning and start all over

Questions 65 through 68

  (A) buspirone
  (B) trazodone
  (C) monoamine oxidase inhibitors
  (D) lithium carbonate
  (E) fluoxetine
  (F) chlordiazepoxide

Match the clinical statement with the appropriate medication.

65. Used to prevent recurrent attacks of mania

66. Used in treating delirium tremens

67. Cheeses, wine, and liver may produce paradoxical hypertension

68. May lead to serious hyperpyrexia when given with tricyclic antidepressants

Questions 69 through 72

(A) REM sleep
(B) spike and domed waves 3 per second
(C) lowered EEG frequency and amplitude
(D) evoked cortical potential

Match the clinical diagnosis with the correct electroencephalographic finding.

69. Petit mal (absence) seizures

70. Hypothyroidism

71. Excludes deafness in autistic child

72. Narcoleptic attack

Questions 73 through 78

(A) primary prevention of mental retardation
(B) secondary prevention of mental retardation
(C) tertiary prevention of mental retardation

Match the treatment procedures with the appropriate prevention level.

73. Teenage sex counseling to reduce the number of pregnancies

74. Vocational training and sheltered workshops

75. Screening of infants for inborn metabolic disorders

76. Public education about causes of retardation

77. Special education classes for the retarded in public schools

78. Genetic counseling

Questions 79 through 83

(A) Alzheimer's disease
(B) Tay-Sach's disease
(C) Huntington's chorea
(D) Autistic disorder
(E) general paresis

Match the neuropathology findings with the correct diagnosis.

79. Loss of nerve cells in putamen and caudate nuclei

80. No demonstrated brain pathology

81. Cortical glial cells markedly reduced, many rod cells, perivascular cuffing

82. Senile plaques and neurofibrillary degeneration

83. Ganglioside accumulation in neurons of brain and retina

Questions 84 through 88

(A) formication
(B) withdrawal convulsions
(C) conjunctival injection
(D) pupillary constriction

Match the abused substance with the appropriate physical finding or symptom.

84. Marihuana

85. Cocaine

86. Diazepam

87. Heroin

Questions 88 through 92

(A) encopresis
(B) trichotillomania
(C) Munchausen by proxy
(D) Tourette's Disorder
(E) conduct disorder
(F) elective mutism, selective mutism
(G) autistic disorder
(H) separation anxiety disorder

Match the clinical description with the most likely childhood disorder.

88. An eight-year-old girl who formerly talked normally, now does not talk to her family or to her teacher but is heard talking to her doll

89. A seven-year-old girl with no eyebrows and bald patches on the right side of her head

90. A ten-year-old boy, suspended from school because of repeated disruptive behavior, refused to obey his mother and recently ran away from home for a day

91. An eight-year-old boy sent home from school because of repeatedly cursing the teacher, shows recurrent shoulder shrugging and face twitching

92. "It's always the same on Mondays"—a mother tells how her nine-year-old son complains of chronic abdominal pains and tiredness especially at the beginning of the week. Recently he has been sent home from school several times because of headaches. On Fridays and Saturdays he is usually fine but on Sunday he often begins to be ill again

Questions 93 through 96

    (A) fluoxetine

    (B) bupropion

    (C) carbamazepine

    (D) amitriptyline

    (E) lithium carbonate

    (F) alprazolam

For each clinical situation described, select the medication most likely to cause the complication.

93. A 42-year-old woman is complaining of stomach upset and loss of appetite. In the last few days she has been bothered with unaccustomed headaches. Two weeks ago her doctor started her on a medication for the crying spells she was having. She does not feel like crying now

94. A 20-year-old student has to sit near the door in his classes as he often has to leave to urinate. Also he has an annoying hand tremor which interferes with his note taking. He has a nasty taste in his mouth and his stomach "just doesn't feel right." Two weeks ago he started taking medication because he was getting "hyper" just like his father does

95. A 10-year-old boy was started on medication for his restlessness, intrusiveness, inability to stay on task, and problems in school. A month later, his mother is concerned because he has become quite constipated. His behavior in school is now much more acceptable but he has been saying that he cannot see the board clearly. He drinks much more now because, he says, his mouth is always dry

Questions 96 through 99

    (A) transsexual

    (B) transvestite

    (C) frotteurism

    (D) fetishism

    (E) pedophilia

    (F) sexual masochism

For each clinical vignette, select the most likely paraphilia diagnosis.

96. A 17-year-old young man asks you to call him "Lisa" and states "I really am a woman." He flatly denies that he is gay

97. A 17-year-old man waits until it is rush hour each day before he goes home from school. He squeezes into crowded busses so that he can press against women he considers attractive. Typically at these times he has an erection and sometimes ejaculates

98. A 17-year-old young man has been accused of child abuse. His two grade-school nieces have told how, on many many occasions when he was their babysitter, he removed their clothes and touched them "down there" on their genitalia

99. A 17-year-old young man has been making his girl friend concerned. He has been asking her to spank him increasingly severely. He has been telling her that this makes him much more aroused sexually and more able to perform—and indeed this does appear to be true

Questions 100 through 103

    (A) carbamazepine

    (B) chlorpromazine

    (C) lithium carbonate

    (D) methlyphenidate

100. Purplish metallic sun tan

101. Exacerbation of Tourette's Disorder

102. Stevens–Johnson syndrome

103. Nephrogenic diabetes insipidus

Answers and Explanations

Answers 1 through 10 deal with the developmental landmarks of normal growth and development. (1:31–4; 2:99–100)

1. **(A)** At about *4 or 5 months of age,* the infant is aware of *strangeness* or differences in situations and people. The child acts afraid and clings more tightly to the mothering person.

2. **(C)** Usually between *12 and 15 months,* the toddler develops a communication vocabulary of three to five words.

3. **(B)** At *10 months* the average child is *saying "dada"* and beginning to learn the use of specific verbal sounds to produce environmental effect. The child realizes that the babbling "da-da-da" brings a gratifying response from the significant male in her life.

4. **(D)** The *two-year-old* youngster is starting to *refer to herself by name,* a manifestation of her increasing self-awareness.

5. **(A)** The newborn infant makes the facial movements of smiling for many reasons but by two months the child is smiling *socially and spontaneously* as a sign of pleasure and to produce pleasure.

6. **(B)** The *ten-month-old* child can *sit alone* quite well, without having to be propped up and without wobbling unduly.

7. **(A)** The *two-month-old infant* is beginning to be more pleasurable to the family as, by this time, he is starting to *coo, gurgle, and laugh.*

8. **(B)** *"Pat-a-cake"* and *"peek-a-boo" games* begin to be exciting and fun for the child about *10 months* of age as she experiments with distance, depth, things there, and things not there.

9. **(D)** The *two-year-old* child carefully and methodically can build a *tower of six or seven blocks* and have the greatest glee at knocking it all down— and then building it again.

10. **(C)** As every mother of a *15-month-old* toddler knows, the youngster by this age is *walking alone* and getting into everything. He has been standing since 9 to 11 months and walking with a supporting hand since about one year of age; at 15 months he is moving well on his own.

Answers 11 through 15 deal with drug interactions and reactions.

11. **(C)** Barbiturate enzyme induction speeds up the metabolism of *diphenylhydantoin.* When barbiturates and diphenylhydantoin are given together over any duration and barbiturates are then discontinued, diphenylhydantoin toxicity is likely to occur due to slowed drug breakdown. *(1:620–1; 2:817–8)*

12. **(B)** Tricyclic antidepressants and *monoamine oxidase inhibitors* are sometimes given concurrently when patients have not improved with other antidepressant treatment. With this combined regimen, there is a high incidence of side effects. The patient may develop restlessness, dizziness, convulsions, hyperpyrexia, and intracranial hemorrhage. Fatalities have occurred. *(1:382; 2:792,802)*

13. **(A)** In patients taking *lithium,* there is increased incidence of thyroid goiter. *(1:853; 2:824–5)*

14. **(E)** Users of *glutethimide,* a once widely used anxiolytic sedative–hypnotic, are liable to develop withdrawal convulsions after prolonged intake. This drug is also prone to cause drug dependency. *(1:622)*

15. **(D)** When the anticholinergic antidepressant *amitriptyline* is given in combination with the anticholinergic neuroleptic thioridazine or comparable drugs, and especially when a further anticholinergic medication, an antiparkinsonian drug, is added severe and potentially fatal urinary retention or paralytic ileus can develop. *(1:619; 2:784–5)*

Answers 16 through 20 deal with diagnostic symptoms.

16. **(C)** In *general paresis, tertiary neurosyphilis,* classically the pupils do not react to light but do react to accommodation—the *Argyll Robertson pupil.* Accommodation Reaction Present—Argyll Robertson Pupil. *(1:269)*

17. **(B)** When patients are given *thioidazine* in doses of more than 800 mg per day (and rarely at lower doses), there is the risk of developing irreversible pigmentary retinopathy. This retinal change can occur in a matter of days and may result in blindness. *(1:642–3; 2:786)*

18. **(E)** *Peripheral neuropathy,* abdominal pain, confusion, and depression may occur together or as discrete symptoms in *acute intermittent porphyria.* *(1:267; 2:283)*

19. **(A)** A greenish-yellow ring encircling the cornea, the *Kayser–Fleischer ring,* is seen in patients with *hepatolenticular degeneration, Wilson's Disease*—a congenital autosomal–recessive defect in copper metabolism. *(1:73; 2:290)*

20. **(D)** Patients who present with *phencyclidine intoxication* are likely to show dilated pupils and vertical or horizontal nystagmus or both, in addition to intense, bizarre emotional and behavioral symptoms. *(1:310–3; 2:343)*

Answers 21 through 30 deal with syndromes.

21. **(F)** *Wernicke's syndrome* occurs in chronic alcoholic and severely malnourished or debilitated patients. These patients have necrosis and hemorrhage in the periaqueductal region and in the mammillary bodies. Symptomatically the patient shows ophthalmoplegia with marked mental confusion or clouding. *(1:290; 2:323,325)*

22. **(C)** The patient with *Munchausen syndrome, chronic factitious disorder with physical symptoms,* most often a male, simulates a wide range of serious or esoteric illnesses and in this way is admitted to a succession of hospitals where he may undergo many procedures, including operative intervention. *(1:480–4; 2:550–1)*

23. **(E)** An X-linked autosomal–recessive defect that is the focus of increasing research is the *Lesch–Nyhan syndrome.* This congenital disorder of purine metabolism, due to the absence of hypoxanthine guanine phosphoribose transferase, occurs in boys who show elevated serum uric acid, mental retardation, and unusual aggressiveness that is self-directed and directed to others. *(1:694; 2:56)*

24. **(A)** In *pseudocyesis* or *false pregnancy,* the woman subject develops the outward signs of pregnancy—absence of menstruation, gradual abdominal distention, breast enlargement, and even labor pains.

   This symptom most often occurs in immature or hysterical females but similar symptoms can be seen in males, usually in fathers-to-be. *(1:26,419)*

25. **(H)** The *Ganser syndrome, the syndrome of the approximate answer,* was first described in the prison population. Typically in stressful situations, such as a prison interrogation, the subject answers questions with a response that is approximate to the correct answer but is not correct. This seems to be an automatic, primitive, not very efficient defense, usually not fully under the patient's control. *(1:425–6; 2:582)*

26. **(G)** *Tourette's Disorder.* The syndrome of motor and vocal tics, commoner in males, occurs in about 1:2000 population. The full syndrome is manifested by multiple tics, explosive utterances, and sometimes coprolalia. Increasingly less obvious symptoms of the syndrome are being diagnosed; the disorder is probably commoner than once thought. *(1:760–3; 2:686–8)*

27. **(D)** *Amphetamine psychosis.* Chronic amphetamine use and abuse, as seen in some long-distance truck drivers who use the stimulant drug to stay awake, may cause a psychotic paranoid syndrome that is very similar to paranoid schizophrenia. *(1:305–7; 2:342–3)*

28. **(H)** *Tardive dyskinesia.* Lip, tongue, jaw, and face movements, choreiform arm and hand gesturing, and recurrent back and neck contractions may develop in patients taking dopamine receptor-blocking medications, most often the neuroleptics but also other drugs that block dopamine receptors. Originally the syndrome was described in patients who had been on long-term neuroleptics, but increasingly these symptoms are being reported in children, adolescents, and adults at every stage of treatment and after the cessation of the medication. *(1:90,644–646; 2:781–3)* .

29. **(A)** Dementia developing insidiously in the middle age and elderly period should suggest the possibility of *Alzheimer's disease.* Memory loss, especially for recent events, personality change, and neurological deterioration all indicate an organic brain syndrome. *(1:249–52; 2:285–7)*

30. **(E)** *Adjustment disorder with depressed mood.* Vasectomy in the male has been a frequent precursor of a postoperative depression, as is hysterectomy in the female. Sleep and appetite disturbances, lack of energy, and tiredness are common manifestations of depression. *(1:494–7; 2:608)*

Answers 31 through 37 deal with situations that would contraindicate the use of a medication or would raise major risk.

31. **(A)** Even within the normal dosage range, *tricyclic antidepressants* cause postural hypotension, tachycardia, and EKG changes in children and adults. These drugs have a quinidine-like effect on the heart and prolong cardiac conduction time. Disturbances of cardiac rhythm may develop but these arrhythmias occur most often where there is cardiac pathology or drug overdose. *(1:666; 2:800)*

32. **(C)** *Lithium*, especially when taken in the first trimester of pregnancy, causes an increased incidence of birth defects. Ebstein's anomaly of the tricuspid heart valve, a relatively uncommon defect, may be caused by lithium during the first trimester *(1:254–5)*

33. **(D)** Hypertensive crisis due to the inhibition of deamination of pressor amines, such as tyramine, is a rare but potentially fatal complication of *monoamine oxidase inhibitor* use. Food rich in tyramine—certain cheeses, beer, some wines, sour cream, chicken liver, avocado, figs—must be avoided with monoamine oxidase inhibitor use. *(1:657–8; 2:802–3)*

34. **(A)** *Interpretive psychotherapy* gives the patient planned insight, through interpretation, into the dynamic basis for her feelings and behavior. Optimally this insight should lead to freeing up of emotions and personality restructuring. *(1:575; 2:859–60)*

35. **(D)** In *supportive psychotherapy*, there is no attempt to change the patient's personality in any profound fashion. Using the strengths and the ways of coping he already has, the patient is helped to manage his life more efficiently. Existing defenses are strengthened and the patient is supported in developing more reasonable ways of managing. *(1:575–6; 2:860–1)*

36. **(B)** In *behavior therapy* the subject is taught better coping behavior by allowing her to learn new patterns and to experience different rewards. Appropriate behavior is rewarded and *reinforced*. Maladaptive behavior produces a negative reaction or is ignored. *(1:595–9; 2:891–905)*

37. **(C)** In *transference neurosis*, which occurs in the course of psychotherapy, the patient develops a strong emotional reaction to the therapist, who is reacted to as if he were a nuclear person in the patient's early life. *(1:186; 2:857)*

Answers 38 through 47 deal with psychological testing. (1:155–70,681–4; 2:225–46,1277–9)

38. **(C)** The *Children's Apperception Test*, an adaptation of the *Thematic Apperception Test*, is a set of pictures of animal characters in ambiguous situations. The child is encouraged to project his feelings and personality onto these *ambiguous stimuli*. *(1:684; 2:1277)*

39. **(B)** The *Bender–Gestalt Test* tests visual–motor coordination and visual recall. *(1:166; 2:1277)*

40. **(B)** The *Bender–Gestalt Test* is a series of *geometric designs* that the subject is asked to copy and sometimes then to draw from memory. *(1:166; 2:1277)*

41. **(A)** The *Vineland Social Maturity Scale* gives a Developmental Quotient based on the child's level of functioning as *reported* by the parents, teachers, or parent surrogates. The test evaluator *does not observe* the child. *(1:682; 2:703–4,1279)*

42. **(B)** The *Bender–Gestalt Test* is used to *evaluate brain damage* in patients. *(1:166; 2:1277)*

43. **(C)** The *Children's Apperception Test* would be one method of revealing a child's private fantasies and motives. *(1:684; 2:1277)*

44. **(D)** The *Thematic Apperception Test* uses a set of ten *ambiguous pictures* as stimuli to elicit the subject's projection. The Rorschach test also uses ambiguous stimuli but the test cards are inkblots. *(1:160–2; 2:241,363)*

45. **(B)** In the *Rorschach test*, several of the inkblot test cards are partially or completely colored to offer *color stimuli* for subjective projection. The Thematic Apperception Test cards are all black and white. *(1:1159–62; 2:234,363)*

46. **(C)** *The Minnesota Multiphasic Personality Inventory (MMPI)* is a set of 550 test questions to which the subject is expected to answer "True," "False," or "Cannot say." *(1:157–8; 2:229–30,362–3)*

47. **(C)** Of these five tests, only the *Minnesota Multiphasic Personality Inventory* can be *computer scored* at present. *(1:157–8; 2:229–30)*

Answers 48 through 50 deal with mental retardation syndromes caused by metabolic defects.

48. **(B)** *Phenylketonuria*. With early diagnosis and a diet low in phenylalanine, the crippling effects of this metabolic disorder can be prevented. *(1:688–92; 2:707)*

49. **(A)** *Maple syrup disease (Menke's Disease)*, an autosomal–recessive disorder, manifests in the first weeks of life. *(1:692–3)*

50. (C) *Galactosemia,* an autosomal–recessive disorder, is caused by a deficiency of galactose-1-phosphate uridyltransferase. *(1:694)*

Metabolic defects are the cause of mental retardation in only a very small percentage of cases, but the clinician must be alert to the more common or easily recognizable syndromes. Early treatment of these disorders may prevent intellectual and physical handicapping. *(1:686–94; 2:706–9)*

Sometimes questions are given to test the candidate's awareness of more tenuous associations. In this group of answers, the question phrase has been deliberately kept more brief so that the examinee must be more careful in selecting the appropriate matching answer.

51. (C) The patient suffering from the binge eating of *bulimia nervosa* commonly self-induces vomiting. Vomiting is often produced by sticking a finger down the throat, and eventually causing calluses on the back of the fingers; the recurrent vomiting may cause dental erosion and parotid gland enlargement. Bulimics often use laxatives or diuretics to produce weight loss. Cardiomyopathy may be produced by ipecac abuse. *(1:746–8; 2:760–3)*

52. (A) The commonest symptom of *narcolepsy* is sleep attacks, when the patient is uncontrollably overpowered by sleep. Many narcoleptics suffer from *catalepsy,* a sudden loss of focal or general muscle tone, often precipitated by an emotion such as laughing. Narcolepsy is a disturbance of REM inhibition. *(1:475; 2:747–8)*

53. (F) *Delirium tremens, alcohol withdrawal delirium* occurs 24 to 48 hours after the alcohol intake of a chronic alcoholic is stopped or reduced. *(1:288–9; 2:323)*

54. (B) *Amphetamine abuse* can cause agitated delirium or a syndrome similar to paranoid schizophrenia.

Bruxism, compulsive teeth grinding, may be a symptom of chronic amphetamine use. *(1:305–7; 2:342–3)*

55. (E) Although the behavior of the people on the other side of the street does not refer in any way to the speaker, he attributes to this behavior some purpose referring to him. This remark is an illustration of an *idea of reference.* *(1:202,219; 2:1254)*

56. (D) Only by massive emotional *denial* could a professional, trained nurse block out of awareness any concern about a rapidly growing breast mass. Denial may have been emotionally necessary as the reality of this lump faced her with intolerable anxiety about her continued existence and femininity. *(1:183; 2:137–8)*

57. (F) The psychotic patient who giggles and laughs as she relates her routine activities is showing *inappropriate affect.* *(1:214; 2:188–9,366)*

58. (B) This adolescent girl is *expressing through a somatic symptom* (vomiting) feelings that she could not express verbally to the controlling parent—she is *somatizing.* *(1:416–8; 2:533)*

59. (A) "Everything seems strange. People are so far away."

In the state of *derealization,* the subject feels that things around him are somehow unreal, almost distant. This feeling occurs occasionally in normal people, especially during childhood and adolescence, but, when the symptom is frequent or incapacitating, it may be a manifestation of developing thought disorder, of schizophrenia. In depersonalization, the subject feels that his body is unreal. *(1:221,433; 2:189)*

60. (B) "My insides are rotting away."

Somatic delusions, especially of a bizarre, malevolent physical process, are characteristic of *involutional melancholia.* These delusions can, of course, occur in other forms of psychotic depression and in other psychotic states. *(1:347– 8,812; 2:190,410)*

61. (F) The subject here is echoing the words of the questioner. *Echolalia* most typically occurs in schizophrenia but can occur in other disorders, such as Tourette's Disorder and organic syndromes. *(1:218,756)*

62. (D) When a reality-based external perception, such as blowing tree branches, is misinterpreted due to the subject's emotional maladjustment, this mistaken interpretation is termed an *illusion.* *(1:221; 2:189)*

63. (C) When the schizophrenic patient coins his own idiosyncratic words, these words are described as *neologisms.* *(1:218; 2:189)*

64. (E) Children in the grade-school years are normally rather compulsive and rule oriented. The youngster described in this question is pathologically bound by his own rigid regulations. His behavior is markedly *compulsive* and is liable to be increasingly handicapping. *(1:218; 2:190,472–3)*

65. (D) *Lithium carbonate* is used to treat manic attacks and, in maintenance treatment, to prevent the *recurrence of manic episodes.* Increasingly, lithium is used to prevent the recurrence of *depression* in *bipolar manic depressive illness.* *(1:382,651–5; 2:430,820–9)*

66. **(F)** *Chlordiazepoxide* is one of the drugs used in treating *delirium tremens, alcohol withdrawal delirium.* Diazepam is commonly used also. *(1:288–9,622–6; 2:324–5)*

67. **(C)** *Monoamine oxidase inhibitors* potentiate the dietary tyramine in foods like cheese, wine and beer, pickled herring, and chicken liver, leading to attacks of *paradoxical hypertension.* *(1:657–8; 2:802–3)*

68. **(C)** *Serious hyperpyrexia* may occur when patients are given *monoamine oxidase inhibitor drugs in combination with tricyclic antidepressants.* *(1:656–8; 2:802)*

Answers 69 through 72 deal with the electroencephalogram in psychiatry.

69. **(B)** *Petit mal epilepsy, absence seizures,* is typically associated with 3-per-second spike and domed waves on the electroencephalogram. *(1:263)*

70. **(C)** In *hypothyroidism* there is usually generally *lowered EEG frequency and amplitude.* *(1:268; 2:525–6)*

71. **(D)** To differentiate *autistic disorder* in childhood from severe *deafness,* it may be necessary to see whether auditory stimuli *evoke cortical potentials* on the electroencephalogram. The autistic child, who can hear, will show evoked cortical potentials in response to a sound though there may be no outward behavioral response. The deaf youngster will show no sound-evoked cortical potentials. *(1:703; 2:716)*

72. **(A)** *REM sleep patterns* on the electroencephalogram are associated with *narcoleptic attacks.* *(1:475; 2:747–8)*

Answers 73 through 78 deal with prevention of mental illness and mental retardation. (1:144,685–98; 2:1155–8)

73. **(A)** Chromosomal defects and obstetric complications are more common in pregnancies of adolescents (and women over 40). The *reduction in adolescent pregnancies* would be one form of *primary prevention* of mental retardation in children. *(1:144,686–94,697; 2:706,1155)*

74. **(C)** *Vocational training and sheltered workshops* would help the retarded live with their handicaps and find a productive role in society.

Helping the handicapped youngster live productively with his or her handicap is an example of *tertiary prevention.* *(1:697–8; 2:709–11,1155)*

75. **(B)** The *screening* of newborn infants for *inborn metabolic disorders* will not prevent the disorder

from occurring *(primary prevention),* but will allow for early treatment of the illness *(secondary prevention). (1:697– 8; 2:706–9,1155)*

76. **(A)** *Public education about the causes* of mental retardation is aimed at preventing the retardation syndromes from occurring *(primary prevention). (1:144,686–94,697; 2:706–9,1155–8)*

77. **(C)** *Special education classes* in the public schools help the retarded develop their limited skills and still remain, as far as possible, members of their appropriate age group. These youngsters are helped to cope with their intellectual handicap as efficiently as possible *(tertiary prevention). (1:697– 8; 2:709–11)*

78. **(A)** *Genetic counseling* to parents who carry a mental retardation-producing gene informs them of the risk to their future offspring. This counseling is planned to prevent the occurrence of hereditary mental retardation syndromes *(primary prevention). (1:686–94,697–8; 2:709–11,1155–8)*

Answers 79 through 83 deal with neuropathology.

79. **(C)** *Huntington's chorea,* a degenerative nervous system disease, is inherited as an autosomal dominant and is characterized by widespread brain atrophy, especially in the caudate and putamen nuclei. *(1:810–1; 2:288–9)*

80. **(D)** *Autistic disorder.* Since 1943, when Kanner first described infantile autism, there has been extensive neuropathological and neurobiochemical research into this syndrome. No pathological brain process has yet been demonstrated in these children. *(1:700–1; 2:712–3)*

81. **(E)** In *general paresis, tertiary neurosyphilis,* there is marked degeneration and disappearance of cortical glial cells, most evident in the frontal cortex. Rod cells are prominent and widely distributed throughout the cortex. Perivascular cuffing with lymphocytes, plasma cells, and mast cells is another manifestation of the chronic syphilitic meningoencephalitis. Wagner von Jauregg was awarded the Nobel Prize in medicine for his discovery of malaria-induced fevers as treatment for general paresis. *(1:269)*

82. **(A)** Pathological examination of the brain in *Alzheimer's disease* shows severe neurone loss, with senile plaques and neurofibrillary tangles. In Alzheimer's disease, the cortical atrophy is widespread but plaques are most often found in the frontal cortex and the hippocampus. *(1:250,810; 2:286–7)*

83. **(B)** *Tay-Sach's disease* is a cerebromacular degeneration, inherited by autosomal recessive dominance. Ganglioside accumulation in the nerve cells of the brain and retina leads to profound mental retardation, convulsions, physical deterioration, and early death. *(1:693; 2:56,61)*

84. **(C)** *Marihuana, cannabis,* causes conjunctival injection, dilated pupils, dry mouth, coughing, tachycardia and appetite increase. *(1:313–5; 2:345–6)*

85. **(A)** *"Cocaine bugs,"* the feeling that insects are crawling in or under the skin has long been recognized as a symptom of cocaine abuse. Formication is a tactile hallucination of a crawling feeling in or under the skin. *(1:220,302–5; 2:338–9)*

86. **(B)** *Withdrawal convulsions* are liable to occur when benzodiazepines are stopped or reduced after chronic use. *(1:296; 2:328–30)*

87. **(D)** *Pinpoint pupils, a manifestation of pupillary constriction* are typically seen in heroin and opioid abusers. *(1:298–9; 2:330–1)*

Answers 88 through 92 deal with psychiatric disorders of childhood. (1:699–786; 2:649–735)

88. **(F)** *Elective mutism, selective mutism,* is one of the few childhood psychiatric disorders that is more common in girls. Typically the young girl, most often first or second grade, refuses to talk in certain social situations while still talking normally in others. *(1:772–3; 2:694–7)*

89. **(B)** *Trichotillomania, compulsive pulling out of one's own hair,* is another childhood syndrome that is more common in girls. The hair is pulled out, usually with the dominant hand, so bald patches will appear on the right-hand side of the scalp in right-handed children. Hair may be pulled from any body area and often is chewed or swallowed, sometimes in a ritualistic way. Stomach or intestinal hair balls (trichobezoars) may occur. *(1:491–3; 2:617–9)*

90. **(E)** *Conduct disorder,* a repetitive and persistent pattern of behavior in which societal norms or the rights of others are violated, is the commonest emotional diagnosis in most child and adolescent psychiatry clinics. Conduct disorder is more frequent in boys. *(1:722–5; 2:664–70)*

91. **(D)** *Tourette's Disorder* is often misdiagnosed by clinicians, teachers, and parents if the diagnosis is not considered. Especially when the syndrome of vocal and motoric tics is developing, the symptoms may be considered to be manifestations of deliberate bad behavior or of a conduct disorder. *(1:760–3; 2:686–8)*

92. **(H)** *Separation anxiety disorder* in childhood is often manifested by *school phobia.* The child develops anxiety and physical symptoms when separated or threatened with separation from the parenting person or home. Often the parent has difficulty separating from the child. School phobia symptoms tend to be worst on Sundays and the beginning of the school week and subside as the week passes. *(1:733–6; 2:673–7)*

93. **(A)** *Fluoxetine,* a phenylpropylamine antidepressant, does not have the anticholinergic side effects of the tricyclic antidepressants but tends to cause nausea, stomach upset and diarrhea. Patients find that they have less appetite and may lose weight. Headache is a common side effect. Antidepressant effect may be noted in one to two weeks but full antidepressant action may not occur until the medication has been given for three to six weeks. *(1:649–50; 2:801)*

94. **(E)** Patients on *lithium carbonate* may show good anti-manic benefit but discontinue the medication because of annoying side effects—a constant nasty taste in the mouth, intention hand tremor, urinary frequency, stomach upset, and a feeling of mental dullness. *(1:651–5; 2:822–6)*

95. **(D)** Tricyclic antidepressants, including *amitriptyline,* are used in the treatment of children with *attention deficit hyperactivity disorder* especially when the psychostimulants are ineffective or contraindicated. Many youngsters find the anticholinergic side effects quite distressing—recurrent constant dry mouth, unaccustomed constipation, and blurred vision. Tricyclics in any dose have to be used with caution with children and adolescents due to possible cardiotoxicity. *(1:666,729; 2:661, 798–9)*

96. **(A)** *Transsexuals, patients with gender identity disorder,* do not like and repudiate their assigned sex and actively seek a change to the other sex. *(1:752; 2:588–91)*

97. **(C)** *Frotteurism* is a paraphila in which typically a male seeks situations where he can rub his genitalia against clothed women and achieve sexual arousal or orgasm. This behavior most often occurs in very crowded social places, especially rush hour busses and trains. *(1:446–7; 2:592–5)*

98. **(E)** A *pedophile* gets sexual arousal and release by having sexual activities with prepubertal children. For this diagnosis, the sexual perpetrator has to be at least five years older than the victim. Most pedophilic acts involve touching or fondling or oral sex. *(1:444–5; 2:592–5)*

99. **(F)** The *sexual masochist* becomes sexually aroused and gains sexual pleasure from being beaten, humiliated, or made to suffer. *(1:445–6; 2:592–5)*

100. **(B)** In the early years of phenothiazine use, it was often easy to recognize which patients were being treated with *chlorpromazine*—these were the patients who had the purplish metallic suntan. Now this side effect is well recognized—and also the tendency to develop severe sunburn—so patients receiving neuroleptics are warned to avoid undue sun exposure. *(1:642; 2:786)*

101. **(D)** *Methylphenidate* may induce or exacerbate the symptoms of Tourette's Disorder. *(1:658–60; 2:993)*

102. **(A)** *Carbamazepine*, an anticonvulsant effective in treating trigeminal neuralgia, is increasingly used in the treatment of mania, bipolar disorder and impulse control disorders. Severe blood dyscrasias and potentially fatal hypersensitivity hepatitis are rare side effects. The *Stevens–Johnson syndrome* of exfoliative dermatitis is also a rare side effect. *(1:634; 2:828)*

103. **(C)** *Lithium*-induced *nephrogenic diabetes insipidus* can result in markedly increased urinary output. Vasopressin has no effect on the polyuria which can be treated with chlorothiazide. *(1:652–3; 2:822–3)*

CHAPTER 10

One-Best-Answer
Questions

INTRODUCTION

This is the traditional, most often used question format. A statement or question is followed by three to five options. The examination candidate is required to select the one best answer to the question. The other options may be partially correct but there is only one best answer for this type of question.

DIRECTIONS: Each of the numbered items or incomplete statements in this chapter is followed by lettered answers or completions of the statement. Choose the ONE lettered answer or completion that is BEST in each case.

1. All of the following statements about suicide rates are correct *except*

    (A) lower in African Americans
    (B) higher in foreign-born Americans
    (C) higher in males
    (D) higher in divorced
    (E) highest in adolescence

2. The incidence of suicide is higher in all of the following *except*

    (A) Protestants than in Catholics in America
    (B) psychiatrists than other medical specialists
    (C) patients who are mentally ill
    (D) rural than urban communities
    (E) patients who are physically ill compared with those who are well

3. Imipramine is used in treating all of the following syndromes *except*

    (A) opioid abuse
    (B) attention deficit hyperactivity disorder
    (C) major depression
    (D) agoraphobia
    (E) functional enuresis, enuresis

4. All of the following statements about teenage girls with anorexia nervosa are correct *except*

    (A) likes to prepare meals
    (B) has a male pubic hair configuration
    (C) is active and energetic
    (D) has amenorrhea
    (E) feels fat even when quite thin

5. Females develop anorexia nervosa

    (A) after a difficult labor
    (B) with a craniopharyngioma
    (C) as a manifestation of major depression
    (D) after dieting for previous real or fancied obesity
    (E) most often before age sixteen

6. Insomnia is a manifestation of all of the following *except*

    (A) depression
    (B) aging
    (C) anxiety
    (D) narcolepsy
    (E) caffeine intoxication

7. Which of the following describe lithium blood levels?

    (A) therapeutic level 1.2 to 1.6 mEq/L serum
    (B) inversely related to phenothiazine levels
    (C) reduced with increased salt intake
    (D) wider therapeutic–toxic margin than most psychotropic drugs
    (E) reduced by excessive sweating

8. Under voluntary commitment, all of the following are correct *except*

    (A) patient may request admission
    (B) once admitted, patient may request discharge
    (C) after discharge is requested, patient may only be held several days without judicial commitment
    (D) judicial commitment of such a patient can then be for only six months
    (E) after discharge is requested and commitment procedures are underway, patient can request voluntary admission again

9. Testamentary capacity is the

    (A) ability to act as court witness
    (B) capability of filing suit for damages
    (C) knowledge of right and wrong
    (D) competency to make a will
    (E) ability to give informed consent

10. As evidence of legal capacity to make a will, the person making the will must fulfill all of the following requirements *except*

    (A) know to whom he would be expected to leave his property
    (B) leave a reasonable sum to his nearest kin
    (C) be substantially aware of what he owns
    (D) know that he is making his will
    (E) mental disorder does not impair judgment

11. In differentiating a conversion symptom from an organic paralysis, which of the following is diagnostically significant?

    (A) paralysis does not fit anatomic distribution
    (B) patient seems unduly lacking in concern
    (C) immature theatrical personality
    (D) absence of organic factors
    (E) patient is female

12. Which of the following antidepressant medications is most liable to cause delayed intracardiac conduction?

(A) Bupropion

(B) Trazodone

(C) Fluoxetine

(D) Desipramine

(E) Phenelzine

13. In severe depression, which of the following is correct?

(A) depression less in morning but worsens toward evening

(B) patient wakens early in morning

(C) delusions and illusions do not occur

(D) anxiety and panic attacks would indicate another diagnosis

(E) often complicated by alcohol abuse

14. The suicide rate for African American males is

(A) higher than for white males

(B) lower in urban areas

(C) increasing in recent years

(D) lower than for African American females

(E) highest in 15 to 19 age group

15. Imipramine side effects include all of the following *except*

(A) worsening of narrow angle glaucoma

(B) cardiac arrhythmias

(C) induction of mania in bipolar disorder

(D) hypertensive crisis when alcohol is ingested

(E) weight gain

16. In Alzheimer's disease there is a loss of cholinergic neurones in

(A) vermis of the cerebellum

(B) locus ceruleus and nucleus basalis

(C) pineal body

(D) hippocampus and fornix

(E) frontal cortex

17. With a schizophrenic patient, the lasting benefits of therapy are measured by all of the following *except*

(A) ability to work

(B) job turnover

(C) capacity for making and holding friends

(D) stability of residence

(E) early discontinuation of medication

18. The prognosis in schizophrenia is more liable to be favorable if all of the following factors are present *except*

(A) obvious external precipitating factors

(B) older age at onset

(C) acute onset

(D) low level of anxiety

(E) depressive symptoms

19. In autistic disorder, the prognosis is more favorable if

(A) the child is bowel and bladder trained

(B) there are no autistic siblings

(C) the child is neat and tidy in his ways

(D) the youngster is physically healthy

(E) the child has obvious language ability

20. All of the following apply to reserpine-induced depression *except*

(A) it is dose related

(B) it usually clears when drug is discontinued

(C) when persistent it is relieved by electroconvulsive therapy

(D) it occurs during first week of drug treatment

(E) it may lead to suicide

21. All of the following statements about chronic lead poisoning of childhood are correct *except* it

(A) is seen mainly in urban ghetto families

(B) is caused by sniffing gasoline

(C) is most often diagnosed in grade school children

(D) produces chronic intellectual retardation

(E) is caused by fumes from burned batteries

22. In acute intermittent porphyria, all of the following statements are applicable *except*

(A) barbiturates bring symptomatic relief

(B) the disease is more common in women

(C) the illness produces an acute toxic psychosis

(D) motor paralyses may be life threatening

(E) recurrent colic may lead to surgical operations

23. In the management of the chronic alcoholic, all of the following measures may be useful *except*

(A) disulfiram

(B) phenelzine

(C) group psychotherapy

(D) halfway houses

(E) vocational training

24. Temporary memory defects are likely to result from treatment with

    (A) propanolol
    (B) phenothiazines
    (C) tricyclic antidepressants
    (D) electroconvulsive therapy
    (E) buspirone

25. In treating the toxic delirious patient, all of the following may be useful *except*

    (A) frequent family visits
    (B) haloperidol intramuscularly
    (C) monitor electrolyte balance
    (D) installation of night light
    (E) low dose of phenobarbital at bedtime

26. In operant conditioning, which of the following is correct?

    (A) the response originates with the subject
    (B) unacceptable thoughts are repressed
    (C) intermittent reinforcement is ineffective
    (D) the underlying causative factors are revealed
    (E) the longer the time interval before reinforcement, the more efficient the learning

27. In the general population, the lifetime risk for developing schizophrenia is

    (A) 0.2%
    (B) 1%
    (C) 5%
    (D) 8%
    (E) 10%

28. Behavior therapy is based on all of the following concepts *except*

    (A) treatment is directed at specific problems
    (B) treatment goals should be clearly defined in advance
    (C) behavior is due to underlying dynamic motivations
    (D) behavior develops in response to rewards
    (E) progress should be able to be measured

29. A male therapist is treating a 32-year-old married woman in intensive psychotherapy. She sends him a beautiful wristwatch for his birthday. The psychotherapist returns the watch and tries to discuss with her why she sent the gift. She forgets to come to the next session and then has to go to a dentist appointment at the time of the following treatment hour. The psychotherapist is dealing with which of the following with this patient?

    (A) therapeutic alliance
    (B) resistance
    (C) secondary gain
    (D) reaction formation
    (E) introjection

30. All of the following statements are applicable to migraine patients *except*

    (A) often family history of migraine
    (B) frequently achievement-oriented family background
    (C) hostility tends to be repressed
    (D) usually narcissistic and insensitive
    (E) hypnosis may be useful treatment

31. In the management of the migrainous patient you may want to use all of the following *except*

    (A) psychotherapy
    (B) biofeedback
    (C) ergotamine
    (D) electroconvulsive therapy
    (E) propanolol

32. Affect is

    (A) the emotions experienced by the patient
    (B) the patient's emotions observed by the examiner
    (C) the patient's level of cooperation
    (D) the motor restlessness shown by the patient
    (E) the way the patient produces responses in others

33. All of the following statements about mental retardation are correct *except*

    (A) highest diagnosed incidence age 10 to 14
    (B) most are borderline or mildly retarded
    (C) severe mental retardation less common in elderly
    (D) electroencephalograms are usually non-specific
    (E) slightly more common in women than men

34. All of the following statements about phantom phenomena are correct *except*

    (A) normally occur after limb amputation in adults
    (B) occur after mastectomy
    (C) phantom tends to shrink and disappear with time
    (D) accentuated and perpetuated by delayed wound healing
    (E) indicate emotional maladjustment

35. It is suspected that one hour ago the teenage patient smoked two marihuana joints. All of the following symptoms would confirm this suspicion *except*

    (A) he feels very hungry
    (B) his eyes are bloodshot
    (C) his pulse is slow and regular
    (D) he is relaxed and sleepy
    (E) he tells you he is feeling "paranoid"

36. Depression with melancholia could be manifested by all of the following *except*

    (A) difficulty falling asleep
    (B) loss of appetite
    (C) feels worse in the morning
    (D) believes she is the worst sinner
    (E) nothing cheers her up

37. Which of the following statements commonly apply to ulcerative colitis patients?

    (A) tend to be sensitive and intelligent
    (B) are often emotionally dependent
    (C) higher family incidence
    (D) never learned to handle rage and frustration productively
    (E) tend to manifest hystrionic personality traits

38. In managing the renal patient on a long-term hemodialysis program, the psychiatrist may be aware that all of the following statements are correct *except*

    (A) high risk of suicide
    (B) magical expectations for renal transplant
    (C) marked financial and emotional drain on family
    (D) potential for violent or aggressive behavior
    (E) high incidence of sexual problems

39. All of the following predispose to the development of combat neuroses and post-traumatic stress disorder in front-line soldiers *except*

    (A) inadequate group leadership
    (B) married with dependents at home
    (C) inactivity under fire
    (D) high unit losses
    (E) loneliness

40. All of the following statements about premature ejaculation are correct *except*

    (A) most common in lower socioeconomic groups
    (B) treated by the squeeze technique
    (C) not affected by circumcision

    (D) may be caused by organic factors
    (E) not a manifestation of a specific emotional disorder

41. Which of the following anxiolytics has the longest response time?

    (A) chlordiazepoxide
    (B) diazepam
    (C) buspirone
    (D) clonazepam
    (E) chlorazepate

42. All of the following side effects have been reported with thioridazine *except*

    (A) retrograde ejaculation
    (B) withdrawal convulsions
    (C) pigmentary retinopathy
    (D) postural hypotension
    (E) constipation and paralytic ileus

43. Which of the following statements about attention deficit hyperactivity disorder is correct

    (A) equal incidence in preschool boys and girls
    (B) diagnosed most often in preschool-age children
    (C) symptoms lessen and disappear by mid to late adolescence
    (D) frequently coexists with conduct disorder
    (E) symptoms do not develop until at least age two

44. Which of the following statements about electroconvulsive therapy is correct?

    (A) for therapeutic effect it is necessary to produce an obvious muscular convulsion
    (B) the patient frequently loses weight during treatment
    (C) hypertension is a contraindication
    (D) amenorrhea for two or three months may commonly result
    (E) should not be given to elderly patients

45. The risk of suicide is greater in all of the following situations *except*

    (A) when there has been a previous attempt
    (B) during Christmas or holiday seasons
    (C) when there is a family history of suicide
    (D) when the patient has no close family
    (E) when the patient is over 60 years old

46. In dealing with former hospital patients, examples of tertiary prevention include all of the following *except*

    (A) Alcoholics Anonymous
    (B) sheltered workshops
    (C) halfway houses
    (D) genetic counseling
    (E) vocational placements

47. Programs designed for the primary prevention of emotional disorders in children and adolescents might include

    (A) well-baby clinics
    (B) readily accessible day-treatment centers
    (C) guidance in normal child development for teenage parents
    (D) teenage sex education
    (E) rubella vaccination

48. Previously hospitalized chronic psychotic patients are usually readmitted for all of the following reasons *except*

    (A) their families do not want them
    (B) they do not want to return to former homes
    (C) they have no useful job skills
    (D) they do not know how to function comfortably in normal social groups
    (E) they develop disabling medication side effects

49. All of the following statements about Developmental Reading Disorder (Dyslexia) are correct *except*

    (A) it is usually obvious by second grade
    (B) it often leads to low self-esteem and depression
    (C) it is usually associated with borderline intelligence
    (D) there is a higher incidence of reading disorders in other family members
    (E) it is found in children with visual–motor perceptual handicaps

50. Behavior therapy would be an appropriate form of treatment for all of the following *except* a

    (A) middle-aged male with focal paranoid delusion
    (B) mute autistic six-year-old child
    (C) young adult woman with fear of enclosed spaces
    (D) 23-year-old male fetishist
    (E) regressed 40-year-old chronic schizophrenic

51. A five-year-old boy is suddenly hospitalized with acute appendicitis. To minimize lasting emotional trauma, the doctor should do all of the following *except*

    (A) encourage the parents to bring the youngster's pajamas, toys, and favorite blanket for his room
    (B) explain to the child before the operation what will happen and what it will be like postoperatively
    (C) sedate the child before his admission so he does not become anxious at what is happening
    (D) encourage the mother to remain with the child during the day and, if possible, overnight
    (E) make sure that the staff introduce themselves by name to the child

52. All of the following statements about suicide in adolescence are correct *except*

    (A) suicide attempts are three times more common in girls than in boys
    (B) suicide is the third most common cause of death in the 15 to 19 age group
    (C) successful suicide is three times more common in boys than in girls
    (D) suicide is less common in college student population
    (E) suicide incidence is highly associated with drug and alcohol abuse

53. A patient reacts to the clinic doctor she has never seen before as if the clinician were disinterested and rejecting. The patient's reaction to the doctor is an example of

    (A) displacement
    (B) rationalization
    (C) transference
    (D) reaction formation
    (E) splitting

54. To evaluate a child's personality, the examiner may use all of the following *except*

    (A) playing with clay
    (B) Rorschach Test
    (C) Draw-a-Person Test
    (D) Children's Apperception Test
    (E) Stanford–Binet Test

55. As an adjustment disorder in reaction to temporary stress, a four-year-old may show all of the following *except*

    (A) tantrums
    (B) nightmares
    (C) recurrent tics

(D) dyslexia

(E) enuresis

56. All of the following statements are valid for infant intelligence testing *except*

(A) infants respond well to appropriate test instructions

(B) low validity in predicting intelligence level in adolescence and adulthood

(C) rely mainly on motor–sensory functioning

(D) little applicability to later verbal and abstract ability

(E) useful in detecting severe retardation

57. A 40-year-old woman had overdosed on Amitriptyline. She is now flushed, has a dry skin and dilated pupils, and is tachycardic. She is confused and appears to be responding to visual hallucinations. To bring about symptomatic improvement, your medication of choice would be

(A) thioridazine

(B) atropine

(C) physostigmine

(D) naloxone

(E) chlordiazepoxide

58. Paranoid psychoses occur commonly in all of the following disorders *except*

(A) bromide intoxication

(B) chronic amphetamine abuse

(C) myxedema psychosis

(D) autistic disorder

(E) cannabis abuse

59. In acute intermittent porphyria

(A) barbiturates are the treatment of choice

(B) chlorpromazine is contraindicated

(C) men are affected more often than women

(D) abdominal pain is a common symptom

(E) autosomal recessive inheritance

60. In which of the following disorders is the incidence significantly higher in women than men?

(A) bipolar disorder

(B) antisocial personality disorder

(C) major depression

(D) schizophrenia

(E) transsexualism

61. All of the following statements about postpartum depression are correct *except*

(A) does not respond to hormone treatment

(B) tends to recur with subsequent pregnancies

(C) more likely that patient's mother had post-partum depression

(D) does not respond well to antidepressants

(E) can be treated with electroconvulsive therapy

62. To protect the fetus of a pregnant addict, which of the following would be the best management?

(A) withdraw the woman from opioids using methadone

(B) maintain the woman on high-dose methadone

(C) maintain the woman on low-dose methadone

(D) withdraw the patient from opioids using clonidine

(E) discontinue opioids and treat withdrawal symptoms

63. After a course of electroconvulsive treatments is complete, which of the following commonly occur?

(A) memory impairment for several weeks

(B) recurrent epileptic convulsions

(C) lactorrhea for one or two months

(D) persistent occipital headaches

(E) chronic lower backache

64. All of the following statements about exhibitionism are correct *except*

(A) equally common in men and women

(B) patients rarely seek treatment voluntarily

(C) psychotherapy alone is often ineffective

(D) compulsive genital exposure to women

(E) sexual arousal in anticipation of stranger's reaction

65. Which of the following statements about binge eaters is incorrect?

(A) consume large amounts of food in a short time

(B) tend to be upset and very guilty about their binge eating

(C) typically binge on smooth-textured, high-calorie sweet foods

(D) patients are usually overweight

(E) frequently binges followed by self-induced vomiting

66. All of the following statements about anorexia nervosa are correct *except*

(A) is often preceded by obesity

(B) is most common in the second decade of life

(C) occurs usually in women

(D) higher incidence of mood disorders in family

(E) loss of appetite is early symptom

67. In treating recurrent manic-depressive depressions, a course of electroconvulsive therapy

    (A) prevents the recurrence of further episodes
    (B) is contraindicated in the elderly
    (C) should not be given during pregnancy
    (D) becomes less effective with succeeding episodes
    (E) is usually effective with 5 to 10 treatments

68. In planning a psychiatric primary prevention program for the elderly, you might do all of the following *except*

    (A) plan a social club for them
    (B) encourage local businesses to employ social security recipients
    (C) set up a "Welcome Wagon" group to introduce new elderly arrivals into the social community
    (D) contract with the local psychiatric hospital for readily available backup facilities
    (E) establish foster grandparent program in local Children's Hospital

69. In child abuse, all of the following conditions are commonly found *except*

    (A) the abuse is often rationalized as necessary discipline
    (B) the male parent is the more frequent abuser
    (C) the abused child is often seen by the parents as being different
    (D) most frequently found in pre-kindergarten children
    (E) abused child is often provocative and disruptive

70. Physical dependence on opioids is shown by

    (A) needle marks and signs of phlebitis
    (B) opioids in urine
    (C) drowsiness and pinpoint pupils
    (D) development of abstinence syndrome on withdrawal
    (E) recurrent euphoric "rush"

71. Delirium may occur due to withdrawal after chronic use of

    (A) chlorpromazine
    (B) heroin
    (C) cocaine
    (D) alcohol
    (E) bupropion

72. All of the following statements about schizophrenia are correct *except*

    (A) equally commonly diagnosed in men and women
    (B) prevalence has increased in last 25 years
    (C) diagnosed more often in lower socioeconomic groups
    (D) typically diagnosed at younger age in men than in women
    (E) non-twin sibling has about 8% likelihood of developing schizophrenia

73. Wife abuse is usually associated with each of the following *except*

    (A) abusing husband comes from abusing home
    (B) battered wife comes from violent and abusing home
    (C) pregnancy causes reduction in battering
    (D) spouse abuse is more frequent in drug-abusing families
    (E) abusing men are immature and inadequate

74. In response to your question about the meaning of "people who live in glass houses should not throw stones," the young man states "you might break the glass." This reply is an example of

    (A) magical thinking
    (B) primary process thinking
    (C) concrete thinking
    (D) autistic thinking
    (E) illogical thinking

75. In preparation for kindergarten, a five-year-old boy is brought for examination because he is not yet speaking. You should consider in your diagnosis all of the following *except*

    (A) bilateral hearing loss
    (B) autistic disorder
    (C) mental retardation
    (D) tongue tie
    (E) acquired aphasia

76. All of the following statements apply to functional enuresis, enuresis, *except*

    (A) it may be a manifestation of regressive behavior
    (B) family difficulties secondary to enuresis may be a greater problem
    (C) imipramine may be effective
    (D) it is found equally in boys and girls
    (E) it occurs during all sleep stages

77. In dealing with enuretic children and their families, the physician should be aware that

    (A) enuresis is usually caused by emotional difficulties
    (B) children always outgrow enuresis
    (C) enuresis often occurs in other family members
    (D) enuresis requires no treatment if there is no physical cause
    (E) enuretic children sleep more soundly than non-enuretic

78. Patients with severe bulimia nervosa who show hypotension, tachycardia, precordial pain, and muscle weakness are most likely suffering from

    (A) laxative abuse
    (B) ipecac intoxication
    (C) hypocalcemia
    (D) diuretic abuse
    (E) magnesium intoxication

79. To treat a 26-year-old woman with a socially incapacitating fear of cats, you may wish to use all of the following except

    (A) gradual desensitization
    (B) flooding
    (C) supportive psychotherapy
    (D) methylphenidate
    (E) hypnosis

80. All of the following syndromes commonly present with anxiety symptoms except

    (A) pernicious anemia
    (B) hyperthyroidism
    (C) pheochromocytoma
    (D) carcinoid syndrome
    (E) hypoglycemia

Answers and Explanations

1. **(E)** *Suicide rates* in the United States are lower for *African Americans,* though the incidence in urban areas is getting nearer the rates for *European Americans. Foreign-born Americans* have higher suicide rates than native born. *Males* commit suicide more often than females, who make more frequent suicide attempts. People who are divorced have higher suicide rates than those who are married. The incidence of suicide tends to increase with increasing age and is not highest in adolescence. Adolescents usually do not die; so, even though the adolescent suicide rate is lower than for succeeding age groups, adolescent suicide is the third most common cause of death at that age. *(1:551–9; 2:1023–5)*

2. **(D)** The *incidence of suicide* in the United States is generally higher in *Protestants* than *Catholics* and is higher in *the mentally ill.* Suicide rates are higher in the physically ill. Several countries, including West Germany, Japan, Denmark, and Sweden, have higher suicide rates than the United States.

    Suicide is more common in urban populations when compared with rural populations. *(1:551–9; 2:1024)*

3. **(A)** *Imipramine* is not used to treat opioid abuse or withdrawal. *(1:297–301,663; 2:330–7,792–3)*

4. **(B)** Usually a teenage girl with *anorexia nervosa* has *amenorrhea* (the lack of this symptom makes anorexia nervosa more difficult to diagnose in the male). Patients with anorexia nervosa are usually *active* and *energetic* and enjoy collecting recipes and preparing meals for others. Anorexia nervosa patients do not have a male pubic hair configuration but may have *lanugo hair* (like the newborn) on the arms and the legs. *(1:743–6; 2:755–9)*

5. **(D)** Females with *anorexia nervosa* often give the history of developing the illness *after dieting for real or fancied obesity.*

    After a difficult labor, especially with marked blood loss or infection, pituitary necrosis may occur with resultant hypopituitarism. A cranio-pharyngioma may cause pituitary hypofunction by local effects. Hypopituitarism produces a very different symptom pattern. Anorexia nervosa is not associated with psychotic depression though anorexia is a very common symptom of depression. The commonest age of onset of anorexia nervosa is late adolescence and early adulthood. Anorexia nervosa is rare before age ten and is not very common in early adolescence. *(1:743–6; 2:755–9)*

6. **(D)** The elderly need less sleep and have markedly reduced deep sleep; thus, older patients often complain of *insomnia.* Depressed patients tend to waken during the night and then stay awake or sleep only fitfully. Anxious subjects have difficulty falling asleep. Caffeine and stimulant intoxication will cause insomnia. *Narcolepsy is manifested by excessive daytime sleepiness, hypersomnia. (1:470–5; 2:743–8)*

7. **(C)** Lithium blood levels vary inversely with salt intake; toxicity is potentiated by reduced salt use. The therapeutic serum level of lithium is usually stated as 0.8 to 1.2 mEq/L, though even this range allows toxic reactions in some patients; 0.7 to 1.0 mEq/L may be safer. As manic symptoms subside, toxic effects may occur at a lower blood level.

    Lithium has a narrower therapeutic-toxic margin than most psychotropic drugs, and the blood levels are not related to phenothiazine blood concentration. Excessive sweating is likely to cause lithium intoxication. *(1:651–5; 2:820–8)*

8. **(D)** Under *voluntary commitment procedures,* a patient may *request admission* to a mental hospital. Once admitted, he *can request discharge* and *can only be held for several days without judicial commitment* (the specific number of days varies from state to state). However, even when commitment procedures are underway, a patient can request voluntary admission status again. Judicial commitment of a previously voluntary patient will be for a specific period, according to state law, but this period of commitment can be extended with further judicial hearings if the patient's condition warrants continued hospitalization. *(1:823–4; 2:1071–3)*

9. **(D)** *Testamentary capacity* is the *competency to make a will.* *(1:825–6; 2:1069–70)*

10. **(B)** As evidence of *legal capacity to make a will* (testamentary capacity), the subject should know the *natural objects* of his bounty—who are his next of kin. He should know the *nature and extent* of his property—what he owns. (He should also know he is *making a will.*) He does not have to leave anything to anyone. The subject can be hospitalized in a mental hospital and still have full testamentary capacity provided that the mental illness did not interfere with his informed understanding. *(1:825–6; 2:1069– 70)*

11. **(A)** Many *conversion reactions* develop in addition to, or are superimposed on, some organically based symptom. Pseudoseizures are commonest in epileptic patients.

   In diagnosing a conversion reaction, it is helpful diagnostically when the paralysis clearly *does not fit anatomic distribution.* (But some physically injured patients have nerve regrowth that does not fit the usual anatomical distribution.) When the patient shows *undue lack of concern,* this may be *la belle indifference* of the patient with a conversion disorder or it may be a stoical response in a person from a stoical family or culture so this reaction is in no way diagnostic. While conversion disorders are diagnosed more frequently in females, this disorder can also present in males.

   Conversion reactions are more likely to occur in *patients who have immature personalities,* and this supports a diagnosis of conversion disorder. By itself, however, personality immaturity would not necessarily indicate conversion disorder. Organic disorders can affect the immature and the mature equally. *(1:418–20; 2:535–40)*

12. **(D)** *Desipramine* like other tricyclic antidepressants has a quinidine-like effect on the heart. Before patients are started on tricyclic antidepressants, electrocardiographic studies should be done. Periodic EEGs may be indicated at all ages. *(1:666; 2:799–800)*

13. **(B)** In severe depression the subject is apt to *waken early* in the morning, when she *feels worse,* but the *depression may lift* somewhat *during the day.* Typically the depressed person has a *poor appetite* and shows *weight loss.* Anxiety and panic symptoms are common in depressed patients. Depression is more common in drug abusers. Delusions of failure, destructiveness, and evil are common in marked depression, and illusions of a corresponding nature are frequent. Somatic delusions are often seen. Severe depression does occur in preadolescents. Prior to adolescence, depression occurs equally in boys and girls; only in adoles-

cence and older is depression more common in females. *(1:363–82; 2:403–41)*

14. **(C)** The *suicide rate* for *male African-Americans* is *lower* than the rate for *European-American males* but higher than the rate for African-American females. The suicide rate is higher for *urban African-Americans* than for those in rural areas. African-American male suicide rates in the elderly and in the 20- to 30-year-old group are higher than the adolescent 15 to 19 age level. The black male suicide rate is *tending to rise* nearer the level of white Americans. *(1:575; 2:1023–5)*

15. **(D)** Tricyclic antidepressants, such as *imipramine,* cause a worsening of narrow-angle glaucoma due to their anticholinergic effect. Imipramine may cause changes in the electrocardiogram of even physically healthy patients; in an overdose, cardiac arrhythmias occur, sometimes with fatal results. Tricyclic and monoamine oxidase antidepressants, when given together, may precipitate twitching, restlessness, convulsions, hyperpyrexia, and even death. Imipramine can precipitate mania in patients with bipolar disorder. Adolescents given tricyclic antidepressant for affective or other disorders may develop manic symptoms as the first manifestation of a life-long bipolar disorder. Weight gain is common in patients receiving tricyclic antidepressants.

   As drug abusers have noted, imipramine and the tricyclic antidepressants potentiate the sedative effect of alcohol; in combination these drugs do not produce a hypertensive crisis. *(1:662–7; 2:798–801)*

16. **(B)** In *Alzheimer's Disease* there is a loss of cholinergic neurones in the locus ceruleus and the nucleus basalis. *(1:250; 2:286–7)*

17. **(E)** *Therapeutic benefits* in treating a *schizophrenic* patient are measured by *ability to work* and to *hold a job* (job turnover); *capacity for making and keeping friends;* and *stability of residence:* the capability of finding a place to stay and of remaining socially stable. Many chronic schizophrenic patients maintain social and vocational competence provided they remain on their medication. The medication should be maintained at the lowest therapeutic level to minimize short-term and long-term side effects but pressure merely for the discontinuation of medication may be premature and untherapeutic. *(1:332; 2:368–70)*

18. **(D)** Where there are *obvious external precipitating factors* and an *acute onset,* the prognosis for the *schizophrenic* is *more favorable.* The prognosis is poorer with earlier age of onset. Patients who develop schizophrenia at a later age are more

likely to have developed adult coping skills and support systems.

A prepsychotic *schizoid* personality and a *low level of anxiety* would be indicators of a *poorer prognosis*. Depressive symptoms are usually indicative of a better prognosis. *(1:332; 2:368–70)*

19. **(E)** Most *autistic children* are *physically healthy* and have *no autistic siblings*. Often the autistic child is *easy to toilet train*. Undue neatness and a need for sameness is a symptom of the autistic disorder. However, where the child has no obvious *language ability by the age of five,* the prognosis is unfavorable. *(1:699–704; 2:711–7)*

20. **(D)** *Reserpine* may induce a depression that is dose-related in severity and usually clears when the drug is discontinued. Reserpine-induced depression may result in suicide. Sometimes the depression may persist after the reserpine is stopped and antidepressant treatment, including electroconvulsive therapy, may be indicated. Reserpine-induced depression usually does not occur during the first week of reserpine treatment. *(1:569)*

21. **(C)** *Chronic lead poisoning* of childhood is usually seen in *young preschool children and infants* living in *urban poverty ghetto areas*. These children *eat lead-containing* paint or plaster from the walls of old or dilapidated houses. Lead poisoning also occurs when patients are exposed to fumes from burning batteries. Older children who sniff, "huff," lead-containing gasoline or solvents can develop lead poisoning.

Chronic lead poisoning can lead to *brain damage* and *mental retardation. (1:692,740; 2:707,680)*

22. **(A)** *Acute intermittent porphyria* is more common in *women* and may present with an *acute toxic psychosis, potentially life-threatening motor paralyses,* or a combination of both. Because they present with acute, recurrent abdominal colic and pain, many of these patients have exploratory surgery before the metabolic disorder is diagnosed.

Barbiturates are absolutely *contraindicated* as barbiturates may precipitate an acute attack. *(1:267; 2:283)*

23. **(B)** In managing the *chronic alcoholic, group psychotherapy, halfway houses,* and *vocational training* are useful treatment procedures.

If the alcoholic wishes to stop drinking, *disulfiram (Antabuse),* can be used to maintain aversion therapy. Chronic alcoholics should avoid the use of monoamine oxidase inhibitors such as phenelzine; many alcoholic beverages contain tyramine which could produce a severe reaction. *(1:284–92,657–8; 2:319–40)*

24. **(D)** *Electroconvulsive therapy.* Propanolol, buspirone phenothiazines, and tricyclic antidepressants do not cause memory loss. After several electroconvulsive treatments, the patient is likely to show amnesia, especially for recent events. This memory loss usually clears completely in 1 to 2 months. *(1:673; 2:840)*

25. **(E)** In treating the *toxic delirious patient, diazepam, haloperidol,* and *chloral hydrate* are all used beneficially.

Barbiturates often produce increased confusion and delirium. Frequent family visits during the day and night, and a night light will help keep the patient oriented. *(1:241–5; 2:282–4)*

26. **(A)** In *operant conditioning,* the *response originates with the subject* and, when this response is the *desired behavior,* it is rewarded or *reinforced.* There is no attempt to elicit underlying causative factors and no effort is made to produce repression. Intermittent reinforcement is effective but the longer the periods between the reinforcements, the less effective the reinforcement of the desired behavior. *(1:110–2; 2:157–8)*

27. **(B)** The lifetime prevalence for *schizophrenia* in the general population is about 1%. *(1:321; 2:374–6)*

28. **(C)** *Behavior therapy* is based on the concepts that *behavior* is *learned* and develops in *response* to rewards. For efficient treatment, problems should be clearly designated and goals defined in advance. There is no attempt to elicit or understand supposed underlying dynamic motivations. *(1:595–9; 2:891–2)*

29. **(B)** By forgetting to come to one appointment and later scheduling a conflicting appointment, the patient is showing her *resistance* to uncovering the reasons for the gift to the psychotherapist. The extent of her resistance confirms that the motives for the gift were not totally logical but were a manifestation of *transference:* she has transferred onto the therapist feelings from an earlier significant relationship. *(1:571–4; 2:857–61)*

30. **(D)** *Migraine* patients more often come from *achievement-oriented families* with a *history of migraine*. Frequently family members show a tendency to *repress or internalize hostility*. These patients are not usually unduly narcissistic and often are very sensitive to others. Hypnosis may be beneficial in producing symptomatic relief. *(1:507; 2:891)*

31. **(D)** *Psychotherapy* is often useful in helping *migraine patients* become less tense and less prone to attacks. *Biofeedback* and relaxation procedures are effective in producing improvement in mi-

graine patients. *Ergotamine* is still an effective drug to treat migraine.

Electroconvulsive therapy would not be beneficial in uncomplicated migraine. *(1:507; 2:900)*

32. **(B)** In dealing with patients, *affect* is the term used for the emotions observed by the examiner. The patient's *mood* are the emotions felt by the patient. *(1:214–7; 2:188)*

33. **(E)** The highest reported incidence of mental retardation is in the 10 to 14 age group, when even borderline retardates are having difficulty in school with academic work. After they leave school, most borderline or mildly retarded teenagers and adults find socially productive occupations and live healthy normal lives and are no longer considered mentally retarded.

Skull x-rays and electroencephalograms are usually normal or show non-specific changes. Severe mental retardation is less common in the elderly because the patients with severe retardation are more likely to die in childhood or earlier adulthood. Mental retardation is more common in males at every age level. *(1:685–6; 2:705–6)*

34. **(E)** *Phantom phenomena* normally occur *after amputation* of any body part including breasts or teeth in *adults;* typically the phantoms tend to *shrink* and *disappear* with time, though they can reappear. Delayed wound healing tends to maintain the phantom. Phantom phenomena are not manifestations of wish fulfillment nor are they usually painful. Phantom phenomena do not indicate emotional maladjustment or illness. Children born with congenital amputations do not have a phantom. *(1:520)*

35. **(C)** In cases of *marihuana (cannabis) intoxication,* the subject is likely to show dry mouth, conjunctival injection, and tachycardia, not bradycardia. He is liable to feel relaxed and sleepy—"mellow"—and hungry. Many cannabis users show an ability for self-observation even while they are becoming intoxicated; paranoid symptoms are common with marihuana intoxication. *(1:313–5; 2:345–9)*

36. **(A)** Patients with *depression with melancholia* fall asleep without too much difficulty but then awaken during the night and either cannot get back to sleep or find they have unsettled sleep. These patients feel worse in the morning and tend to feel better as the day progresses. They suffer from depressive delusions—believing she is the worst sinner—and sometimes show somatic delusions. Typically nothing seems to relieve the burden of depression with these patients; efforts to cheer them up often seem to burden them further. *(1:366–7; 2:410)*

37. **(E)** Patients who develop *ulcerative colitis* are usually *sensitive, intelligent,* but basically *dependent* emotionally. Typically they have *never learned how to handle rage and frustration* productively and tend to express their feelings in their symptoms.

These subjects are often rather *compulsive.* Many of their personality traits may have been produced by the disabling, unpredictable chronic illness which may be exacerbated by any strong emotions, sometimes including happy emotions. They usually do not show hystrionic personality traits. *(1:506; 2:513–5)*

38. **(D)** *Long-term renal hemodialysis patients* have a *high risk of suicide* due in part to this continuing *marked financial and emotional drain* on them and their families. Many of these patients have sexual problems. Many of these patients and their families have *magical expectations* about receiving a *renal transplant* and about what such a kidney transplant might do for them.

These patients tend to become depressed and subdued rather than violent or aggressive. *(1:519–20)*

39. **(B)** Front-line soldiers are liable to develop disabling *post-traumatic stress disorders, combat neuroses,* when they are *lonely, under fire but unable to react actively,* and *lacking competent, trustworthy group leadership. High unit losses* tend to undermine morale and accentuate individual and group anxiety. Soldiers who are married and have dependents are emotionally more able to withstand the combat stresses. *(1:409; 2:479–83)*

40. **(A)** *Premature ejaculation,* where the male recurrently ejaculates before he wishes to do so, is more commonly diagnosed in the college-educated population—possibly because this social group is more concerned with partner gratification. Premature ejaculation is not a manifestation of emotional disorder though the subject may become distressed by the symptom. Circumcision has no effect, either causative or therapeutic, on premature ejaculation. Organic factors may cause or accentuate premature ejaculation. The Masters and Johnson squeeze technique is used to treat this symptom. *(1:454,459; 2:599–600)*

41. **(C)** *Buspirone* takes two to four weeks to have the full anxiolytic response. This delayed response may be unacceptable to patients who wish more rapid anxiety relief. Buspirone is not associated with abuse or addiction. *(1:630–1; 2:812–3)*

42. **(B)** *Thioridazine* may cause *retrograde ejaculation* and, in high doses, over 800 mg per day, irreversible *pigmentary retinopathy.*

Thioridazine is highly anticholinergic and

causes postural hypotension and constipation, sometimes to the point of paralytic ileus. *Withdrawal convulsions* do not occur with thioridazine withdrawal but occur more typically following withdrawal in chronic users of barbiturates, benzodiazepines, alcohol, or meprobamate. *(1:642; 2:779–87)*

43. **(D)** *Attention deficit hyperactivity disorder* is more common in males at all ages. Increasingly this disorder is being diagnosed in infants and very young children and recognized and treated in adolescence and adulthood. Attention deficit hyperactivity disorder frequently coexists with conduct disorder. *(1:725–30; 2:651–64)*

44. **(B)** With *electroconvulsive therapy,* the patients should be warned that *moderate weight gain* is common after treatment and women often have *amenorrhea* for a period of *two or three months.*

    An obvious muscular convulsion is not necessary for therapeutic effect: muscle relaxants are used to minimize the convulsive effect of the treatment. For elderly depressed patients, electroconvulsive therapy may be the safest and most efficient treatment, even with depressed patients who have mild dementia. Hypertension is not a contraindication to electroconvulsive therapy where good anesthetic care is available. *(1:669–73; 2:836–41)*

45. **(B)** The *risk of suicide* is greater in the elderly subject over 60 years of age with no close family but with a family history of suicide, and where there has been a previous suicide attempt. There is not an increased risk of suicide at Christmas or over holidays. *(1:551–9; 2:1021–35)*

46. **(D)** *Tertiary prevention* aims to minimize the chronic handicapping effects of an illness. In dealing with formerly hospitalized psychiatric patients, this could include *sheltered workshops, halfway houses,* and suitable *vocational placements.* For the chronic alcoholic, contact with *Alcoholics Anonymous* may help maintain productive functioning. Genetic counseling would be an example of primary prevention, prevention of a disorder or disability occurring. *(1:144; 2:1155)*

47. **(B)** *Primary prevention* is planned to prevent the occurrence of an illness.

    To prevent the appearance or production of emotionally disturbed children, *well-baby clinics* and *parental education* in normal child development and child rearing would be useful. *Rubella vaccination* would prevent the birth of infants with congenital rubella. Child development classes for adolescent parents can help prevent parental mismanagement by adolescent mothers and fathers. Teenage sex education can help prevent unwanted pregnancies and pregnancies for which the mother is not prepared emotionally or socially.

    Day treatment centers deal with the disturbed youngster when primary prevention has failed and would be an example of either secondary or tertiary prevention. *(1:144; 2:1155)*

48. **(E)** *Previously hospitalized chronic psychotic* patients usually have to be *readmitted* because the family does not want them (they have nowhere to go), they have no useful job skills, and they do not know how to function comfortably in normal social groups. They may not wish to return to their former homes or communities. Usually the patients are only discharged from hospital when the medications and the side effects are stabilized so readmission is usually not due to further side effects. Even if the patient does develop annoying or disabling medication side effects, these symptoms usually can be managed on an out-patient basis. The reasons for hospital readmission are thus more *social* than due to any recurrence of the illness. *(1:144–5; 2:1145–52)*

49. **(C)** *Developmental reading disorder, dyslexia* is more common in *boys.* It is found in children with *visual–motor perceptual handicaps* but is not specifically associated with borderline retardation. After years of failure, these children often feel failures themselves with resultant *low self-esteem* and *depression.* There is a higher incidence of reading disorders in other family members. *(1:711–3;2:720–4)*

50. **(A)** Behavior therapy has been used effectively with *mute autistic children, phobic* women, male *fetishists,* and regressed *chronic schizophrenics.*

    Paranoid delusional males would usually be unwilling to participate in behavior therapy. They tend to be resistant to any therapeutic intervention. *(1:595–9; 2:892–904)*

51. **(C)** To help a *young child* cope with the stress of *emergency surgery,* the child should have the reality situation *explained* in terms he can understand; it is most helpful if the *mother can stay* with the child, especially over the operative period. The child should be permitted and encouraged to bring his pajamas and favorite toys with him to this unfamiliar and scary environment. The staff should introduce themselves to the child by name so that they are seen as supportive human beings.

    The child should not be needlessly sedated before coming to the hospital so that he does not have to cope with a threatening environment through foggy, drugged perception with numbed, sedated coping skills.

    If the child is not prepared or given added emotional support, an immediate acute adjustment reaction and long-term post-traumatic psychological difficulties may result. *(1:409–12; 2:479–83)*

52. **(D)** Suicide is more common in *college students* than in their peers in other social settings. *Suicide attempts* are three times more common with teenage girls than with boys but *successfully completed suicide* is three times more common with the male adolescent. There is a strong association between drug and alcohol use and teenage suicide. Suicide is the *third most common cause* of death in the 15 to 19 age group. *(1:551–9; 2:1029–31)*

53. **(C)** The patient reacted to the physician based on feelings prompted by earlier relationships. These feelings from an earlier important relationship were transferred onto the clinician—an example of *transference*. Transference occurs in all relationships. *(1:573; 2:139–40)*

54. **(E)** To evaluate a *child's personality*, the examiner may use *playing* with clay, dolls, or other toys. The *Children's Apperception Test* is a modification of the Thematic Apperception Test for use with children. The *Rorschach Test* can be used as a projective test, especially with other children and teenagers, while the *Draw-a-Person Test* gives useful information from the preschool years onward. The Stanford–Binet Test is used for intelligence testing and is not usually used to evaluate personality. *(1:683–4; 2:238–42,703)*

55. **(D)** *Tantrums, bed wetting (enuresis), recurrent tics,* and *nightmares* may all be symptoms of an *adjustment reaction of childhood*. The youngster shows signs of emotional maladjustment under stress and regresses, but returns to previous level of psychological adaptation and growth when the stress is relieved.
   Dyslexia is not a temporary response to stress. *(1:711–3; 2:720–4)*

56. **(A)** *Infant intelligence testing* has *little predictive* ability in foretelling the later level of intelligence of the subject in adolescence or adulthood. Such testing evaluates mainly *motor–sensory functioning* that is usually adversely affected by *severe retardation*. Verbal and abstract ability are only minimally evaluated: these factors are much more important in the intelligence measured in older children. Infant testing is mainly based on observation by others; the infants are usually given little test instruction. *(1:682–3; 2:703)*

57. **(C)** *Amitriptyline* is a potent anticholinergic. The patient has developed anticholinergic toxicity for which *physostigmine* is the specific antidote. Physostigmine has potentially life-threatening side effects so must be used with caution. *(1:619; 2:784–5,788–9)*

58. **(D)** *Paranoid psychoses* are commonly seen in *bromide intoxication*, in *chronic amphetamine abuse*, in *cannabis abuse*, and in *myxedema (hypothyroid) psychosis*.
   The myxedema patient has blunting of perception, increasing deafness, and slow cerebration due to the metabolic disorder. There may be no obvious outward reason for these changes. The subject feels something is happening to him or her and tends to deal with the anxiety by external projection—by paranoid distortion and delusions.
   Autistic children are usually too self-centered to be concerned about external influences. Paranoid projection implies a higher level of awareness of outside factors. *(1:348,701–4; 2:394–5,712–3)*

59. **(D)** *Acute intermittent porphyria*, an *autosomal dominant* metabolic disorder, occurs more often in *women*. *Barbiturates* (and alcohol) may precipitate an acute attack and are contraindicated. *Chlorpromazine*, or other neuroleptics, is usually the best symptomatic treatment.
   Abdominal pain is a very *common symptom* in this disease. *(1:267; 2:283)*

60. **(C)** *Major depression* occurs more commonly in women than in men. Before puberty, major depression occurs equally in males and females but during adolescence the female preponderance is established. Antisocial personality disorder and transsexualism are both diagnosed much more frequently in men. Bipolar disorder and schizophrenia are approximately evenly associated with the sexes. *(1:321,364; 2:409–10)*

61. **(D)** *Postpartum depression* is more common in women whose mothers had postpartum depression and is liable to recur with subsequent pregnancies. The depression can indeed be treated effectively with *antidepressants* or with *electroconvulsive therapy*. The depression does not respond symptomatically to hormone treatment. *(1:359–60)*

62. **(C)** Opioid withdrawal with a pregnant addict can precipitate fetal death or miscarriage. To maintain the pregnancy and to produce a minimally addicted infant, the pregnant addict should be maintained on low-dose methadone until delivery. *(1:301; 2:331)*

63. **(A)** Following a course of *electroconvulsive therapy*, there is often *memory impairment* for several weeks. In women *amenorrhea* of one to two months often occurs but lactorrhea is not a side effect of electroconvulsive therapy. There should not be recurrent seizures. Persistent occipital

headaches and lower back pain are not normal residual effects. Immediately after a treatment, there may be some muscle aching, but this usually clears in a matter of hours. *(1:672–3; 2:840–1)*

64. **(A)** *Exhibitionism* is still primarily a male syndrome. Even in this era of women's liberation, women are less frequently arrested for exhibitionism, which is the act of public *genital exposure, often compulsive,* in order to achieve *sexual excitement* or gratification.

These patients rarely seek treatment voluntarily and psychotherapy alone is often, probably usually, ineffective. Exhibitionists are *not easily treated by psychotherapy.* These patients may have little wish to modify this behavior but are often forced into a form of psychotherapy under legal pressure. *(1:445; 2:592–5)*

65. **(D)** *Binge eaters consume large amounts of food, typically smooth-textured, high-calorie, in a short time* and tend to be *upset* and *guilty* after their gorging. Frequently binges are followed by self-induced vomiting—that may produce calluses on the back of the hand from forcing fingers down the throat (Russell's sign) or dental enamel erosion. The vomiting may be induced to relieve abdominal discomfort or the guilt about over-eating.

Binge eaters tend to be within the normal weight range. *(1:746–9; 2:760–1)*

66. **(E)** *Anorexia nervosa* occurs usually in *women,* is most common in the *second decade* of life, and often is preceded (or alternated) by *obesity.* Studies of the families of patients with anorexia nervosa have shown an increased incidence of mood disorders.

In spite of the name anorexia nervosa, anorexia (loss of appetite) is a late symptom in this syndrome. Many of these patients are still hungry while they are starving themselves. *(1:743–6; 2:755–9)*

67. **(E)** A course of *5 to 10 electroconvulsive treatments* usually *relieves the guilt* and *suicidal* impulses in the depression of manic–depressive illness and leads to *social recovery* in the majority of cases.

Electroconvulsive treatment can be given usefully during *pregnancy and in the elderly* when good anesthesia supervision is available.

One course of electroconvulsive therapy will not prevent future episodes of recurrent depression, but this treatment can be used to abort or minimize the severity of later attacks. Electroconvulsive therapy does not become less effective with succeeding episodes. *(1:669–73; 2:636–41)*

68. **(D)** *Primary prevention* aims to prevent the development of emotional illness in elderly patients.

Prevention should be planned to reduce or eliminate factors that predispose to psychiatric difficulties.

An appropriate *social club, employment opportunities, volunteer work such as Foster Grandparents* and *"Welcome Wagon"* introductions all help prevent isolation, loneliness, and frustration that could lead to emotional illness. Back-up hospital facilities are not planned to prevent psychiatric decompensation but are needed to treat illness after primary prevention has failed. *(1:145; 2:1155–9)*

69. **(B)** In *child abuse* cases, the abuse is often *rationalized as being merely necessary discipline* and the *abused child* is often seen by the parents as being in some way *different.*

More often the abusing parent is the *mother.* The highest incidence of child abuse is in children *under age three.* Abused children are often *provocative, disruptive, and intrusive.* *(1:784–6; 2:1082–3)*

70. **(D)** Needle marks, signs of phlebitis, opiates in the urine, drowsiness, pinpoint pupils, and the history of experiencing repeated "rushes" may all indicate that the subject is self-administering opioids, but they do not necessarily prove physical dependence.

Physical dependence is proved when the subject develops an *abstinence syndrome* on *withdrawal* of the drug. *(1:300–1; 2:330–7)*

71. **(D)** *Delirium* may occur in drug withdrawal after chronic use of *alcohol.* *(1:288–9; 2:323–4)*

72. **(B)** The prevalence of schizophrenia has not increased in the last 25 years. Studies have suggested that the prevalence may be actually decreasing. Schizophrenia is diagnosed with about equal frequency in men and women though the syndrome tends to be diagnosed at a later age in women. Schizophrenia is diagnosed more often in the lower socioeconomic groups though in part this may be due to the social downward drift due to the socially incapacitating effect of the disorder. The lifetime prevalence of schizophrenia in the general population is about 1% but this rises to an 8% risk in non-twin siblings. *(1:321–8; 2:374–7)*

73. **(C)** The risk for *spouse abuse* increases with pregnancy. Abusing husbands tend to come from abusing homes and wives who are abused typically come from an abusing background also. The family background is similar where there is husband abuse by the wife. Abusing men tend to be immature and emotionally inadequate. There is a strong association between spouse abuse and drug abuse. *(1:464; 2:643–4)*

74. **(C)** This patient is showing *concrete thinking,* thinking that is very literal and does not take into account the abstract dimensions of a situation. Some very normal people are very concrete or matter-of-fact in their thinking. With other people, concrete thinking indicates deterioration in thinking ability, due to a process such as a developing thought disorder or a dementia. *(1:222; 2:190)*

75. **(D)** *Tongue tie* does not cause marked delay in talking.

This speech delay, however, could be due to *bilateral severe hearing loss, autistic disorder, acquired aphasia,* or *profound mental retardation.* Often there are multiple factors producing delay or absence of language in children. *(1:713–20; 2:724–8)*

76. **(D)** *Functional enuresis, enuresis,* is more common in boys.

The symptom may in some patients be a manifestation of *regressive behavior. Enuresis occurs during all sleep stages.* The *shaming* and *punitive treatment* these enuretic children often face may emotionally *handicap* them much more than the enuresis itself. *Imipramine* will usually produce symptomatic improvement in the symptoms of enuresis but tolerance to the medication effect typically occurs in several weeks. The patient's symptoms are likely to recur when the medication is stopped. *(1:765–7; 2:690–2)*

77. **(C)** *Functional enuresis, enuresis,* often occurs in other *family* members. Functional enuresis may occasionally be a symptom of the child's *emotional* difficulties but enuresis is usually not caused by emotional problems.

Children tend to outgrow this symptom but any army or college physician can testify that children do not always outgrow enuresis. Bedwetting may continue into late adolescent and adult years.

Enuretic children do not sleep more deeply than non-enuretic children.

Enuresis should always be evaluated to see what treatment and preventive measures are necessary, even if there is no demonstrable physical cause. Underlying psychological stresses may need treatment. The clinician should plan the management of the enuresis so that children are helped to deal productively with their symptoms and are not burdened by shame, frustration, and resentment. *(1:765–7; 2:690–2)*

78. **(B)** *Bulimia nervosa* patients are prone to self-induce vomiting and to abuse purgatives and diuretics in order to lose weight after binge eating. Ipecac intoxication may lead to hypotension, tachycardia, and precordial chest pain due to ipecac-induced cardiomyopathy which may be fatal. Abuse of laxatives and diuretics is likely to lead to dangerous electrolyte imbalance and dehydration. *(1:746–8; 2:760–3)*

79. **(D)** *Ailurophobia, an unrealistic fear of cats,* a form of *simple phobia, specific phobia* can effectively be treated by gradual, systematic desensitization, by flooding (an intense, total exposure to the feared object), and by hypnosis. Psychotherapy can be used as the primary treatment for the phobia and to support and integrate the other treatments. Methylphenidate usually has no beneficial effect with phobias. *(1:400–4; 2:468–72)*

80. **(A)** While many medical disorders may present with or cause anxiety, *pernicious anemia* most often manifests with depressive symptoms. Pancreatic carcinoma often presents with depression, sometimes as the initial symptom.

Hyperthyroidism, pheochromocytoma, carcinoid syndrome, and the syndromes that cause *hypoglycemia* all will present with anxiety symptoms. *(1:517–8; 2:454–5)*

CHAPTER 11

Case Histories
Questions

INTRODUCTION

In many examinations, the student is asked questions based on one- or two-paragraph case histories. Typically there are three to five questions for each case history, though there may be fewer questions, or, less commonly, a longer list of questions. The given case history may appear unrealistic or forced because the examiner wishes to focus on specific issues. Similarly, the answers offered for selection may sometimes be limited in scope or skewed, as the candidate is expected to respond to one particular cue.

These case history questions are often used to test the trainee's ability to synthesize. Thus, there are no specific reference chapters for this section as a whole.

DIRECTIONS (Questions 1 through 10): Each group of items in this section consists of lettered headings followed by a set of numbered items. For each numbered item, select the ONE lettered heading that is most closely associated with it. Each lettered heading may be selected once, more than once, or not at all.

Questions 1 through 4

(A) primary prevention
(B) secondary prevention
(C) tertiary prevention

You have diagnosed a chromosome translocation syndrome in a 15-year-old girl with moderate mental retardation and mild congenital physical anomalies. You undertake certain measures. Match each numbered procedure with the correct level of prevention.

1. You advise the teenager and her parents about the likelihood of her passing on these handicaps.

2. You check the child recently born to her sister for similar chromosome anomalies.

3. You arrange for vocational training in a sheltered workshop for the teenage patient.

4. At the parents' request, you arrange for contraceptive instruction for the adolescent patient.

Questions 5 through 8

(A) generalized anxiety disorder
(B) somatization disorder
(C) cyclothymia
(D) adjustment disorder with depressed mood
(E) posttraumatic stress disorder
(F) borderline personality disorder
(G) panic disorder
(H) major depression

For each patient described, select the most likely diagnosis.

5. A 29-year-old nurse who gives a ten months' history of recurrent episodes of dizziness, palpitations, difficulty in breathing, and shakiness. During these episodes she feels like she is going to die or that she is going crazy.

6. A 19-year-old girl came home two weeks ago to find her boyfriend unclothed with a neighbor girl. She threw him out of the house and now states that she does not miss him at all. Nevertheless, in the past ten days she has had recurrent "crying spells." She is "off her food" and does not feel like doing very much. She cannot be bothered watching her favorite television soap operas for more than a few minutes at a time.

7. A 35-year-old salesman has always "had his days." For days or weeks at a time he is easy to get along with, the customers love him, and he just seems to keep going and going. Then there are weeks when he is grouchy, irritable, and just drags himself around.

8. A 42-year-old woman comes for a physical examination. In recent months, she has been constantly tired, losing weight, and not able to get a restful sleep. As she describes her symptoms, she begins to cry. Even though she has not had a physical examination for years, she "knows" she has cancer because she can feel something chewing away at her insides. She "knows" that this is a punishment from God since she is such an unforgiveable sinner.

Questions 9 through 10

(A) transsexualism
(B) tranvestism
(C) fetishism
(D) frotteurism
(E) exhibitionism
(F) sexual masochism

For each patient described, select the most appropriate paraphilia diagnosis.

9. A 19-year-old man locks himself in the bathroom where he dresses in his sister's underwear and masturbates.

10. A 19-year-old man waits in a house doorway until he sees an unaccompanied adult woman approaching. Then sexually aroused, he exposes his genitals to this stranger. Usually he masturbates after the exposure episode.

DIRECTIONS (Questions 11 through 118): Each of the numbered items or incomplete statements in this section is followed by answers or by completions of the statement. Select the ONE lettered answer or completion that is BEST in each case.

Questions 11 through 14

A 15-year-old boy is brought to your office by his friends, who say he is "high" on drugs. They are scared of him. As you look at the teenager, you note his sallow complexion and his generally thin appearance. He is constantly restless as he sits in the chair. He grinds his teeth periodically and his eyes shift rapidly as he scans your office. When he talks, his voice sounds thick. You can find no signs of self-injection on physical examination. He admits he is taking "dope."

With some resistance, the adolescent patient responds to your questioning. He reveals a wide range of paranoid thinking and tells how he is planning to "get" those people who are making his life difficult. When you try to sway his ideas by pointing out his lack of logic, he stares suspiciously at you.

11. Your likely diagnosis is

(A) schizophrenia, paranoid type
(B) hallucinogen delusional disorder
(C) amphetamine abuse
(D) heroin abuse
(E) schizophrenia, disorganized type

12. Your diagnosis is confirmed best by

(A) urine testing
(B) Rorschach test
(C) serial sevens test
(D) fasting blood sugar
(E) skull x-ray

13. Your treatment may include all the following *except*

(A) haloperidol
(B) psychotherapy
(C) family counseling
(D) methadone maintenance
(E) hospitalization

14. This illness may be due to the following chronic effect shown on the electroencephalogram

(A) marked increase in REM activity
(B) focal slow waves, especially in temporal lobes
(C) blocking of REM sleep
(D) recurrent 3-per-second spike and wave
(E) triphasic wave pattern

Questions 15 and 16

For almost two months after his wife's death, a 49-year-old man was despondent and somewhat irritable. During this time, according to his daughters, "he just did not eat" and he did not want to "bother" with his family. After this time, he began to be more outgoing, took more interest in his work, and started to go out with his friends. He still had times when he felt lonely and sad.

15. The man was showing

(A) major depression
(B) grief reaction
(C) conversion disorder
(D) reaction formation
(E) learned helplessness

16. According to statistical data, within two years he is most likely to

(A) develop a cardiovascular illness
(B) remarry
(C) commit suicide
(D) become an alcoholic
(E) show signs of early dementia

Questions 17 through 21

An intelligent 5-year-old boy had been the only child in a family until a sister was born. Following the birth, he began to wet his bed after being dry for three years.

17. You should

(A) avoid doing a physical examination since this is an emotional problem
(B) schedule catheterization to test his bladder capacity
(C) take a thorough history and do a careful physical examination
(D) arrange for a battery of intelligence and projective tests including the Rorschach test
(E) reassure the mother that this is a minor adjustment problem

18. Since this is a reaction to the birth of a sister, the parents should

(A) give the patient extra attention and support
(B) hire a babysitter to give him personal care
(C) point out that this bedwetting is very childish
(D) ignore his bedwetting
(E) send him off to the grandparents for a rest

19. Other symptoms that may coexist with the bedwetting include all of the following *except*

(A) nightmares
(B) tantrums
(C) autism
(D) thumb sucking
(E) nail biting

20. All of the following statements are true about functional enuresis, enuresis *except*

   (A) children tend to grow out of the symptom by adolescence

   (B) it is more common in girls than in boys

   (C) often there is a history of enuresis in the parents or close relatives

   (D) bedwetting occurs during all sleep stages

   (E) children are often more handicapped by the shame and ridicule than by the bedwetting symptom itself

21. In the drug treatment of enuresis, the medication presently most effective is

   (A) dilantin

   (B) phenelzine

   (C) chlordiazepoxide

   (D) lithium

   (E) imipramine

Questions 22 and 23

You have been treating a severely depressed 52-year-old woman with tranylcypromine. After three weeks of treatment, her depression appeared to be clearing. One evening she asks to see you because she is "not feeling herself." She feels sick to her stomach, her neck muscles are stiff, and she has a "dreadful headache."

22. You anticipate that she is suffering from

   (A) depressive somatization

   (B) cryptococcal meningitis

   (C) a hypertensive crisis

   (D) early psychotic decompensation

   (E) depression with melancholia

23. When you take a history, you will ask especially about

   (A) head injury

   (B) dietary intake

   (C) recent infections

   (D) family conflicts

   (E) menstrual history

Questions 24 through 28

Father comes home tired from work to find that his two young sons have trampled his rose garden during their ball game. In a fury, he spanks them severely.

24. The younger five-year-old boy stomps out of the house in a rage. He kicks the sleeping dog on the front porch as he goes by. His behavior toward the dog is an example of

   (A) projection

   (B) isolation

   (C) displacement

   (D) reaction formation

   (E) dissociation

25. His eight-year-old brother, hurt and angry, goes down to the basement and spends the next hour chopping wood. This wood chopping is a manifestation of

   (A) identification

   (B) intellectualization

   (C) introjection

   (D) sublimation

   (E) suppression

26. Their little sister watched the spankings anxiously and then ran fearfully into the garden. A few minutes later she was heard laughing loudly at a rather dismal television program. Her laughter was an outward sign of

   (A) conversion

   (B) isolation

   (C) repression

   (D) reaction formation

   (E) rationalization

27. Father is normally a mild-tempered man who does not like to get angry. He is upset because he lost control of his feelings. Later that evening, he develops a pounding headache, an example of

   (A) regression

   (B) incorporation

   (C) conversion

   (D) undoing

   (E) somatization

28. Mother's parents fought all through her childhood so she does not like any family conflict. Though the noise of the spankings has been clearly audible through the house, somehow mother in the next room has not noticed the tumult. Her reaction is a manifestation of

   (A) negativism

   (B) denial

   (C) autism

   (D) dissociation

   (E) projection

Questions 29 through 33

A 40-year-old farm worker is hospitalized for an infectious pneumonitis. He seems to be responding well to antibiotics but on the third day of his hospital stay he becomes restless, irritable, and wants to leave. He appears to be confused. A psychiatrist is called in consultation. The psychiatrist notes from the chart that the patient is a widower, a veteran who lives by himself. The history states that he has been in good general health, with no accidents, and that he smokes and drinks moderately. His physical examination is essentially negative apart from the clearing bronchopneumonia. "There is no history of previous emotional illness" according to the hospital record. The man is lying in bed with arm and leg restraints. He is sweating profusely and the bed is in disarray. He does not acknowledge the doctor's presence but is anxiously watching what he claims to be "little lizards over there in the corner"; he says he sees these lizards climbing up the wall.

29. The most likely diagnosis with this patient is

  (A) schizophrenia, paranoid type
  (B) conversion disorder
  (C) delirium tremens, alcohol withdrawal delirium
  (D) delusional paranoid disorder
  (E) pathological intoxication

30. The preferred treatment for this disorder includes all of the following *except*

  (A) high-calorie, high-carbohydrate diet
  (B) intramuscular chlorpromazine
  (C) parenteral fluids
  (D) chlordiazepoxide intramuscularly
  (E) multivitamin supplement

With treatment, the patient becomes less disturbed but the nursing staff is still concerned. The patient is physically healthy, spends his time walking around the unit, but does not seem to recognize his surroundings. Even though he is told repeatedly that he is in a hospital, a few minutes later he appears to have forgotten. He states he is in a hotel, on vacation from his work in a local automobile factory. He is just waiting to go home to his wife. His general mood is friendly and cooperative.

31. He is now showing

  (A) la belle indifference
  (B) perseveration
  (C) thought blocking
  (D) confabulation
  (E) flight of ideas

32. This symptom is a manifestation of

  (A) Korsakoff's syndrome
  (B) acute porphyria
  (C) malingering
  (D) Capgras' syndrome
  (E) schizophrenia, undifferentiated type

33. Other symptoms that may develop as part of this illness include all of the following *except*

  (A) acute pancreatitis
  (B) hepatic coma
  (C) pellagra
  (D) Wernicke's encephalopathy
  (E) splenic infarction

Questions 34 through 36

Parents bring their five-year-old son to you, complaining that he spends all his time winding and rewinding an old beaten clock and becomes most upset if disturbed. Though he does not talk or make communicating sounds yet, he can take apart and put together intricate clock mechanisms; the father says he himself could not do so well. The youngster does not play with other children, but may sit for long periods in front of the television rocking quietly to the music. The little boy is a healthy-looking child. When you lift him up, he hangs heavily in your arms.

34. Your likely diagnosis is

  (A) autistic disorder
  (B) moderate mental retardation
  (C) congenital deafness
  (D) avoidant disorder
  (E) elective mutism

35. Your most effective treatment is likely to be

  (A) electroconvulsive therapy
  (B) behavior modification
  (C) child psychoanalysis
  (D) long-term residential treatment
  (E) methylphenidate

36. This syndrome was first described by

  (A) Anna Freud
  (B) B. F. Skinner
  (C) C. Jung
  (D) E. Bleuler
  (E) L. Kanner

Questions 37 through 39

You are called to the local police station to evaluate a 26-year-old man who has suddenly assaulted a life-long neighbor. He claims that the neighbor has been spying on him and just recently trained his dog to dig up his roses. When you are introduced to the patient, he mutters something like "He sent you."

The man is unwilling to sit down. He paces around restlessly and refuses to be touched. Periodically he stops and seems to talk quietly to himself. At other times he appears to be listening to some private sounds or voices.

37. This disturbed man attacked his neighbor to prevent what he believed to be the neighbor's spying. The emotional mechanism whereby he justified his assault is

    (A) dissociation
    (B) rationalization
    (C) projection
    (D) displacement
    (E) undoing

38. The most likely diagnosis of this patient is

    (A) homosexual panic
    (B) bipolar disorder, manic type, acute
    (C) delusional disorder
    (D) schizophrenia, paranoid type
    (E) antisocial personality disorder

39. His present symptoms are best treated by

    (A) imipramine
    (B) haloperidol
    (C) clonidine
    (D) pemoline
    (E) chlordiazepoxide

Questions 40 through 43

A 49-year-old housewife is admitted to the hospital because she is having a "nervous breakdown." She is restless, weepy, and states repeatedly that she is destined for the fires of hell. All her life she has been a hard-working woman, caring for her family, with no physical or emotional illnesses. In recent months she has been increasingly anxious and irritable. She was hospitalized when she refused to go upstairs in her home, claiming that men were waiting up there to kill her.

40. The most likely diagnosis is

    (A) early Alzheimer's disease
    (B) depression with melancholia
    (C) adjustment disorder with depressed mood
    (D) schizophrenia, paranoid type
    (E) somatization disorder

41. The treatment that would produce the quickest symptomatic relief for the patient would be

    (A) fluoxetine, orally
    (B) electroconvulsive therapy
    (C) chlordiazepoxide intramuscularly
    (D) intensive psychotherapy
    (E) propanolol, orally

42. As longer-term maintenance treatment, the following would be appropriate

    (A) diazepam
    (B) meprobamate
    (C) carbamazepine
    (D) chlordiazepoxide
    (E) sertraline

43. This patient's statement that she deserves to die and go to hell, and her fear of going upstairs lest she be killed, are examples of

    (A) dissociation
    (B) undoing
    (C) autism
    (D) ambivalence
    (E) isolation

Questions 44 through 47

A previously healthy eight-year-old boy is hospitalized with a malignancy that is diagnosed as inoperable and rapidly progressive. When you go to visit him, you find that he is located in a small, isolated room, around a corner from the rest of the inpatient unit. The nurses tell you that the patient was moved to this location to allow him peace and comfort. The nurses are upset about this boy's illness and find it very difficult to cope with his approaching death.

44. Their reason for his isolation is an example of

    (A) undoing
    (B) sublimation
    (C) dissociation
    (D) rationalization
    (E) compulsion

You find that one nurse has not kept away from the boy. Indeed she is in and out to see him every 15 minutes, to the point of tiring the youngster. You learn that last year the father of this nurse died of a similar malignancy.

45. The nurse's behavior can be considered as

    (A) counterphobic
    (B) schizoid
    (C) cyclothymic

(D) projecting

(E) hysterical

When you visit the eight-year-old patient, he is showing marked weight loss, an intravenous infusion is running, and his mother seems to be wiping away tears. The boy greets you with a feeble smile and within minutes, is talking with you about the summer trip he plans to take next year.

46. He is handling the stress of his illness by

(A) conversion

(B) denial

(C) regression

(D) sublimation

(E) isolation

These medically knowledgeable parents appreciate that their son is receiving the best possible care. Nevertheless, when you leave the patient, you find the boy's father loudly abusing a nurse about the incompetent treatment his son is getting. You help to calm the father and later you explain to the nurse how the father is handling the normal mourning anger.

47. He is handling his normal mourning anger by

(A) dissociation

(B) reaction formation

(C) suppression

(D) projection

(E) displacement

Questions 48 through 53

A 20-year-old male has just been convicted a second time for possession of heroin. He has been addicted for three years and on several occasions has unsuccessfully attempted to break the habit. He is put on probation on the condition that he undergo treatment for his addiction.

48. Withdrawal from heroin is best carried out as an

(A) outpatient with supportive psychotherapy

(B) outpatient with methadone cover

(C) inpatient with heroin antagonist

(D) inpatient with methadone cover

(E) inpatient with immediate withdrawal and no drug coverage ("cold turkey")

49. A major danger of recurrent self-injections is

(A) diabetes

(B) tuberculosis

(C) hepatitis

(D) syphilis

(E) enteritis

50. In spite of the patient's denials, the physician is suspicious of continued heroin self-administration. All of the following signs would indicate self-injection *except*

(A) recently thrombosed veins

(B) recurrent skin abscesses

(C) septicemia

(D) hepatitis

(E) syphilis

51. In heroin addiction, withdrawal symptoms include all of the following *except*

(A) runny nose, watery eyes

(B) vomiting and diarrhea

(C) muscle and stomach cramps

(D) repeated seizures

(E) recurrent yawning

52. When the addict is withdrawn cold turkey from an addicting opiate, established abstinence symptoms appear in

(A) 30 to 60 minutes

(B) 3 to 6 hours

(C) 12 to 24 hours

(D) 2 to 3 days

(E) 1 to 2 weeks

53. Heroin abstinence symptoms clear within

(A) 12 to 24 hours

(B) 1 to 3 days

(C) 4 to 8 days

(D) 7 to 14 days

(E) 2 months

Questions 54 and 55

A 35-year-old married woman comes to see you because she is "tired out and draggy." She has no energy. She has put on 30 pounds in weight, her "complexion is a mess" and "life is just not worth living." She received some tranquilizing pills from her local doctor but this medication only made her feel worse. As you look at her, she is indeed droopy. She sits hunched in her chair, her round, fat face wet with tears. She talks in a low monotonous voice.

54. Your most likely diagnosis is

(A) bipolar disorder, depressed

(B) acute intermittent porphyria

(C) Cushing's syndrome

(D) somatization disorder

(E) dependent personality disorder

55. You would confirm your diagnosis by demonstrating

(A) increased urinary 17-hydroxycorticoids
(B) abnormal focus on electroencephalogram
(C) poor form content on Rorschach
(D) long history of separation anxiety
(E) improvement with electroconvulsive therapy

Questions 56 and 57

A 46-year-old woman is hospitalized because she attempted to assault the local mayor, who, she claimed, was poisoning her water. On examination the woman weeps quietly but profusely. She thinks she may have been mistaken about the mayor, but she is not sure. She has been so confused lately, so tired, and so full of aches and pains. She states she is not good for anything, the children just want to get rid of her, and she cannot even sing in the choir. Her hearing is not what it used to be. She is just old and worn out.

She does indeed look tired and droopy. Her face is sallow, her skin dry, and her hair lifeless. She talks slowly, rather deliberately, and in a dull monotone.

56. Your likely diagnosis will be

(A) amphetamine abuse
(B) major depression
(C) histrionic personality disorder
(D) schizophrenia, paranoid type
(E) hypothyroidism

57. The specific treatment required would be

(A) thioridazine orally
(B) electroconvulsive therapy
(C) thyroid extract
(D) chlordiazepoxide
(E) estrogen replacement

Questions 58 and 59

The psychiatrist is called to see a 26-year-old former mental hospital patient. Two days previously the patient was involved in a motorcycle accident. Though he was probably drunk at the time, he was only dazed and shaken up by the crash. His neighbors have now brought him to the emergency room because they found him wandering around his yard, confused and half naked. His previous hospital history is not available. He is disoriented as to time and place. His speech is slow and rather slurred. He is annoyed by all this "fussing" and wants to go home, though he cannot say where his home is. The physical examination is unremarkable apart from superficial skin abrasions from his accident.

58. The most likely diagnosis is

(A) schizophrenia, paranoid type
(B) subdural hematoma
(C) toxic psychosis due to hallucinogens
(D) moderate mental retardation
(E) schizophrenia, catatonic type

59. The diagnosis is confirmed by

(A) CSF colloidal gold curve
(B) computer tomograms of the head
(C) Rorschach test
(D) urine toxicology screen
(E) serial sevens testing

Questions 60 through 65

60. An eight-year-old boy attends a special education class in school. Since he is said to be of borderline intellectual functioning, his intelligence quotient would be in the range

(A) 30–70
(B) 71–84
(C) 71–95
(D) 61–75
(E) 80–100

61. Though he is teased mercilessly by other children on the school bus, he does not appear to mind. Indeed he seems to invite their teasing so he can act the fool. His behavior is an indication of

(A) fixation
(B) isolation
(C) undoing
(D) reaction formation
(E) displacement

62. Following a minor fight in school, he develops weakness of his right leg. No physical cause can be shown for the leg weakness, which becomes so marked that he cannot go to school. He is now showing a

(A) depersonalization disorder
(B) dissociative disorder
(C) phobia
(D) anxiety disorder
(E) conversion disorder

63. His outward lack of concern is categorized as

(A) autism
(B) la belle indifference
(C) denial
(D) ambivalence
(E) displacement

64. This leg weakness has allowed him to avoid the unpleasant school teasing. This result is the

(A) primary gain
(B) primary process
(C) secondary process
(D) illusion
(E) rationalization

65. After two weeks he is assigned a homebound teacher and his family continues to be very kind and supportive. It will be difficult to remove his emotionally based weakness due to increasing

(A) negativism
(B) malingering
(C) secondary gain
(D) autistic thinking
(E) suppression

Questions 66 and 67

In the early evening a 23-year-old man is brought to the hospital emergency room. He is a high school teacher attending a professional convention. He has been working so hard at the convention all day that he has only had time for a coffee break. He had been planning to relax with his colleagues over the evening banquet.

During the afternoon, his fellow teachers found him to be increasingly unstable. His comments seemed at times strange or out of context. Eventually he became quite confused—as another visiting teacher stated, "almost drunk," though he had drunk just one beer.

The young man is restless, sweating, and disoriented to time and place. Physically he is in excellent condition, though there may be needle marks on his thigh.

66. The most likely diagnosis is

(A) heroin withdrawal
(B) acute hypoglycemia
(C) acute anxiety disorder
(D) delirium tremens
(E) methadone intoxication

67. The diagnosis would be confirmed by

(A) electroencephalogram
(B) urine testing
(C) nalorphine, intramuscularly
(D) blood sugar estimation
(E) intramuscular haloperidol

Questions 68 through 71

In your small town, you are aware that a 37-year-old man has been visiting out-of-town specialized clinics since his accident last year. When you knew him in school, this man was even then a "loner," rather sensitive and irritable. He went on through college and married, but his marriage ended several years ago. He was involved in a minor car accident a year ago, has never been back to work and, as you know, has two or three lawsuits pending against the local highway department, the driver of the other car, and the mayor.

He comes to see you with the complaint of back pain. He begins his history by telling you how incompetent all his previous doctors have been—but he knows you are very capable. As you do your physical and psychiatric examination, he makes scathing comments about several of your town acquaintances. You find no evidence of physical disability.

68. In your psychiatric diagnosis, you are most likely dealing with

(A) bipolar disorder, depressed type
(B) schizophrenia, paranoid type
(C) paranoid personality disorder
(D) conversion disorder
(E) malingering

69. The patient asks your opinion of his previous medical examiner and his examination. You should

(A) agree that the examination was poor and the examiner incompetent since you know that the other physician is incompetent
(B) state that you cannot give an opinion since you did not see the patient yourself at that time and you do not know the findings or recommendations
(C) tell the patient directly that he is a troublemaker and you are not going to be part of his schemes
(D) ignore his question and begin talking about another safer topic
(E) advise him to contact the local medical society

70. In dealing with this patient, you should

(A) do a limited examination and refer him to a psychiatrist
(B) carry out a thorough examination and note all findings and recommendations clearly on the patient's record
(C) begin to set up regularly scheduled appointments, at least twice a week
(D) start him on a fairly strong analgesic for the back pain he complains of
(E) refuse to see him again

71. This man's emotional condition is

(A) likely to stay the same

(B) a precursor of senile dementia

(C) probably going to lead to a florid schizophrenia

(D) a manifestation of underlying depression

(E) likely to become completely normal as he grows older

Questions 72 and 73

"Like a vise crushing my skull" was the symptom a 26-year-old married woman used to describe why "she never slept a wink at night" and never could eat anything. She brought a written list of physical complaints. She said she was constantly tired and exhausted by her two children, though she did manage to go out to Bingo several evenings each week.

Physical examination is negative and indeed the lady seems to be in excellent physical condition, though slightly overweight. She talked freely about herself and her family.

72. Her diagnosis is likely to be

(A) bipolar disorder, depressed type

(B) factitious disorder with physical symptoms

(C) somatization disorder

(D) conversion disorder

(E) schizophrenia, disorganized type

73. All of the following statements about this disorder are correct *except*

(A) benefit from individual psychotherapy

(B) more common in women

(C) usually begins in teens and twenties

(D) male relatives have higher incidence of alcoholism

(E) much higher mortality rate than general population

Questions 74 through 75

Because she has seen many stories about community violence on local television, a 26-year-old married woman is too scared to travel alone on the local city bus service. She insists that her husband go with her each time to buy groceries.

74. The fact that her husband does accompany her each time and she enjoys his attention may prolong this phobia due to

(A) reinforcement of the phobia

(B) secondary gain

(C) primary gain

(D) rationalization

(E) displacement

75. Though they have a car and used to shop near home, she now insists on doing all her shopping downtown and always going by bus. This behavior is an example of

(A) intellectualization

(B) sublimation

(C) fixation

(D) counterphobic reaction

(E) suppression

Questions 76 through 80

You are asked to see an 18-year-old girl hospitalized because of recurrent nocturnal convulsions. You find her in her hospital room, surrounded by cards, pictures, and flowers, with her boyfriend solicitously holding her hand. Physical examination and laboratory tests have all been normal.

You ask the boyfriend to leave the room. The young girl is friendly, cooperative, and seemingly not too worried about her illness. She had her first seizure when her boyfriend was walking her home from a movie three weeks ago. Since that time the convulsive episodes have tended to recur about the time of day when he is liable to be with her. She tells you that she comes from a devoutly religious family. Her 19-year-old boyfriend is hard-working and good-looking. With some more direct questions, she does admit that she and her boyfriend did almost "get carried away" in their embracing a month ago but they both decided "they were too young."

76. The most likely diagnosis is

(A) malingering

(B) histrionic personality disorder

(C) conversion disorder

(D) multiple personality disorder

(E) simple phobia

77. Her symptoms were produced by

(A) feelings of anger toward her boyfriend

(B) the wish for a closer sexual relationship with her boyfriend conflicting with moral prohibition

(C) unresolved Oedipal feelings

(D) counterphobic reaction

(E) identification with mother

78. The defense whereby her conflict is repressed and expressed symbolically in a physical symptom is an example of

(A) displacement

(B) intellectualization

(C) conversion

(D) isolation

(E) rationalization

79. The fact that she is now the focus of so much care and solicitude by her family and boyfriend may make her illness more difficult to treat. This factor is called

(A) identification with the aggressor

(B) fixation

(C) regression

(D) secondary gain

(E) narcissism

80. To produce a rapid symptomatic improvement you may use

(A) electroconvulsive therapy

(B) interpretive psychotherapy

(C) hypnosis

(D) propanolol

(E) fluoxetine

Questions 81 and 82

A 19-year-old, previously healthy female student is referred to you because of "seizures." She is just two months into her first year at college. These episodes began two weeks after she came to the university. Typically the attacks occur just after she has had breakfast at the dormitory, before she can go to classes. She becomes weak and giddy, her heart beats rapidly, she cannot breathe properly, her hands go numb and tingle, and her legs give way under her. Her friends tell her she is pale and sweating. She wonders if she has heart trouble, a brain tumor, or "something." Physical examination is normal.

81. The likely diagnosis is

(A) schizophreniform disorder

(B) major depression

(C) panic disorder

(D) psychomotor epilepsy

(E) depersonalization disorder

82. The diagnosis may be confirmed by asking the subject to

(A) take the Minnesota Multiphasic Personality Inventory

(B) overbreathe for 2 minutes

(C) do push-ups for 15 minutes

(D) consume sugar during an attack

(E) have an electroencephalogram

Questions 83 through 85

An 18-year-old girl is referred for evaluation because of marked weight loss. A year ago she was somewhat overweight, weighing 160 pounds; now she weighs 78 pounds, due to the strict dieting she has been maintaining. Though she claims she has a good appetite, she meticulously limits her food to very small portions. She always makes sure her brothers have extra food and she likes to cook for the family. She started limiting her food when her boyfriend teased her about being "well rounded." Her menses started when she was eleven but stopped four months ago. She is active, energetic, and considers herself healthy.

83. The most likely diagnosis is

(A) hypopituitarism

(B) anorexia nervosa

(C) somatization disorder

(D) conversion disorder

(E) major depression

84. On physical examination, in addition to her weight loss, it will be noted that she has

(A) feminine pubic hair distribution

(B) masculine pubic hair distribution

(C) no pubic hair

(D) masculine pubic hair and chest hair

(E) loss of hair pigmentation

85. All of the following statements about this syndrome are correct *except*

(A) it occurs predominantly in women

(B) it rarely has coexistent bulimia nervosa symptoms

(C) the peak age of onset is 15 to 20

(D) there is high incidence in ballet and modeling professions

(E) sisters are more likely to have similar symptoms

Questions 86 and 87

In school the teacher notes that an eight-year-old boy confuses letters and words as he reads. He sees *saw* for *was*, *b*'s for *d*'s, and *p*'s for *g*'s. He really can only read when the book has many pictures. He is becoming frustrated with school. You examine the youngster physically. He is somewhat awkward but is in good physical condition.

86. Your likely diagnosis is

(A) mild mental retardation

(B) attention deficit hyperactivity disorder

(C) separation anxiety disorder, school phobia

(D) developmental reading disorder

(E) overanxious disorder

87. Your optimum treatment would then be

    (A) supportive psychotherapy
    (B) methylphenidate
    (C) remedial teacher
    (D) transfer to another school
    (E) imipramine

Questions 88 and 89

A six-year-old boy is brought to you by his mother at the request of his schoolteacher. He is said to be "totally out of control" in school.

Apparently he spends his time wandering about the classroom, sometimes aimlessly, sometimes talking to other children. He hardly ever sits still, even for their in-school television programs. His mother states he has always been "on the go" but in their farm home he is usually outside with the animals. His parents worry about his being up at all hours of the night. Group testing in school gives this boy an average intelligence quotient.

88. Your diagnosis is likely to be

    (A) autistic disorder
    (B) oppositional defiant disorder
    (C) conduct disorder, undifferentiated type
    (D) attention deficit hyperactivity disorder
    (E) overanxious disorder

89. In treating this patient you would use all of the following *except*

    (A) pemoline
    (B) imipramine
    (C) methylphenidate
    (D) amphetamine
    (E) haloperidol

Questions 90 and 91

As student mental health consultant you are asked to interview a 21-year-old girl because she is "crazy." Apparently she has been bothering her classmates by her disheveled appearance and her loud laughter during class study periods. When you see her you note that she is indeed a messy dresser. She smiles rather fatuously as she talks, but she is cooperative. As she begins to tell what she is doing, she stops and seems to listen momentarily. She admits readily that she is listening to "her voices" and that she often hears these voices. She continues to talk about her classes, but you find her conversation difficult to follow. Periodically she giggles to herself.

90. Of the following, the most likely diagnosis is

    (A) histrionic personality disorder
    (B) borderline personality disorder
    (C) schizophrenia, disorganized (hebephrenic) type
    (D) schizophrenia, catatonic type
    (E) schizoid personality disorder

91. In your immediate treatment you may want to include all of the following *except*

    (A) haloperidol
    (B) family counseling
    (C) hospitalization
    (D) carbamazepine
    (E) behavior therapy

Questions 92 through 94

A 32-year-old woman is brought to the hospital by her distraught husband. In the past three days she has been on a shopping spree and has charged several thousand dollars on various charge accounts. In this time she has bought three fur coats. At home she has cleaned the house daily. Last night at 4:00 A.M. she decided to retile the kitchen floor so she phoned all her neighbors to ask them to help. She talks and jokes constantly. The husband says she has had three episodes like this before but "this is the worst."

92. It is likely this woman has

    (A) passive–aggressive personality disorder
    (B) pathological intoxication
    (C) schizophrenia, disorganized type
    (D) bipolar disorder, manic type
    (E) psychogenic fugue

93. All of the following statements about this disorder are correct *except*

    (A) about equally prevalent in men and women
    (B) untreated episode tends to last three months
    (C) better prognosis than unipolar depressive disorders
    (D) commonly runs in families
    (E) tends to start at younger age than unipolar depression

94. In managing this patient you should plan to use

    (A) interpretive psychotherapy
    (B) family therapy
    (C) outpatient electroconvulsive therapy
    (D) supportive psychotherapy
    (E) hospitalization with drug therapy

Questions 95 through 97

You are asked to see a 25-year-old man in the hospital emergency room. Physical examination and laboratory tests have shown nothing abnormal, but he is said to be "acting queer." When you see him, he is sitting on a bench looking straight ahead. His face is motionless and he does not seem to notice the hustle around him. When you talk to him, he does not answer. You raise his arm, which then remains in an outstretched position.

95. Your most likely diagnosis is

(A) delirium tremens

(B) psychogenic amnesia

(C) conversion disorder

(D) paranoid personality disorder

(E) schizophrenia, catatonic type

The patient is hospitalized for further evaluation. Laboratory tests are still normal. Two days later he becomes acutely agitated, shouting and screaming almost incoherently. He seems unable to sit still, has torn his bed sheets and mattress into shreds, and has hit two staff members.

96. He is now showing

(A) panic disorder

(B) catatonic excitement

(C) bipolar disorder, manic type

(D) catastrophic reaction

(E) explosive personality

97. Your treatment should be

(A) propanolol orally

(B) lithium carbonate orally

(C) barbiturates intramuscularly

(D) haloperidol intramuscularly

(E) chlordiazepoxide orally

Questions 98 and 99

A 49-year-old lawyer is brought by his wife for examination. She states that he has not been eating much lately. He sleeps poorly and gets up in the middle of the night and stays up. The man looks much older than his age. He walks slowly and appears tired. With little prompting, he tells you that "it is hopeless." He has tried very hard but he knows he has failed to stop the rising murder rate in the community. He has been feeling lately that he deserves to be executed for all the killings.

99. He is likely to be suffering from

(A) schizophrenia, paranoid type

(B) major depression with mood *congruent* psychotic features

(C) major depression with mood *incongruent* psychotic features

(D) borderline personality disorder with depression

(E) dysthymia

99. The appropriate management includes all of the following *except*

(A) hospitalization

(B) electroconvulsive therapy

(C) levodopa

(D) fluoxetine

(E) haloperidol

Questions 100 and 101

You have been called in consultation to see a 45-year-old widower. He is weepy, depressed, and unable to do his work as company accountant. From the family history, you note that his sister committed suicide. You are concerned that he might be suicidal.

100. You should

(A) avoid mentioning suicide in case you cause him to begin thinking about it

(B) directly raise the question as to whether he has thought of killing himself

(C) talk first with other family members to see if they have seen signs of suicidal intent

(D) arrange to see him for a series of appointments so you can raise the question at an appropriate time

(E) avoid distressing him now with pointed questions about suicide but start him on antidepressant medication

101. The patient admits that he is profoundly depressed and is thinking seriously about killing himself. You should

(A) point out that his religion considers suicide to be a mortal sin

(B) send him home with family members to get his clothes so that he can be admitted to hospital that day or the next

(C) institute or maintain high dose of antidepressants; set up daily outpatient appointments

(D) admit him directly to the hospital from your office. Be sure he is closely accompanied to the hospital unit

(E) arrange contact for him with one of the suicide prevention groups, like "Rescue." They will provide good community support

Question 102 and 103

A 26-year-old woman has been limited to her home for the past ten months. She is fearful of venturing beyond her front gate even to mail a letter. She feels sure that if she goes out she will have an anxiety attack and no one would understand or be able to help her.

102. The most likely diagnosis is

   (A) simple phobia, specific phobia
   (B) dependent personality disorder
   (C) agoraphobia
   (D) dysthymia
   (E) somatization disorder

103. Appropriate treatment could include all of the following *except*

   (A) systematic desensitization
   (B) flooding
   (C) family therapy
   (D) methylphenidate
   (E) imipramine

Questions 104 and 105

An eight-year-old boy has been sent for evaluation because, at the most inappropriate times, he make "animal noises or barking" in the classroom. The teacher says he is fidgety and restless. He is a nice boy, according to the teacher, very conscientious and very neat.

104. The most likely diagnosis of this youngster is

   (A) attention deficit hyperactivity disorder
   (B) oppositional defiant disorder
   (C) separation anxiety disorder
   (D) Tourette's Disorder
   (E) autistic disorder

105. Appropriate treatment for this disorder could include all of the following *except*

   (A) pemoline
   (B) pimozide
   (C) haloperidol
   (D) clonidine
   (E) group therapy

Questions 106 and 107

A 14-year-old girl has been losing weight in the last six months. She has gone down from 110 to 70 pounds. Her menses stopped three months ago. She is described as always having been close to her father and somewhat of a tomboy. This weight loss started one week after she broke up with her boyfriend.

   She is a pert, friendly girl who seems to like her tall,

thin appearance. Apart from her thinness, physical examination is normal except for a moderate right-sided papilledema.

106. Your most likely diagnosis is

   (A) anorexia nervosa
   (B) intracranial tumor
   (C) conversion disorder
   (D) obsessive–compulsive disorder
   (E) bulimia nervosa

107. Your diagnosis might be confirmed by

   (A) fasting blood sugar
   (B) computer tomograms of the head
   (C) Rorschach test
   (D) serial sevens test
   (E) serum amylase

Questions 108 and 109

A 49-year-old woman is brought to the surgical emergency clinic because of recurrent abdominal pain and severe constipation. Her husband states that she has not been feeling well for several months. Indeed, three weeks ago she was started on medication by her family doctor because she had been having crying spells, feeling bad about herself, and not eating. In the last week or so she has been cheerier and showing more energy but then she developed these symptoms. On examination, she is flushed, her skin is dry, and her temperature is 38°C (100.4°F). She says she feels a little "mixed up."

108. Select the the medication most likely to be causing these symptoms

   (A) fluoxetine
   (B) phenelzine
   (C) amitriptyline
   (D) lithium carbonate
   (E) diazepam

109. To relieve these symptoms, the most effective medication would be

   (A) atropine
   (B) benztropine
   (C) diphenhydramine
   (D) physostigmine
   (E) valproic acid

Questions 110 through 112

For the past five months a 40-year-old woman has been seeing a succession of physicians about her stomach trouble and eventually she is referred for psychiatric consultation. She knows she has a big deep ulcer—"at least the size of your fist"—that has eaten away her stomach and is now "working on her liver." She can feel the gnawing and biting so she knows. Generally she feels "just no good" and she states she just cannot go on this way. She is no use to anyone. It is just as well her husband died last year and she thinks her children should put her away. She admits she has thought of killing herself and, as God knows, she well deserves to go to hell but she cannot get up the courage. She feel that no one can help her.

Previously she had no history of emotional illness. Extensive physical and laboratory studies are normal.

110. Your diagnosis is likely to be

(A) panic disorder
(B) major depression
(C) schizophrenia, hebephrenic type
(D) bipolar disorder, depressed type
(E) conversion disorder

111. When she talked further about her abdominal discomfort, she described how there was "something like germs in there with teeth, chewing." This symptom is an example of

(A) conversion
(B) phobia
(C) projection
(D) phantom phenomenon
(E) somatic delusion

112. Your treatment might include all of the following *except*

(A) electroconvulsive therapy
(B) reserpine
(C) psychotherapy
(D) haloperidol
(E) desipramine

Questions 113 and 114

A twelve-year-old boy recently moved to a new neighborhood and started a new school. About that time he began to complain of bitemporal headaches. When the patient's history is taken carefully, it is noted that these headaches typically start on a Sunday, recur on Mondays and Tuesdays, and clear by the end of the week. The headaches never occur at the start of holidays. In recent weeks, the headaches have been so marked that the boy has been staying home from school. All medical examinations have been given normal findings.

113. The psychiatric diagnosis most likely to explain these symptoms is

(A) adjustment disorder with depressed mood
(B) bipolar disorder, depressive type
(C) separation anxiety disorder
(D) hypochondriasis
(E) somatization disorder

114. The most effective way to manage this disorder would be

(A) to arrange for a homebound teacher to ensure he does not fall behind academically
(B) the immediate return to school even if he only studies in the counselor's office
(C) immediate intensive psychotherapy to deal with the underlying problem prior to returning to school
(D) to arrange for the parent to take over the teaching responsibilities at home
(E) frequent family therapy involving the boy, his parents, and his siblings.

Answers and Explanations

Questions 1 through 4 deal with prevention in dealing with the mentally retarded. (1:144,697–8; 2:711,1155–8)

1. **(A)** *Genetic counseling* to prevent the birth of other mentally retarded children is an example of *primary prevention.*

2. **(B)** If the newborn child has chromosome defects, it is now too late to prevent the disability from occurring. *Early treatment* can be instituted to minimize the development of handicaps—*secondary prevention.*

3. **(C)** Specialized training in sheltered workshops will help the retarded child to function more productively as a member of society—*tertiary prevention.*

4. **(A)** *Contraceptive instruction* may help reduce the chances that a retarded adolescent will become pregnant and give birth to retarded offspring—*primary prevention.*

5. **(G)** *Panic disorder* is characterized by periodic spontaneous attacks of acute anxiety. Often the attacks come on over several minutes and last usually less than 30 minutes. The subject experiences intense anxiety with a feeling of doom, imminent death or loss of control, with sweating, dizziness, tachycardia, and difficulty breathing. Mental status examination may show preoccupation with the feelings and difficulty concentrating and remembering. *(1:394–400; 2:444–7)*

6. **(D)** An *adjustment disorder* is a transient, maladaptive reaction occurring within three months of an identifiable stress. The implication of this diagnosis is that the maladaptive reaction is temporary and, within a relatively short period, the subject will return to the previous level of emotional functioning. It must be noted that this is a return to the previous level of functioning, no matter whether that prior level of emotional competence was efficient or inefficient.

   The patient in this instance is showing *depressive* symptoms in reaction to the infidelity of her boyfriend—an *adjustment reaction with depressed mood. (1:494–7; 2:605–10)*

7. **(C)** Subjects with *cyclothymia* go through life showing recurrent affective ups and downs, a mild form of bipolar disorder. About 30% of cyclothymic patients have a positive family history for bipolar disorder, the same level as patients with bipolar disorder. Many patients with cyclothymia go on to develop bipolar disorder. *(1:386–8; 2:414–5)*

8. **(H)** The patient is showing a *major depression with mood congruent psychotic features.* Her belief that something is chewing at her insides is a *somatic delusion. (1:366–74; 2:411–2)*

Questions 9 and 10 deal with the paraphilias, sexual deviations. (1:443–8; 2:592–5)

9. **(B)** *Transvestism, transvestic fetishism,* usually begins during childhood or adolescence. The transvestite, almost always a male, cross-dresses in female clothing to cause sexual arousal and to produce orgasm. *(1:446; 2:592)*

10. **(E)** The *exhibitionist,* usually a male, achieves sexual arousal in anticipation and as a result of exposing his genitals to strangers. The person most in danger from these encounters is usually not the shocked woman stranger but the exhibitionist who is likely to find himself chased, beaten, or injured by infuriated victims and others. *(1:445; 2:592)*

Questions 11 through 14 deal with amphetamine abuse. (1:305–7; 2:342–3)

11. **(C)** This patient shows the typical symptoms of *amphetamine abuse.* His presenting emotional symptoms are paranoid in nature. While paranoid schizophrenia cannot be totally excluded, this form of schizophrenia usually occurs in the late 20s or the 30s. The teenager does not show the bizarre mannerisms, thinking disorganization, grossly inappropriate affect, and regressed behavior of the disorganized schizophrenic. Hallucinogen intoxi-

cation may produce a paranoid syndrome and chronic drug ingestion can produce this debilitated state; however, hallucinogen toxicity usually leads to greater disruption of reality contact.

Heroin abuse is usually manifested by needle marks, phlebitis, and other signs of self-administration. Very often, of course, the amphetamine abuser takes the drug by intravenous injection and may have all the signs seen with heroin abuse.

Abuse of any stimulant, including cocaine, will produce symptoms similar to those with amphetamine abuse.

Bruxism is the term for the compulsive teeth grinding shown by this patient.

12. **(A)** The diagnosis is best confirmed by *urine testing* for amphetamines and other drugs.

The Rorschach test would show the patient's emotional state as a paranoid psychosis. The test does not diagnose the etiology. The serial sevens test is too nonspecific an evaluation and tests a subject's ability to maintain a train of thought.

Fasting blood sugar levels and skull x-rays should be normal.

13. **(D)** Methadone maintenance is not used in the treatment of amphetamine addiction or abuse. Methadone is used in treating opioid abuse.

The teenager with an amphetamine psychosis requires *hospitalization. Haloperidol* or a similar antipsychotic may be necessary to control anxiety or disruptive behavior. During and following the acute symptoms, *psychotherapy* may help the patient, and *family counseling* may be indicated both for the patient and his family.

14. **(C)** *Amphetamines block REM sleep.* Amphetamine psychosis may be related to this electroencephalogram effect. After the withdrawal of barbiturates and other REM-blocking drugs, there is an increase in REM activity, sometimes with nightmares.

Focal slow waves, especially in the temporal lobes, are characteristic of psychomotor epilepsy.

Recurrent 3-per-second spike-and-wave EEG readings are diagnostic of petit mal (absence) seizures.

A triphasic wave pattern on the electroencephalogram is seen in about 25% of patients with hepatic failure.

Questions 15 and 16 deal with normal mourning and grief. (1:58–61; 2:299–300)

15. **(B)** This middle-aged man is showing a normal grief reaction with sadness, some anger, and eventual emotional reinvestment. The major work of mourning is usually complete within three months. Mourning is liable to start when it is rec-

ognized that the ill person is dying and the process of mourning does not necessarily wait until death occurs.

16. **(B)** Statistically it has been shown that a middle-aged widower is likely to remarry within two years of his spouse's death.

Questions 17 through 21 deal with functional enuresis, enuresis. (1:765–7; 2:690–2)

17. **(C)** In any case of *enuresis,* a thorough physical and psychological examination should be carried out by the clinician. Where there is a physical symptom, a physical examination is always necessary. Since this boy was previously toilet trained and has an obvious psychological reason for behavioral regression, more traumatic physical examinations can be delayed. Catheterization should be one of the last evaluation procedures and used only when a physical etiology is strongly suspected. A child may be traumatized by excessive psychological testing just as much as by overzealous physical examinations. Projective tests and especially the Rorschach test have little value with a five-year-old patient. Intelligence testing offers little in the diagnosis of functional enuresis.

Until the clinician is sure of the diagnosis and the etiology of any symptom, reassurance is premature and may be counterproductive.

18. **(A)** The child (or patient of any age) showing an *adjustment reaction* benefits best by *increased emotional support.*

Passing the youngster over to a babysitter or grandparents can be felt as an even more total rejection by a young child. The youngster may blame himself for being in some way unacceptable to his parents.

To stigmatize the bedwetting as "childish," without giving extra emotional support and understanding for those reasons he has to be childish, would merely shame the child and burden him further emotionally.

Bedwetting is a form of communication. While the enuresis should not provoke a punitive rejecting reaction, the message and the behavior should not be ignored.

19. **(C)** Autism is a sign of profound emotional maldevelopment; it is *not a temporary adjustment reaction.*

Regressive behavior like nightmares, tantrums, thumb sucking, and nail biting can be temporary. When the stress is relieved, the symptoms clear.

20. **(B)** *Enuresis, bedwetting,* is more common in *boys.*

Enuresis does tend to *disappear by adolescence* but in some cases persists into adulthood.

Children are often more handicapped by the *shame* and *ridicule* they face than by the symptom itself.

Enuresis frequently occurs in *families* so there is often a history of enuresis in parents or close relatives.

Bedwetting occurs during *all stages of sleep*. Children with functional enuresis do not sleep more soundly than non-enuretic children.

21. **(E)** *Imipramine* usually produces symptomatic improvement in enuretic children but this improvement tends to disappear in a month or two. When the imipramine is discontinued, the enuresis tends to recur. Imipramine does have significant side effects—many youngsters dislike having a dry mouth, constipation, visual blurring, mental fogginess, and hypotension.

Questions 22 and 23 deal with monoamine oxidase toxicity. (1:656–8; 2:802–3)

22. **(C)** This case vignette describes a patient with some of the early symptoms of a *hypertensive crisis*.

23. **(B)** *Dietary intake.* Patients receiving monoamine oxidase inhibitors should be warned that foods containing tyramine—cheeses, wines, chicken liver—may induce a disabling and potentially fatal vasopressor reaction. (The majority of patients on monoamine oxidase inhibitors will not have a hypertensive crisis even when these foods are eaten.)

Questions 24 through 28 deal with defense mechanisms. (1:183–4; 2:136–8)

24. **(C)** The five-year-old cannot express his anger toward his father but he displaces his rage onto a more acceptable focus—*displacement*. The emotion remains the same but it is displaced onto a more acceptable object. *(1:184; 2:127)*

25. **(D)** The eight-year-old boy partially represses his anger and no longer directs it at his family. Rather, he redirects his aggressive tensions into socially more acceptable behavior. He chops wood—an example of *sublimation*. *(1:184; 2:138)*

26. **(D)** Their little sister is scared and upset. Her inappropriate laughter is an overreaction, a manifestation of *reaction formation*. She laughs *too much*. *(1:405; 2:136)*

27. **(E)** The father does not or cannot totally repress his conflictual anxiety about his temper outburst. He is hurting and his hurt is manifested by direct somatic expression of his feeling state. He has *somatized*. *(1:183–4; 2:533)*

28. **(B)** The mother's ability to block out disturbing external reality is an example of *denial*. She manages not to hear, though she is not deaf. *(1:182; 2:137–8)*

Questions 29 through 33 deal with delirium tremens, alcohol withdrawal delirium (a favorite examination topic). (1:288–9; 2:323–5)

29. **(C)** Visual hallucinations are more typically seen in a toxic psychosis like delirium tremens and would be uncommon in paranoid schizophrenia. The paranoid schizophrenic usually has fairly circumscribed paranoid delusions but may function well socially and intellectually.

The patient with delusional paranoid disorder does not have prominent or sustained hallucinations and is well organized; the subject has a relatively fixed delusional system without other signs of thought disorder.

In a patient with a conversion disorder, an emotional conflict is symbolically expressed by a physical symptom involving the voluntary musculature or the special senses. Visual hallucinations are not considered visual conversion symptoms. Some of the hysterical dissociative states, including the latah, amok, and berserk states, may be manifested by agitated frenzy, but marked visual hallucinations would usually not be present. Pathological intoxication is a term infrequently used now. Often the syndrome is a manifestation of a dissociative disorder. Pathological intoxication occurs when the subject is taking, or has just taken, alcohol and there is an excessive intoxication reaction to the alcohol.

30. **(B)** *Intramuscular chlorpromazine* would be contraindicated in chronic alcoholic patients with delirium tremens. Chronic alcoholics are likely to have chronic liver damage; chlorpromazine has hepatotoxic effects. Chlorpromazine lowers the seizure threshhold; in patients with delirium tremens, treatment is planned to avoid seizures.

The *restraints* should be *removed* if possible or the patient may exhaust himself in a struggle to be free. Chlordiazepoxide is often used to produce sedation.

Parenteral fluids with *vitamin* supplements and a *high-calorie, high-carbohydrate* diet are usually part of the immediate and long-range treatment.

31. **(D)** *Confabulation* is the automatic falsification of recall to fill gaps in memory—as is described in this question. *La belle indifference*, classically seen in conversion disorder, is an unusual lack of reasonable anxiety in face of disabling or usually distressing symptoms. This symptom is not indicative of any syndrome as it can occur in stoical people. *Perseveration* is present when the subject gives the

same response to different and unconnected questions.

Thought blocking or *thought deprivation* is the sudden stopping of the flow of thought. "My mind just went blank" can occur normally, but when this symptom is prominent it may be a sign of schizophrenia.

A *flight of ideas* typically occurs in hypomanic or manic states where the subject shows a very rapid flow of thinking, sometimes so fast that the connections are no longer obvious.

32. (A) *Confabulation* is a typical manifestation of *Korsakoff's syndrome.* (1:255,290; 2:293,323)

33. (E) Syndromes that can occur as part of *chronic alcoholism* include acute *pancreatitis, hepatic failure, coma, pellagra,* and *Wernicke's encephalopathy.* Splenic infarction is not typically a manifestation of the alcoholic syndromes.

Questions 34 through 36 deal with autistic disorder. (1:699–704; 2:711–7)

34. (A) Your likely diagnosis is *autistic disorder.* When you lift up the child, he does not respond to you—he just hangs. The autistic child may resist being lifted as this is an intrusion into his private existence, but he will not respond to your lifting by "moulding" his body to your body. Unless the retarded child is autistic, he will show a moulding or resisting response. The other youngsters typically would react to you as a person.

The preoccupation with moving mechanisms, the *self-rocking,* and the *anxious reaction when disturbed* are characteristics of the autistic child.

The deaf child, who is not autistic, may not communicate in words, but he interacts with sounds and gestures.

The children showing elective mutism, selective mutism, are able to talk but selectively refuse to speak to certain people or in certain situations. Elective mutism is more common in girls.

Avoidant disorder is a diagnosis that is being dropped from DSM IV.

35. (B) In general, no treatment has been very effective with autistic youngsters. *Behavior modification* is the therapeutic approach that has given most predictable improvement by more efficient use of (usually limited) treatment resources. *Electroconvulsive therapy* has no long-range beneficial effect. *Methylphenidate* may make the patient more distressed or disturbed. If the youngster is showing attention deficit hyperactivity symptoms, methylphenidate may produce some symptomatic improvement.

Long-term institutional care usually leads to profound social and intellectual retardation in autistic children. Classical *child psychoanalysis* is ineffective with the autistic child. *Modified child psychotherapy* can sometimes successfully intrude into the child's private world and help him emerge. However, results of even many years of psychotherapy tend to be rather poor.

36. (E) The syndrome of *infantile autism*, now called autistic disorder, was first described by *Leo Kanner* in 1943.

Questions 37 through 39 deal with schizophrenia, paranoid type. (1:334–5; 2:371)

37. (C) This disturbed patient justified his assaultive behavior on the basis of his paranoid *projections.* He *projected* his own unacceptable and intolerable thoughts onto his neighbor and then attacked the neighbor with the justification of these projections.

38. (D) The most likely diagnosis is *schizophrenia, paranoid type* in a man with fairly circumscribed paranoid delusions and auditory hallucinations.

Hallucinations do not occur in patients with *antisocial personality disorder*. The gross reality distortion manifested by the hallucinations and the paranoid delusions would not support a diagnosis of *homosexual panic,* a diagnosis that may have little validity.

This patient does not show the incessant driven quality of the *manic.* His affect is inappropriate and contradictory. The emotional state of the manic is excessive rather than grotesque or idiosyncratic. While the most likely diagnosis is that of paranoid schizophrenia, a manic state is not totally excluded. The patient with a *delusional disorder* has a fairly fixed but circumscribed delusion system, most often paranoid in nature. These patients do not show other manifestations of thought disorder.

39. (B) This patient is best treated with *haloperidol* or similar antipsychotic in adequate doses.

Questions 40 through 43 deal with major depression with melancholia (involutional melancholia). (1:366–8; 2:410–11)

40. (B) This is the typical history of a patient with *major depression with melancholia—involutional melancholia*—a life-long, conscientious, hard-working woman in the involutional period of life, presenting with depression and bizarre self-accusatory delusions.

Alzheimer's disease would usually manifest with greater confusion and memory loss. A thorough medical evaluation is always indicated when dementia is suspected.

A patient with an *adjustment disorder with depressed mood* would not manifest these bizarre delusions.

A patient with a *somatization disorder* will express emotions through physical symptoms but not to this delusional degree; nor is such a patient profoundly depressed.

Paranoid schizophrenia would not manifest with this exaggerated affect but would present with inappropriate paranoid projection, often with overt auditory hallucinations.

41. **(B)** *Electroconvulsive therapy* is most effective in treating first episodes of major depression with melancholia. Recurrent bouts do not respond quite as well.

42. **(E)** *Sertraline* or other antidepressant medications may be used to maintain the patient at a comfortable level of emotional adaptation. Supportive psychotherapy should be combined with long-term maintenance drug therapy to facilitate prevention or early detection of symptomatic recrudescence.

43. **(D)** *Ambivalence* is the presence of contrasting and conflicting thoughts or emotions: the wish and need to die coexisting with the fear of death and the wish to live. Patients with major depression with melancholia may act on one side of the ambivalence and commit *suicide*. Suicide is a definite risk in this syndrome.

Questions 44 through 47 deal with the management of the dying child. (1:60; 2:299–300)

44. **(D)** The reality that this boy is dying faces the nurses with intolerable feelings. They deal with their problem by isolating the boy and then explain their seemingly illogical behavior by outwardly logical intellectual reasons—by *rationalization. (1:184; 2:1265)*

45. **(A)** For very understandable causes, this nurse would naturally be made anxious and upset by this patient. She handles her inner conflicts and tension by overdoing the very thing she fears—a specific form of *reaction formation* where the phobic object is sought after rather than avoided—*counterphobic* behavior. *(1:400–1; 2:1247)*

46. **(B)** The eight-year-old boy copes with the intolerable life situation by blocking out certain parts of reality—by *denial*. This is a normal way of adapting to dying and should be supported as much as the patient and family need the denial. *(1:183; 2:137–8)*

47. **(E)** As part of normal mourning, these parents are angry. They are angry at their little son for leaving them, they are angry at God or Fate for giving them such pain, and they may well be angry with themselves for not in some way preventing this illness. They cannot express this anger at the cause of their rage so they handle it in part by displacing it onto a more acceptable target, in this situation the nurse—*displacement*. Sometimes the doctors and the nurses become an acceptable focus for displaced anger because they appear so strong and competent and thus able to tolerate the anger. *(1:184; 2:127)*

Questions 48 through 53 deal with heroin drug dependence. (1:297–302; 2:330–7)

48. **(D)** *Withdrawal from heroin*, detoxification, is best carried out in an *inpatient* setting with *methadone cover*.

   No matter how much the patient promises or intends, it is almost impossible to withdraw the chronic addict from this drug on an outpatient basis.

   Withdrawal without methadone cover would lead to a severe abstinence syndrome.

   Naloxone and other opioid antagonists would precipitate an abrupt abstinence syndrome.

49. **(C)** *Hepatitis* is a major danger in the addict's self-injection. Other illnesses caused by dirty syringes include AIDS, endocarditis and pulmonary emboli. Tuberculosis, syphilis, and enteritis are associated with the addict's living conditions but are not transmitted by dirty or shared syringes.

50. **(E)** *Syphilis* would not usually be an indication of self-injection. *Phlebitis*, skin *abscesses*, *septicemia*, and *hepatitis* all may be caused by repeated self-injections.

51. **(D)** The *abstinence syndrome* in *heroin* withdrawal includes runny nose and watery eyes as in an upper respiratory infection, repeated yawning, vomiting and diarrhea, and muscle and stomach cramps. Seizures do not occur as part of an opioid withdrawal syndrome.

52. **(C)** When an addict is withdrawn from heroin, *abstinence symptoms* build up gradually but are *established* in *12 to 24 hours*.

53. **(C)** Withdrawal *abstinence symptoms* can be expected to *clear* in *four to eight days*. Symptoms persisting longer necessitate further medical or psychiatric evaluation.

Questions 54 and 55 deal with Cushing's syndrome. (1:96,268; 2:292)

   Occasionally there are examination questions focused on physical illnesses presenting as an emotional problem. Even though the examination subjects may be psychiatry and the behavioral sciences, the candidate should not ignore the significance of physical signs or symptoms detailed in any question.

54. (C) This woman presents with the clinical features of *Cushing's syndrome*. She is depressed—"life is not worth living"—but her physical symptoms and hormonal imbalance are likely to have caused this depression.

The clinician must always consider the whole range of medical and psychological diagnoses when considering a problem, even though the patient may be suggesting by the presenting complaints that the difficulty is either physical *or* emotional.

55. (A) The diagnosis of Cushing's disease is confirmed by demonstrating *increased urinary 17-hydroxycorticoids*. The *electroencephalogram* should not show abnormal foci. Poor form content on the *Rorschach test* is a nonspecific finding that must be evaluated in the appropriate clinical context.

Binge eating is symptomatic of a range of disorders, psychological and physical.

If the woman is severely depressed, *electroconvulsive therapy* might give symptomatic relief but this treatment result is not specifically diagnostic of any syndrome.

Questions 56 and 57 deal with hypothyroidism (myxedema). (1:268; 2:525–6)

56. (E) This patient presents with the typical symptoms of *hypothyroidism* (myxedema).

The cerebration of these patients is slow, their perception is blunted, and they feel different. They see no obvious reason for this change so they tend to blame external factors; *paranoia* is a common symptom in hypothyroidism.

Depression also frequently occurs and is precipitated in part by the physical debility and discomfort.

57. (C) The specific treatment for hypothyroidism is thyroid replacement—*thyroid extract* or equivalent.

Hypothyroid patients who are given thyroid may symptomatically get worse before they get better. The body readjustment precipitated by the thyroid intake may exacerbate emotional and physical difficulties.

Questions 58 and 59 deal with the patient who has a subdural hematoma. (1:64,83; 2:255–6). It is important to recognize that patients with emotional disorders can present with non-psychiatric disorders.

58. (B) This is the typical history of a patient who has developed a *subdural hematoma*. Even patients with previous psychiatric hospitalization can develop the whole range of physical illnesses.

59. (B) The diagnosis is confirmed by *computer tomography of the head.*

Questions 60 through 65 deal with the mentally retarded child. (1:685–98; 2:702–11)

60. (B) In the *Diagnostic and Statistical Manual* of the American Psychiatric Association, *borderline intellectual functioning* (intelligence quotient in the range 71 to 84) is included in conditions not attributable to mental disorder. *(1:547–8)*

Level of Retardation	IQ
mild	50–55 to approximately 70
moderate	35–40 to 50–55
severe	20–25 to 35–40
profound	under 20 or 25

(1:686; 2:705)

61. (D) The child who acts the class clown is often showing *reaction formation*. Peer teasing can make a child very anxious and upset, especially when the teasing is based on a realistic reason. One way of coping with such teasing or feelings of vulnerability is to emphasize the vulnerability oneself and flaunt it for the amusement of others. By emphasizing the opposite of his true feelings—reaction formation—the youngster can cope with an otherwise intolerable situation. *(1:184; 2:136)*

62. (E) He is now showing a *conversion disorder*. His emotional conflict has been repressed but has been expressed symbolically through this symptom affecting his voluntary musculature. *(1:418–20; 2:538–9)*

63. (B) His outward lack of concern is called *la belle indifference*, a term coined by Janet, a French neuropsychiatrist. The normal person would naturally be most concerned by a physical paralysis. A patient who has a conversion disorder may show this seeming total lack of concern. *(1:419; 2:539)*

64. (A) The *primary gain* of a symptom is the relief of the conflictual anxiety. This young man was being mercilessly teased. He could not effectively fight back. He could not escape. His leg weakness has allowed him relief from the anxiety. *(1:419; 2:1263)*

65. (C) *Secondary gain* is the reward, the attention, and the care the subject begins to receive because of his illness. Secondary gain will tend to perpetuate the emotional illness because the illness becomes rewarding in itself.

This rather tragic retarded boy is now finding that his leg paralysis brings him all kinds of support, care, and attention—more than he was able to get before he developed the conversion symptoms. This *secondary gain* from his paralysis will make it more difficult for him to give up his paralysis and go back to being a retarded, inadequate eight-year-old. *(1:419; 2:539,1267)*

Questions 66 and 67 deal with the patient who presents with the symptoms of acute hypoglycemia. (1:96–7,518; 2:522)

66. **(B)** The most likely diagnosis is *acute hypoglycemia* in a diabetic young man who is taking insulin.

Hypoglycemia may present with a wide range of emotional symptoms that mimic neurotic, psychotic, or confusional states.

67. **(D)** The diagnosis is confirmed by *blood sugar estimation* to demonstrate the hypoglycemia.

In evaluating the patient, the clinician should **try** to ascertain the previous medical and psychological history. Where the subject has been well adjusted and productive, an acute psychotic reaction, especially with confusion, is likely to be toxic or organic in origin. Thigh needle marks would suggest intramuscular or subcutaneous injections rather than the addict's intravenous "mainlining."

A simple acute anxiety reaction would not manifest with gross confusion or bizarre actions or comments.

Questions 68 through 71 deal with paranoid personality disorder. (1:527–8; 2:630–1)

68. **(C)** This history describes the typical subject with a *paranoid personality disorder*—hypersensitive, suspicious, isolated, often litiginous, and usually very insecure beneath his aloofness.

Though the patient is unusually sensitive, suspicious, and irritable, his behavior and history do not indicate a major break with reality as would be found in a patient with paranoid schizophrenia.

He is angry and aggressive but gives no indication of cyclic depressive swings. This patient is overly involved, anxious, and irritable; the patient with a conversion disorder is more likely to appear blandly unconcerned, only superficially involved, and often theatrical.

You have no indication of deliberate falsification of symptoms or history as would be noted in the patient who is malingering.

69. **(B)** No clinician should be seduced into diagnosing or evaluating in retrospect or from hearsay. If you did not evaluate the patient at the time in question or if you do not have all the findings, you *cannot make a competent evaluation.* At the same time, the patient, even a grossly paranoid patient, merits your full attention and a thoughtful response.

70. **(B)** In dealing with the paranoid patient, the clinician is most helpful to the patient if he deals with immediate reality. The doctor should carry out a thorough examination and keep careful notes of all findings and recommendations, positive and negative. A detailed record of actual history (even quoting the patient's words) and of specific clinical signs allows the doctor to help the patient best and also protects the clinician against later suit.

71. **(A)** This man's *paranoia* is likely to *stay the same.* Treatment should be primarily supportive to help the patient function as productively and tolerably as possible.

Questions 72 and 73 deal with somatization disorder. (1:416–8; 2:544–6)

72. **(C)** The patient with a *somatization disorder* often expresses emotional tension and pain in a somatic ache—by *somatization*—a headache, stomach ache, backache. This is one way of telling others that she is hurting. These symptoms can occur in depressive states but the depressed patient is more likely to show psychomotor retardation, feelings of worthlessness, and more obvious depressive affect.

In patients with conversion disorder, anxiety would be repressed and converted into a physical symptom.

The patient does not show the florid disorder of thinking usually manifested by the patient with disorganized schizophrenia.

73. **(E)** Patients with somatization disorder do not have higher mortality rates than the general population.

Individual psychotherapy and family therapy, can be therapeutically beneficial. Medications should be avoided wherever possible.

Somatization disorder is much more common in women but the male relatives of these patients have a higher incidence of alcoholism than the general population.

Questions 74 through 75 deal with phobia. (1:400–4; 2:458–72)

74. **(B)** *Secondary gain* is the emotional reward that comes with being ill—the extra attention, the added support and understanding, and the reduction of responsibility. Secondary gain tends to maintain the illness as the subject becomes reluctant to give up these new gratifications. This woman's phobia is liable to be perpetuated by all the attention her husband now gives her. *(1:185; 2:1267)*

75. **(D)** When the phobic individual insists on experiencing the feared situation repeatedly and unnec-

essarily, this behavior is termed a *counterphobic reaction.*

Questions 76 through 80 deal with conversion disorder. (1:418–20; 2:535–40)

76. **(C)** With the medical, neurological, and laboratory tests all normal, the most likely diagnosis is that of a *conversion disorder.*

A conversion disorder can occur superimposed on an organic illness, so positive physical and laboratory findings would not exclude this diagnosis. Pseudoseizures are most common in patients who have organically caused seizures also. Equally, conversion disorder patients can develop organic illnesses like anyone else. A prolonged period of observation, usually on an outpatient basis, may be necessary to confirm the diagnosis.

In a conversion disorder, the symptom develops due to emotional factors and is not within the patient's conscious control. *Malingering* involves deliberate planning and conscious deciding.

Too often a *personality disorder* diagnosis merely indicates that the clinician did not like the patient or the patient's lifestyle. Her behavior is not *histrionic,* flamboyant, dramatic and excitable; her relationships are not fleeting and self-centered.

The patient shows an integrated personality, consistent over time. She does not have the irrational focused fear of the patient with a simple phobia, specific phobia.

77. **(B)** This adolescent is basically a good girl with high moral standards. She is a normal adolescent with rising sexual drives. The closeness with her boyfriend brings these strong sexual and moral feelings into *conflict,* producing anxiety that is difficult to manage. The fact that the "seizure" removes her from temptation and so relieves the conflict of these two strong feelings is the *primary gain* produced by the conversion disorder.

78. **(C)** Her conflictual feelings are repressed and expressed symbolically in the physical "convulsive" symptoms. This is an example of a *conversion reaction.*

79. **(D)** The extra caring and gratification the patient receives because she is ill is termed *secondary gain.*

80. **(C)** *Hypnosis* would be one way to produce rapid symptomatic improvement. Conversion disorder symptoms are frequently responsive to hypnotic suggestions, without substitute symptoms developing.

Questions 81 and 82 deal with panic disorder. (1:394–400; 2:443–58)

81. **(C)** The term *"seizures"* can cover a wide range of physical and emotional disorders. This young woman gives a classical history for a *panic disorder*—episodic acute attacks of anxiety with physical manifestations of autonomic activity and a sense of impending doom, imminent death, or loss of control.

Psychomotor epilepsy can produce a wide range of episodic physical and emotional symptoms. Usually a temporal lobe focus on the electroencephalogram can be demonstrated in temporal lobe epilepsy.

82. **(B)** The symptoms of the panic attack can be reproduced by asking the subject to *overbreathe for two minutes.* This is usually the best way of showing the patient the physiological cause and the absence of serious physical pathology. Patients with panic attacks tend to hyperventilate.

In the management of the patient, you would likely wish to *explain* the physiological basis for her symptoms, *explore* the possible factors producing this syndrome, and *offer supportive psychotherapy* if indicated.

Question 83 through 85 deal with the anorexia nervosa patient. (1:743–6; 2:753–9)

83. **(B)** The most likely diagnosis is *anorexia nervosa.* There are no indications of the generalized endocrine deficiency seen in hypopituitarism.

84. **(A)** The patient with anorexia nervosa has *sex-appropriate secondary characteristics.* This patient would show feminine pubic hair distribution.

85. **(B)** *Anorexia nervosa* occurs predominantly in *women* and is uncommon in men. The peak age of onset of anorexia nervosa is late adolescence. The syndrome can occur in other family members; sisters of patients with anorexia nervosa are more likely to have anorexia nervosa. Symptoms of anorexia nervosa frequently coexist with symptoms of bulimia nervosa.

Anorexia nervosa is more common in occupations where thinness is preferred—in ballet dancers and fashion models.

Questions 86 and 87 deal with strephosymbolia—dyslexia—developmental reading disorder. (1:711–3; 2:720–4)

86. **(D)** *Strephosymbolia,* reversal of letters, is one manifestation of *developmental reading disorder, dyslexia.* The youngster does not show school phobia or school refusal, but untreated dyslexia may make the school experience anxiety-provoking and unrewarding. Continued school failure and the inability to read the books the other children are reading are likely to make the youngster restless

and aimless in class. Many of these children feel stupid though intellectually they are not retarded.

Medical examination of children with dyslexia is usually noncontributory, but a physical evaluation should be performed to make absolutely certain that this common symptom is not an uncommon manifestation of a serious illness like a brain tumor.

87. **(C)** The optimum treatment for dyslexia is *remedial teaching.*

Psychotherapy may help with some patients, especially with youngsters who are developing a poor self-image due to repeated failure, and who are rejecting school work because the work offered is impossible to do. Methylphenidate is not therapeutically beneficial unless the child has co-existing attention deficit hyperactivity disorder. Imipramine would worsen the child's ability to perform.

Transfer to another school will not solve the problem without specific remedial education.

Questions 88 and 89 deal with attention deficit hyperactivity disorder. (1:725–30; 2:651–64)

88. **(D)** This clinical picture of excessive activity, distractibility, and restlessness is characteristic of the child with *attention deficit hyperactivity disorder.* These high-energy children are liable to cause anxiety in present-day structured school programs.

The *autistic disorder child* does not relate meaningfully to other people, is preoccupied with his own inner world, and often is fascinated by moving mechanisms.

89. **(E)** *Haloperidol* should not be used to treat children with attention deficit hyperactivity disorder. Haloperidol will certainly slow the hyperactive child motorically but the neuroleptic is likely to slow the child's cognition also. The long-range side effects of needless and excessive use of neuroleptics to bring about behavior control in children is yet to be seen; tardive dyskinesia is being diagnosed with increasing frequency in preadolescent children who have been treated with antipsychotic medications. *Methylphenidate, pemoline, imipramine,* or the amphetamines, are the drugs usually used in treating children with attention deficit hyperactivity disorder.

Questions 90 and 91 deal with disorganized (hebephrenic) schizophrenia. (1:332–4; 2:371)

90. **(C)** The layman's concept of being "crazy" is the *disorganized schizophrenic,* and this young woman presents with the symptoms of disorganized schizophrenia. Her behavior is regressed, bizarre, and poorly controlled; her emotions are inappropriate;

and she has obvious distortion of reality contact. Patients with hysterical or schizoid personality disorder do not show hallucinations or similar major signs of loss of reality contact. Patients with borderline personality disorder will show so-called "mini-psychoses" when the patient briefly erupts with primitive, reality-distorting and often reality-disruptive behavior and reactions; these episodes are short-lived and not persistent and pervasive as with the patient with disorganized schizophrenia.

91. **(D)** Carbamazepine is ineffective in the immediate treatment of the symptoms of disorganized (hebephrenic) schizophrenic who may be helped by haloperidol, hospitalization, family therapy, and behavior therapy. Carbamazepine is used for treating patients with manic symptoms and who show impulsive, aggressive behavior.

Questions 92 through 94 deal with bipolar disorder, manic type. (1:363–82; 2:412–41)

92. **(D)** The pressured activity and speech and the elation of this woman are characteristic of a *manic state.* The history of at least three prior episodes points to the cyclical quality of the disorder. Usually, the manic patient is brought for evaluation and treatment because her behavior has become intolerable to the people around her.

The behavior of this woman is certainly not passive, not even the intrusive demanding passivity of the passive–aggressive personality. In personality disorders there is not this excessive affect.

The symptoms of pathological intoxication may be largely due to the uncovering of an underlying schizophrenia by the sedating effect of alcohol. The patient described in this question manifests a pathological excess of affect rather than the toxic, sometimes confused, state seen in pathological intoxication. This patient does not show the primitive bizarre behavior of the disorganized schizophrenic nor the dissociative emotional splitting of psychogenic fugue.

93. **(C)** Patients with bipolar disorder have a worse prognosis than patients with unipolar depressive disorders. Without treatment, manic attacks tend to clear in about three months. Bipolar disorders tend to run in families and are likely to start at an earlier age than unipolar depression.

Bipolar disorder is about equally prevalent in men and women whereas unipolar depression is twice as common in women compared with men.

94. **(E)** The patient with an acute manic state usually has to be hospitalized and treated with drugs or electroconvulsive therapy. In the patient's disturbing, uncontrolled state, outpatient electroconvulsive therapy may not bring the symptoms under control quickly enough. The manic patient may be

unwilling or unable to cooperate with outpatient treatment.

Psychotherapy—interpretive, family, or supportive—has only minimal value until the patient's symptoms are brought under control.

Questions 95 through 97 deal with the catatonic schizophrenic patient. (1:334; 2:371–2)

95. (E) The mutism, immobility, and waxy flexibility shown by this young man are characteristic of *catatonic schizophrenia.*

These symptoms do not occur in psychogenic amnesia, conversion disorder, or in a paranoid personality disorder. The patient does not show the toxic delirium and confusion of delirium tremens. A neuroleptic overdose or a toxic psychosis are more common causes for this kind of catatonic state.

96. (B) The patient is now showing *catatonic excitement*—a state of psychomotor hyperactivity.

97. (D) Immediate intensive treatment of catatonic excitement is necessary before the patient injures himself or those around him or before he collapses from exhaustion. *Haloperidol,* parenterally, or *electroconvulsive therapy,* or sometimes both together, should be used to produce symptomatic relief. Intramuscular lorazepam will help lower the manic excitement and facilitate symptom alleviation with the neuroleptic, often in lower dosage.

Questions 98 and 99 deal with the patient with major depression. (1:363–82; 2:403–41)

98. (B) The patient is showing symptoms of *major depression*—insomnia, loss of appetite, loss of energy, psychomotor retardation, and marked depressive affect. His feeling of guilt is delusional but *congruent* (consistent) with the severe depression he is experiencing.

99. (C) Patients who have depression of this severity, especially with suicidal ruminations, should be hospitalized for their own protection and to allow rapid intensive antidepressant treatment. An antipsychotic medication, such as haloperidol, should be used to bring the psychotic symptoms under control. Fluoxetine or other antidepressant medication should be initiated immediately after any initial physical and laboratory pre-screening. Electroconvulsive therapy would produce the most rapid symptomatic relief of the suicidal depression, with the fewest side effects.

Levodopa would be contraindicated in this patient. Not only does the medication not treat the symptoms of severe depression but the drug may cause either depression or mania as side effects.

Questions 100 and 101 deal with the suicidally depressed patient. (1:551–9; 2:1021–35)

100. (B) If the clinician *suspects* that the patient is *suicidal,* it is usually best diagnostically and therapeutically to *ask the patient directly* in a gentle fashion if he is thinking about killing himself.

No one else—not even his family—can really say if he is actively suicidal. The prescription of antidepressant medication may merely provide the patient with a drug he can use to kill himself.

If the patient is actively suicidal, he may not be able to delay his suicide until the clinician finds an "appropriate" time to ask the direct question at later appointments. Most patients are relieved when they can talk openly about their suicidal impulses, wishes, and fears. A direct question tends to decrease their inner fears.

101. (D) Once the patient admits directly that he is seriously thinking about killing himself, he needs total protection and support at all times. If he is left without support—to get his clothes, to go by himself to the hospital, to contact suicide prevention groups—he may be unable to delay suicidal impulses. When the clinician, family, or society leaves the overtly suicidal patient without support and protection, the subject may feel isolated or impelled to act suicidally. To confront the suicidal patient about his "sin" is merely to increase his emotional burden. The patient should be *admitted to hospital, with responsible accompaniment* to get him there.

Questions 102 and 103 deal with the agoraphobic patient. (1:394–400; 2:456–61)

102. (C) *Agora* is the Greek word for *marketplace. Agoraphobia* is the fear of being in public places, away from home, without company—fear of being in a situation from which there is no easy escape. Typically these subjects fear being in stores, theaters, public transportation, or even waiting in line.

103. (D) Appropriate treatment would include an antidepressant such as imipramine, behavior therapy including systematic desensitization and flooding, and family therapy to facilitate family understanding and appropriate management.

Methylphenidate and other stimulants would be likely to increase anxiety symptoms.

Questions 104 and 105 deal with the diagnosis and management of patients with Tourette's Disorder. (1:760–3; 2:786–8)

104. (D) Patients with *Tourette's Disorder* often are first thought to be disruptive, inattentive, and provocative. They are likely to be punished or treated inappropriately for behavior later found to be symptoms of the disorder. Tourette's Disorder most often begins in the grade school years, is more common in boys (3:1), and may be preceded by symptoms of impulsivity and hyperactivity. These patients often have compulsions and obsessions. Symptoms wax and wane over the months. With effort, most patients can temporarily control the symptoms—a school child may control his tics until he can escape to the bathroom where he can release a burst of tics.

105. (A) *Pemoline* is used in the treatment of patients with attention deficit hyperactivity disorder and would not be used for the management of uncomplicated Tourette's Disorder. If the patient with Tourette's Disorder had symptoms of attention deficit disorder also—which commonly occurs—the pemoline might be a suitable additional treatment. The treatment for uncomplicated Tourette's Disorder could include *pimozide, haloperidol* and *clondine. Group therapy* of patients who have this disorder can be very helpful.

Questions 106 and 107 deal with the patient with an intracranial lesion where this illness might be mistaken for a psychiatric disorder. (1:266–7; 2:270–1)

106. (B) The subject may be living in the most stressful environment, have a history of gross deprivation and emotional trauma, and produce the most markedly pathological psychological testing—none of these will produce papilledema, a manifestation of increased intracranial pressure.

   All causes of *increased intracranial pressure* including an *intracranial tumor* must be investigated.

107. (B) *Computer tomography of the head* would be most likely to confirm or further the diagnosis.

Questions 108 and 110 deal with anticholinergic toxicity. (1:618–9,666; 2:798–9)

108. (C) *Amitriptyline* is a tricyclic antidepressant with major anticholinergic side effects. Especially when a tricyclic antidepressant is given with an anticholinergic neuroleptic and an anticholinergic to minimize neuroleptic side effects, anticholinergic toxicity is likely to be produced. With the use of a medication that has anticholinergic effects, often the initial symptoms of the patient appear to improve but then the patient develops new and different symptoms—the manifestations of anticholinergic toxicity. Typically these patients are flushed with a mild fever, dry mouth and dry skin, and showing agitation, confusion, and hallucinations. Seizures and coma may develop.

109. (D) Symptoms of anticholinergic toxicity can be treated with *physostigmine* (which itself has potentially dangerous side effects).

Questions 110 through 112 deal with the diagnosis and treatment of major depression. (1:363–82; 2:403–41)

110. (B) *Major depression* manifests with marked depression (often suicidal), feelings of guilt and worthlessness, and loss of pleasure. These patients show anorexia, weight loss, markedly decreased energy, insomnia, and psychomotor retardation. Sexual interest is reduced or absent and the patient is likely to be impotent. Thinking is slowed and decision making is difficult. Delusions and hallucinations may be present. There is no previous history of mood swings or cyclic emotional decompensation that would suggest a bipolar disorder. The patient shows exaggerated affect, seen in an affective psychosis, rather than the personality fragmentation of the schizophrenic. Thought disorder occurs early in a schizophrenic disorder. In depression, thinking slowly and indecisively may occur early but severe thinking disorder occurs only with severe depression.

   Delusions do not occur in panic disorders.

111. (E) This symptom is an example of a *somatic delusion.*

112. (B) *Reserpine* would tend to increase this patient's depression and has been known to precipitate suicide. Depression caused by reserpine appears to be dose related.

   A psychotic depressive reaction can be treated with *electroconvulsive therapy* or *desipramine* for the depression, *haloperidol* for the psychotic symptoms, and psychotherapy for support and *rehabilitation.* The patient should be *hospitalized.*

Questions 113 and 114 deal with separation anxiety disorder. (1:733–6; 2:673–7)

113. (C) *Separation anxiety disorder* can occur at any age but is common around age 10 to 12. Separation anxiety symptoms are produced by anxiety over separation from mother, parents, home, and familiar surroundings. Homesickness is usually a mild form of separation anxiety. Symptoms tend to develop in anticipation of separation—thus, on the day before the first school day of the week—and subside when the separation is ended or coming to an end. This anxiety may manifest with a range of physical complaints, usually pain, discomfort, or weakness. Physical examination will show no cause for these symptoms. Often the child's separation anxiety is matched by the parent's difficulty separating from the child. Thus, sometimes minimal laboratory or physical findings may be used by the family to justify the child's staying at home.

114. **(B)** The longer the child stays out of school, the more the youngster becomes socially separated from his peer group and the more he is likely to fall behind in his studies. The longer the child stays out of school, the harder it is to return. So the child with separation anxiety, school phobia, should return to school immediately if possible—even if this means just going into the school building and staying in the counselor's or principal's office.

CHAPTER 12

Practice Test
Questions

Carefully read the following instructions before taking the Practice Test.

1.   This examination consists of 120 questions, covering areas listed in the Table of Contents.

2.   The Practice Test simulates an actual examination in question types and integration of subject areas.

3.   You should set aside two hours of *uninterrupted,* distraction-free time to take the Practice Test. This averages out to one minute per question.

4.   Be sure you have a clock (to time and pace yourself) and an adequate number of No. 2 pencils and erasers.

5.   You should tear out and use the answer sheet that is provided on page 181 and 182.

6.   Be sure to answer all of the questions, and be sure the number on the answer sheet corresponds to the question number in the Practice Test.

7.   Use any remaining time to review your answers.

8.   After completing the Practice Test, you can check all of your answers on pages 169 through 178. A score of 65% to 70% or higher should be considered as a passing score (78 to 84 correct answers).

9.   After checking your answers and your score, you can analyze your strengths and weaknesses on the Practice Test Subspecialty List on page 179. To do this, you should check off your incorrect Practice Test answers on the Subspecialty List. You may find a pattern developing. For example, you may find you do well on the definitions but poorly on adult psychopathology. In such an instance, you can go back and review the adult psychopathology section of this book and supplement your review with your texts and with the references cited in the adult psychopathology section.

DIRECTIONS (Questions 1 through 82): Each of the numbered items or incomplete statements in this section is followed by answers or by completions of the statement. Select the ONE lettered answer or completion that is BEST in each case.

1. Tolerance is the clinical term for

    (A) the unconsciously motivated inability to discuss certain topics in psychotherapy

    (B) the psychological splitting off of mental functions from the rest of the personality

    (C) the declining effect of the same dose of a drug on repeated administration

    (D) the physical symptoms that develop on the withdrawal of a drug on which the subject is physically dependent

    (E) the ability to maintain in psychological awareness directly conflicting or opposing emotions about the same object

2. The defense mechanism whereby the subject emphasizes the opposite of his or her true feelings is

    (A) suppression

    (B) denial

    (C) repression

    (D) rationalization

    (E) reaction formation

3. Akathisia is

    (A) the reduction in frequency and amplitude of voluntary movements

    (B) continuous involuntary orofacial and lingual movements

    (C) repetitive involuntary muscle spasm, especially involving the neck, face, or tongue

    (D) inner restlessness with the inability to keep still

    (E) isolated tremor of tightly pursed lips

4. The Bender–Gestalt Test is

    (A) a series of nine geometrical designs that the patient copies

    (B) an inventory of 550 statements to which the subject has to respond

    (C) a standard set of ten inkblots to which the patient associates

    (D) a set of ambiguous pictures about which the patient gives a story

    (E) a series of standardized subtests measuring verbal and performance abilities

5. Secondary gain is

    (A) the reduction of emotional conflict and anxiety

    (B) the logical, reality-based thinking that promotes sublimation

    (C) the benefits that come from deliberate malingering

    (D) the sympathy, attention, and rewards that come from being ill

    (E) the process whereby unacceptable emotional drives are converted into socially acceptable behaviors

6. Electroconvulsive therapy is most effective in

    (A) amphetamine intoxication

    (B) major depression

    (C) disorganized schizophrenia

    (D) borderline personality disorder

    (E) conversion disorder

7. To treat the child with attention deficit hyperactivity disorder, you are most likely to use

    (A) lithium carbonate

    (B) fluoxetine

    (C) phenelzine

    (D) methylphenidate

    (E) diphenhydramine

8. When a patient who is being treated with a tricyclic antidepressant develops confusion, disorientation, and visual hallucinations, you are most likely dealing with a

    (A) hypertensive crisis

    (B) paradoxical reaction

    (C) anticholinergic psychosis

    (D) neuroleptic malignant syndrome

    (E) catastrophic reaction

9. An example of primary prevention would be

    (A) the development of halfway houses

    (B) repainting inner-city homes

    (C) early return of a phobic child to school

    (D) use of depot neuroleptics

    (E) initiation of a crisis hotline telephone service

10. You are called to the emergency room to see a 23-year-old schizophrenic male. You find him lying on a bed, mute, with his head arching backward and his eyes turned up. Your best immediate treatment would be

    (A) intramuscular haloperidol

    (B) intramuscular amytal

    (C) reassurance and "talking down"

    (D) intramuscular benztropine

    (E) intramuscular physostigmine

11. As they take a shortcut through a graveyard at night, two young men laugh and sing loudly. Their behavior is a manifestation of which defense?

    (A) dissociation
    (B) displacement
    (C) counterphobic
    (D) undoing
    (E) regression

12. Electroconvulsive therapy should not be used where there is

    (A) hypertension
    (B) previous myocardial infarction
    (C) increased intracranial pressure
    (D) cervical spondolisthesis
    (E) pregnancy in third trimester

13. Average intelligence is the Intelligence Quotient range

    (A) 80–100
    (B) 100–120
    (C) 70–90
    (D) 90–110
    (E) 90–100

14. Neologisms are most often indicative of

    (A) mental retardation
    (B) dementia
    (C) multiple personality (dissociative identity disorder)
    (D) malingering
    (E) schizophrenia

15. A 26-year-old woman is afraid to leave her home. She fears that she will have an acute anxiety attack, lose control or have something horrible happen and not be able to escape from the situation. Her most likely diagnosis is

    (A) borderline personality disorder
    (B) agoraphobia
    (C) post-traumatic stress disorder
    (D) social phobia (social anxiety disorder)
    (E) conversion disorder

16. A 30-year-old woman consults her physician because of recurring crying spells, feelings of hopelessness, inability to do her work efficiently, and difficulty in getting a good night's sleep. He starts her on a medication. Within a few days she begins to note recurrent headaches. She finds that her stomach "does not feel right" and her appetite has "disappeared."

The medication most likely to be causing these side effects is

    (A) phenelzine
    (B) lithium carbonate
    (C) nortriptyline
    (D) fluoxetine
    (E) clonidine

17. A conscientious secretary who has been with the company many years is now approaching retirement. Her fellow workers have been noting lately that she is unkempt, almost sloppy, and increasingly forgetful. She surprises her staid employer one day by addressing him as "darling." Her recent annual physical examination showed no evidence of drug or medication use. In your evaluation you would anticipate finding evidence of

    (A) developing depression
    (B) incipient dementia
    (C) latent schizophrenia
    (D) histrionic personality
    (E) chronic delirium

18. Paranoia is produced by the emotional mechanism of

    (A) reaction formation
    (B) repression
    (C) projection
    (D) displacement
    (E) undoing

19. Transference is the

    (A) return to an earlier pattern of coping and behaving
    (B) therapist's illogical feelings based on previous experiences
    (C) patient's past relationship feelings transferred onto a new object
    (D) redirection of feeling onto a more acceptable or safer object
    (E) channeling of otherwise unacceptable drives into productive directions

20. The patient with a passive–aggressive personality disorder is

    (A) neat, methodical, perfectionistic
    (B) aloof, indifferent to others with few friends
    (C) lacking self-confidence and lets others make decisions
    (D) stubborn, delaying, forgetful
    (E) unpredictable, intense, impulsive

21. A delusion is

   (A) an irrational fear
   (B) a misinterpretation of a perceptual stimulus
   (C) a recurrent, intrusive distressing thought
   (D) a false perception
   (E) a false, fixed belief

22. Amphetamine delusional disorder often presents with symptoms similar to

   (A) major depression with psychosis (with psychotic features)
   (B) disorganized schizophrenia
   (C) paranoid schizophrenia
   (D) early Alzheimer's disease
   (E) acute intermittent porphyria

23. Mania may be treated on a long-term basis with

   (A) cimetidine
   (B) carbamazepine
   (C) lorazepam
   (D) trazodone
   (E) hydroxyzine

24. Testamentary capacity is the

   (A) measure of ability to stand trial
   (B) measure of criminal responsibility
   (C) measure of competency to make a will
   (D) measure of ability to handle one's own affairs
   (E) measure of ability to act as a witness

25. Electroconvulsive therapy is very effective in treating

   (A) recurrent agoraphobia
   (B) chronic paranoid schizophrenia
   (C) fugue state (dissociative fugue)
   (D) acute mania
   (E) autistic disorder

26. Symptoms of the rabbit syndrome are

   (A) improved by antiparkinsonian medication
   (B) masked by increased dosage of neuroleptics
   (C) worsened by antiparkinsonian medication
   (D) relieved by physostigmine
   (E) worse after neuroleptics are stopped

27. Pigmentary retinopathy may occur after high doses of

   (A) trifluoperazine
   (B) thioridazine
   (C) nortriptyline
   (D) phenelzine
   (E) alprazolam

28. A nine-year-old boy is referred for evaluation because of increasingly disruptive behavior in class. In the teacher's referral letter, she notes that "at any time without warning, he will shout out in class." He is a polite boy, always very neat, but he just seems to be "restless and jumpy." The most likely diagnosis of this child's symptoms is

   (A) separation anxiety disorder, school phobia
   (B) oppositional defiant disorder
   (C) Tourette's Disorder
   (D) conduct disorder, undifferentiated type (conduct disorder)
   (E) developmental reading disorder

29. In sleepwalking, all of the following are true *except*

   (A) occurs during stage 3–4 sleep
   (B) most common at age 6–12
   (C) if awakened, subject is confused and disoriented
   (D) a manifestation of disturbing anxiety
   (E) subject amnestic for sleepwalking behavior when awakened later

30. With Huntington's chorea, all of the following statements are true *except*

   (A) personality changes may precede neurological symptoms
   (B) sexes equally affected
   (C) suicide risk is increased
   (D) autosomal recessive inheritance
   (E) genetic screening now available

31. Tactile hallucinations are commonly associated with all of the following conditions *except*

   (A) cocaine intoxication
   (B) alcohol withdrawal delirium
   (C) opiate withdrawal
   (D) amphetamine intoxication
   (E) lysergic acid diethylamide hallucinosis

32. Monoamine oxidase inhibitor side effects include the following conditions *except*

   (A) hypertensive crisis with specific foods
   (B) postural hypotension
   (C) insomnia
   (D) neuroleptic malignant syndrome
   (E) seizures, coma with meperidine

33. Hallucinations occur in each of the following syndromes *except*

(A) delirium

(B) bipolar disorder, manic

(C) paranoid personality disorder

(D) anticholinergic psychosis

(E) chronic disorganized schizophrenia

34. Because his wife is threatening to leave him unless he gives up his chronic heroin use, a 23-year-old man decides to stop completely, "cold turkey." Without treatment for his drug withdrawal, he is liable to experience all of the following symptoms *except*

(A) vomiting, cramps, diarrhea

(B) recurrent seizures

(C) muscle spasms

(D) insomnia, restlessness

(E) spontaneous ejaculation

35. All of the following statements are true about bulimia nervosa *except*

(A) episodic binge eating

(B) high-calorie, sweet, easily eaten foods

(C) terminated by abdominal pain, sleep, or induced vomiting

(D) subject recognizes that binge eating is abnormal

(E) little interest in sex

36. All of the following statements are true about transvestism *except*

(A) more commonly diagnosed in males

(B) subject dresses in the clothes of the opposite sex

(C) subject wishes to change anatomical sex

(D) behavior used to promote sexual arousal or gratification

(E) tends to begin in childhood or adolescence

37. In Tourette's Disorder all of the following occur *except*

(A) coprophagia

(B) coprolalia

(C) echolalia

(D) multiple tics

(E) childhood onset

38. With functional enuresis (enuresis) all of the following statements apply *except*

(A) more common in boys

(B) treated with conditioning devices

(C) may benefit from psychotherapy

(D) occurs only during non-REM sleep

(E) frequent family history of enuresis

39. All of the following statements apply to lithium treatment *except*

(A) tremor often helped by propranolol

(B) therapeutic level in elderly 0.6 to 1.0 mEq/L

(C) polyuria and polydipsia may cause noncompliance

(D) postural hypotension, worse in morning

(E) often causes diarrhea, may be worse with long-acting compound

40. A 32-year-old business woman comes for treatment. For the past two years she has had a compulsive need to wash her hands for up to an hour after using the toilet. If she tried to shorten the hand washing, she would find herself becoming increasingly tense. The skin on her hands and arms is becoming dry in some areas and soggy in others, thickened and cracked. Appropriate treatment for this patient would be

(A) clozapine

(B) clonidine

(C) clomipramine

(D) pemoline

(E) pimozide

41. Which of the following statements about disulfiram therapy is correct?

(A) it is indicated where hepatic cirrhosis present

(B) it is used where patient will not comply with other treatment regimens

(C) it is beneficial when patient has Korsakoff's syndrome

(D) patient may get toxic reaction with use of aftershave

(E) patient may get toxic reactions with pyridoxine

42. All of the following statements about psychogenic amnesia are correct *except*

(A) no impairment of consciousness

(B) amytal interview may recover inaccessible memories

(C) difficulty making and retrieving new memories

(D) recovery of memory is typically abrupt and total

(E) hypnosis may be used to retrieve memory

43. In treatment of alcohol withdrawal delirium, delirium tremens, all of the following would be appropriate treatment measures *except*

    (A) chlordiazepoxide 25 to 50 mg every 2 to 4 hours as required
    (B) chlorpromazine 50 to 100 mg every 4 to 6 hours as needed
    (C) high-calorie, high-carbohydrate diet
    (D) multivitamin supplement
    (E) fluid and electrolyte replacement

44. An embarrassed, anxious, and upset 35-year-old man consults you because of recent priapism. Several weeks ago his physician started him on a medication "to boost his spirits." The medication most likely to cause this side effect is

    (A) buspirone
    (B) clonazepam
    (C) trazodone
    (D) clonidine
    (E) fluoxetine

45. Panic attacks may produce symptoms similar to all of the following syndromes *except*

    (A) pheochromocytoma
    (B) hypoglycemia
    (C) hyperthyroidism
    (D) acute intermittent porphyria
    (E) carcinoid syndrome

46. All of the following statements about paranoid personality disorder are correct *except*

    (A) more common in deaf
    (B) persistent persecutory delusions present
    (C) subjects rarely seek treatment
    (D) hypersensitive to fancied slights
    (E) often question spouse's fidelity

47. Six weeks ago, the 23-year-old son of a 48-year-old woman was killed in a car accident. She consults her physician now because she is still having crying spells. She feels tired and has no energy. She keeps thinking about her son and what he was planning to do. She has little interest in her work. The most likely diagnosis is

    (A) major depression
    (B) normal grief
    (C) somatization disorder
    (D) dysthymia
    (E) posttraumatic stress disorder

48. Studies of the brains of Alzheimer's disease patients have shown

    (A) decreased cholinergic cells in nucleus basalis of Maynert
    (B) loss of dopaminergic cells in nigrostriatal tract
    (C) reduced serotonergic neurones in upper pons and midbrain
    (D) fewer histaminergic cells in the hypothalamus
    (E) decreased GABA-ergic cells in the substantia nigra

49. All of the following statements about diazepam are correct *except*

    (A) plasma half-life increased by disulfiram
    (B) longer half-life in elderly
    (C) may cause retrograde amnesia
    (D) may persist longer in obese
    (E) antacids decease absorption

50. All of the following statements apply to abused children *except*

    (A) the child is most likely to be under age three
    (B) the parents rationalize the abuse as necessary discipline
    (C) the parents state the child is different from the other siblings
    (D) one or both of the parents is psychotic
    (E) the child is likely to be irritating or intrusive

51. Dementia may be caused by all of the following *except*

    (A) autoimmune deficiency syndrome
    (B) multiple sclerosis
    (C) normal pressure hydrocephalus
    (D) acute intermittent porphyria
    (E) Huntington's chorea

52. Recent research has suggested an association between violent and suicidal behavior and reduced levels of cerebrospinal fluid metabolites of which of the following central nervous system transmitters?

    (A) dopamine
    (B) serotonin
    (C) norepinephrine
    (D) acetylcholine
    (E) histamine

53. A child with autistic disorder has a more favorable prognosis when

    (A) the child is easily toilet trained
    (B) the child is organized in his play

(C) the youngster has an interest in mechanical objects

(D) the child is able to converse

(E) the child can dance to music

54. A 56-year-old woman is brought to the emergency room because she is restless and confused. She appears to be having visual and auditory hallucinations. She complains of a dry mouth. Her pupils are dilated, reacting only sluggishly, and her skin is warm and dry. She has a tachycardia. This clinical state is most likely caused by

(A) amitriptyline

(B) reserpine

(C) alprazolam

(D) sertraline

(E) carbamazepine

55. A ten-year-old boy is increasingly rebellious at home. In school he curses at the teachers and gets into fights with other children. Twice in the past two months he did not go to school. His parents worry because he is staying out at night with companions who are known drug users. The most appropriate diagnosis for this boy is

(A) separation anxiety disorder

(B) oppositional defiant disorder

(C) conduct disorder

(D) attention deficit hyperactivity disorder

(E) Tourette's Disorder

56. After discharge from hospital where he had been admitted due to recurrent violent rage episodes, a 16-year-old boy consults you. He does not like the medication he has been on—he admits that he is calmer now—but he always has a nasty taste in his mouth, his stomach feels unsettled, his hand shakes, and he has to leave his classes periodically to urinate. The medication most likely to cause these side effects is

(A) lithium carbonate

(B) propanolol

(C) carbamazepine

(D) methylphenidate

(E) valproic acid

57. All of the following statements about lorazepam and oxazepam are correct *except*

(A) acute onset of withdrawal symptoms

(B) may produce sedation two or more weeks after stopping

(C) fewer problem side effects in the elderly than diazepam

(D) metabolized by hepatic glucuronidation

(E) withdrawal liable to produce rebound insomnia

58. In differentiating delirium from dementia you would look for

(A) thought disorder

(B) memory deficits

(C) disturbance of orientation

(D) clouding of consciousness

(E) fluctuation over the day

59. When a patient presents with mutism, negativism, rigidity, and waxy flexibility, your differential diagnosis should include all of the following *except*

(A) major depression

(B) encephalitis

(C) schizophrenia

(D) borderline personality disorder

(E) neuroleptic toxicity

60. In considering the use of lithium with pregnant women, you recognize that all of the following apply *except*

(A) lithium passes through the breast milk to the nursing infant

(B) lithium in the last trimester can cause neonatal toxicity

(C) lithium produces a higher incidence of fetal cardiac deficits

(D) lithium causes an increased incidence of Turner's syndrome

(E) lithium renal clearance is increased during pregnancy

61. In considering patients with mental retardation, which of the following statements apply?

(A) the highest incidence is in early childhood

(B) most of the retarded subjects have I.Q. of 35 to 50

(C) the encephalogram typically confirms the diagnosis

(D) it is most often diagnosed in teenagers

(E) mental retardation is most often due to brain damage

62. Under the stress of parental separation and divorce, a four-year-old child may show all of the following responses *except*

(A) thumb sucking

(B) enuresis

(C) tantrums

(D) encopresis

(E) autism

63. Which of the following statements apply to anorexia nervosa?

    (A) feels guilty and anxious when does not eat
    (B) tends to overestimate body size
    (C) usually very active sexually
    (D) does not occur in males
    (E) early loss of appetite

64. In the management of anorexia nervosa, all of the following statements are correct *except*

    (A) later age of onset has better prognosis
    (B) may have recurrent eating binges
    (C) patients are often deceitful about food
    (D) laxative abuse may precipitate electrolyte imbalance
    (E) patients tend to be compulsive and perfectionistic

65. Suicidal risk is increased with all of the following factors *except*

    (A) history of previous suicide attempts
    (B) patient is female
    (C) patient is elderly
    (D) patient is divorced
    (E) patient is alcohol or drug abuser

66. All of the following statements about Rett's disorder are correct *except*

    (A) occurs primarily in boys
    (B) normal development early in infancy
    (C) delay in language development
    (D) ataxia and difficulty with gait
    (E) stereotypic hand movements

67. A 19-year-old woman overdoses on about 2000 mg amitriptyline. When she is seen in the hospital emergency room that evening, her pupils are dilated, her mouth is dry, she has a tachycardia and her bowel sounds are absent. She is disoriented to person, place, and time, and she may be having visual hallucinations. The medication of immediate benefit would be

    (A) diazepam
    (B) atropine
    (C) benztropine
    (D) physostigmine
    (E) propanolol

68. At the request of the school authorities, a seven-year-old boy has been referred to you for evaluation. To an increasing extent he has been missing school on Mondays and Tuesdays each week because of recurrent abdominal pain. Physical and laboratory examinations have been normal. In your management of this youngster you recommend

    (A) that he go to school regularly each day
    (B) homebound schooling with a tutor
    (C) a change of school teacher
    (D) methylphenidate in the morning and at lunch time
    (E) low dose pimozide at bedtime

69. All of the following are associated with obsessive–compulsive disorder *except*

    (A) magical thinking
    (B) undoing
    (C) somatization
    (D) isolation
    (E) ambivalence

70. All of the following statements about depression in the elderly are correct *except*

    (A) it may produce symptoms similar to dementia
    (B) it has a higher incidence of suicide
    (C) it may coexist with dementia
    (D) it responds poorly to antidepressants
    (E) it may be treated with electroconvulsive therapy

Questions 71 through 73

A middle-aged female patient whom you have been treating for some months with depot haloperidol comes to you complaining of "just not feeling well." Her temperature is 38°C and she says her face and leg muscles feel stiff.

71. You should be concerned that she may be developing

    (A) hypertensive crisis
    (B) acute dystonic reaction
    (C) early tardive dyskinesia
    (D) drug-induced catatonia
    (E) neuroleptic malignant syndrome

72. Your diagnosis will be best confirmed by laboratory tests to show

    (A) increased cerebrospinal fluid protein
    (B) elevated serum creatine phosphokinase
    (C) lowered blood sugar
    (D) high blood eosinophils
    (E) high blood neuroleptic levels

73. In your treatment you would likely use

    (A) physostigmine
    (B) naloxone
    (C) disulfiram

(D) bromocriptine

(E) propranolol

Questions 74 and 75

A 62-year-old society matron is involved in a car accident. She is hospitalized for the treatment of her fractured femur. She has no known physical or psychiatric problems. On the day after her hospitalization, she is restless, sweating; her blood pressure is 150/100 and her pulse rate is raised.

74. In a more detailed history taking, you anticipate

   (A) long-standing bulimia

   (B) chronic alcohol abuse

   (C) spending sprees and hypersexuality

   (D) lifelong compulsive behavior

   (E) recurrent panic attacks

75. Your treatment would include all of the following *except*

   (A) benzodiazepines

   (B) chlorpromazine

   (C) parenteral vitamin B complex

   (D) high-calorie, high-carbohydrate diet

   (E) supportive psychotherapy

Questions 76 and 77

A 48-year-old man, found wandering in the streets, is brought to the emergency room by the police. He is unkempt and looks much older than his age. Though he is unsteady on his feet, physical examination shows no gross defects. He cannot recall how he came to be in the hospital. You are called away momentarily and, on your return, you find that he has forgotten your name and cannot remember the questions you asked.

76. Diagnostically you are probably dealing with

   (A) Korsakoff's syndrome

   (B) Ganser syndrome

   (C) Capgras' syndrome

   (D) Munchausen syndrome

   (E) Klinefelter's syndrome

77. When another physician comes into the examining room, though the patient has never met him before, the patient talks at length about having been treated by this doctor in a nearby town. The patient is now showing

   (A) rationalization

   (B) confabulation

   (C) la belle indifference

   (D) intellectualization

   (E) catastrophic reaction

Questions 78 and 79

Your colleague wishes to refer a child with attention deficit hyperactivity disorder for evaluation.

78. You anticipate that all of the following will be **true** *except*

   (A) the patient is most likely to be male

   (B) the patient is impulsive

   (C) the youngster has difficulty maintaining attention

   (D) the symptoms were first noted in the preschool years

   (E) most children with brain damage are likely to be hyperactive

79. In treating this patient with methylphenidate, you will advise the parents that all of the following statements are correct *except*

   (A) tolerance will develop over several months

   (B) possibility of height and weight retardation

   (C) may induce movement disorder

   (D) weekend and vacation drug holidays may be beneficial

   (E) possible continued benefit from this medication in teenage and adult years

Questions 80 through 82

A 56-year-old man is brought for examination because, in the past month, he has become increasingly socially withdrawn and, for the last two days has hardly moved. He has spent hours staring blankly ahead, occasionally crying quietly. He has been telling his family that he is too old, that he deserves to die, and that they would be better off without him. He has no history of drug or alcohol abuse. Physical examination is normal. His family fears that he might be suicidal.

80. You recognize that all of the following are **correct** about the risk of suicide *except* the risk is

   (A) increased when suicide is discussed with the patient

   (B) greater when there have been prior suicide attempts

   (C) higher in older males like this patient

   (D) increased in widowers

   (E) higher when the patient is beginning to come out of a depression

81. You decide to treat this patient with tricyclic anti-depressants. You advise him and his family of all of the following *except*

    (A) mood improvement is likely to take 2 to 3 weeks of treatment
    (B) dry mouth, constipation, and urinary problems may develop in the first week of treatment
    (C) in patients with bipolar disorder, a manic episode may be induced
    (D) at therapeutic levels, the medication has a quinidine-like effect on the heart
    (E) potentially fatal hypertensive crisis may occur when certain foods are eaten

82. The family asks whether electroconvulsive therapy would be a suitable treatment. You advise them that

    (A) at his age, electroconvulsive therapy is contraindicated
    (B) electroconvulsive therapy has dangerous hypertensive effects
    (C) his symptoms would not be benefitted by electroconvulsive treatment
    (D) electroconvulsive therapy would be a safe and efficient treatment
    (E) electroconvulsive therapy would cause permanent worsening of dementia symptoms

DIRECTIONS (Questions 83 through 120): Each group of items in this section consists of lettered headings followed by a set of numbered words or phrases. For each numbered word or phrase, select the ONE lettered heading that is most closely associated with it. Each lettered heading may be selected once, more than once, or not at all.

Questions 83 through 86

    (A) L-dopa
    (B) carbamazepine
    (C) thioridazine
    (D) lithium
    (E) buspirone
    (F) meprobamate
    (G) benztropine

For each side effect, select the most likely causative medication.

83. Goiter

84. Withdrawal convulsions

85. Pigmentary retinopathy

86. Hypomania

Questions 87 through 89

    (A) akathisia
    (B) akinesia
    (C) rabbit syndrome
    (D) tardive dyskinesia
    (E) acute dystonia

Match the description listed below with the neuroleptic side effect listed above.

87. Grimacing, sucking, choreiform movements

88. Perioral tremor of pursed lips

89. Restlessness, unable to sit still

Questions 90 through 93

    (A) projection
    (B) displacement
    (C) reaction formation
    (D) introjection
    (E) somatization
    (F) conversion
    (G) sublimation

Match the reaction with the correct defense mechanism.

90. The man who is angry with his wife kicks the cat

91. The man who is angry with his wife chops a pile of logs

92. The man who is angry with his wife unexpectedly buys her a piece of jewelry

93. The man who is angry with his wife develops a sudden right-arm paralysis

Questions 94 through 97

    (A) Wilson's disease
    (B) Huntington's chorea
    (C) Tay-Sach's disease
    (D) Alzheimer's disease
    (E) Tourette's Disorder
    (F) Wernicke's syndrome

Match the disorder with the correct neuropathology.

94. Necrosis and hemorrhage in mammillary bodies and adjacent to ventricles

95. Degeneration, cell loss in putamen and caudate

96. No gross neuropathology

97. General brain atrophy, most marked in frontal and temporal lobes

Questions 98 through 101

(A) fetishism
(B) transsexual
(C) transvestite
(D) frotteurism
(E) pedophile
(F) exhibitionist

For each clinical description, select the correct paraphilia diagnosis.

98. Sexual gratification through self-exposure

99. Sexual gratification through dressing in opposite-sex clothing

100. Wish for anatomical sex change

101. Sexual gratification through actual or fantasied activities with children

Questions 102 through 104

(A) amantadine
(B) carbamazepine
(C) diazepam
(D) pemoline
(E) fluoxetine

Match the disorder with the appropriate treatment.

102. Mania

103. Attention deficit hyperactivity disorder

104. Akathisia

Questions 105 through 107

(A) catatonic
(B) residual
(C) schizoaffective
(D) disorganized
(E) paranoid

For each clinical description select the correct schizophrenia subtype.

105. Waxy flexibility, negativism, mutism

106. Silly, giggling, hallucinating

107. Suspicious, litiginous, grandiose

Questions 108 through 110

(A) lithium carbonate
(B) reserpine
(C) nortriptyline
(D) phencyclidine
(E) sertraline

For each clinical description, select the medication most likely to have caused these side effects.

108. Agitation, depression, suicide

109. Finger tremor, slowing of cognition, worsening psoriasis

110. Sedation, worsening of glaucoma, urinary retention

Questions 111 through 114

(A) oppositional defiant disorder
(B) elective mutism (selective mutism)
(C) trichotillomania
(D) autistic disorder
(E) conduct disorder
(F) Tourette's Disorder
(G) separation anxiety disorder
(H) disorganized schizophrenia

For each child or adolescent with an emotional disorder, select the most likely diagnosis.

111. A 13-year-old boy has been skipping school to go fishing. He gets into fights at school and is very disrespectful to his teacher. On two occasions in the past year, he has been caught shoplifting and his mother thinks he is taking money from her purse.

112. A 17-year-old girl reports that when she is "bothered," she will twist her hair around and around and pull it out. She often eats the hair she pulled out, usually the scalp end first. She carefully combs her hair down to hide the bald patch at the side of her head.

113. An 11-year-old girl will be suspended from school if she misses any more classes. For the past six months she has had repeated absences because of recurrent abdominal pain and tiredness—repeated medical examinations have been negative. Somehow these symptoms do not seem to occur on holidays and weekends. The girl says she is worried about the violence in the neighborhood.

114. A four-year-old boy is referred for evaluation because he is not talking yet. He is a healthy-looking child, obviously well cared for and well nourished. He readily comes with you to the examining room. In your office he notices a wind-up toy. As you watch, he winds up the toy and, with obvious interest, lets it run down. He continues to wind up the toy for the next ten minutes. When you try to take the toy away from him, he becomes quite upset and starts an insistent, rather piercing cry.

Questions 115 through 117

   (A) phentolamine

   (B) trazodone

   (C) amoxapine

   (D) meperidine

   (E) maprotiline

Match the medication with the appropriate clinical statement.

115. Antidepressant which may cause akathisia, parkinsonism, and tardive dyskinesia

116. Best emergency treatment for patient who is taking prescribed phenelzine and who develops a hypertensive crisis after snorting cocaine

117. Seizures may occur at the usual or slightly above the usual clinically effective dose

Questions 118 through 120

   (A) major depression

   (B) anorexia nervosa

   (C) narcolepsy

   (D) sleep apnea syndrome (breathing-related sleep disorder)

   (E) somatization disorder

   (F) conversion disorder

For each clinical description select the most likely diagnosis

118. A 38-year-old woman is hospitalized after she stopped eating. She has been spending most of her time during the past few weeks sitting in her bedroom staring at the wall. She says very quietly that she knows that she is condemned by God for her sins. She believes that she is already dead and that her insides are rotting. She has obviously lost a lot of weight and she has started to refuse all fluids.

119. A 47-year-old male has had several accidents at work lately. He has been feeling tired and irritable. His general health is good but he is overweight. His wife reports that he is a restless sleeper and keeps her awake with his snoring.

120. A 17-year-old girl is referred for evaluation. Two nights ago, she came home an hour after her curfew. Her father was very upset with her and accused her of being sexually active with her boyfriend. The girl began to shout back in response to her father's accusations but suddenly lost her voice. The family fear that the intense emotions that everyone was feeling caused this girl to have a stroke.

Answers and Explanations

1. **(C)** *Tolerance* is the declining effect of the same dose of a drug on repeated administration. The subject then has to take a larger dose to get the same effect. *(1:279; 2:314)*

   Resistance is the unconsciously motivated inability to discuss certain conflict bound aspects of psychotherapy. *(1:573–4; 2:173)*

   The psychological splitting off of mental functions from the rest of the personality, as in a fugue state, is the process of *dissociation*. *(1:526–7; 2:558–60)*

   A *withdrawal syndrome* is the substance specific symptom complex that develops when there is a reduction or discontinuation of intake of a psychoactive drug by a regular abuser of this drug. *(1:278–9; 2:1202)*

   Ambivalence is the emotional state when the subject maintains directly conflicting feelings about the same object at the same time, as in a "love–hate" relationship. *(1:405; 2:475)*

2. **(E)** *Reaction formation* is a defense mechanism whereby the person emphasizes the opposite of his or her true feelings, as with the individual who deals with disturbing angry feelings by being outwardly very sweet and polite. *(1:184; 2:136)*

   Suppression occurs when the subject consciously blots out a problem from awareness: "I do not want to think about it."

   In *repression,* unacceptable thoughts or feelings are automatically or unconsciously kept out of awareness. In *denial,* unpleasant realities are emotionally ignored, as is often seen with a life-threatening illness.

   Rationalization is the emotional defense where otherwise awkward or conflicting situations or feelings are given a quasi-plausible intellectual explanation that the subject believes.

3. **(D)** Neuroleptic side effects.

   Akathisia is a feeling of inner restlessness with an inability to remain still. When these patients are questioned closely, they will say that they are not anxious, they just have to keep moving.

   Bradykinesia, or *akinesia,* is the reduction in frequency and amplitude of voluntary movements.

   The patient with *tardive dyskinesia* is most readily diagnosed by visual inspection because he is liable to show continuous, involuntary, repetitious orofacial and lingual movements, with choreic or athetoid movements of other parts of the body.

   Less commonly, patients will show the *rabbit syndrome,* an isolated tremor of tightly pursed lips, parkinsonian in frequency and responsive to antiparkinsonian medication. *(1:643–6; 2:779–84)*

4. **(A)** In the *Bender–Gestalt Test,* the subject copies a series of nine geometrical designs, initially from cards and then from memory. This test is most often used to evaluate the possibility of organically based psychological problems.

   The *Minnesota Multiphasic Personality Inventory (MMPI)* is a collection of 550 statements to which the subject is required to respond.

   The *Rorschach test,* a set of ten inkblot cards, and the *Thematic Apperception Test,* a set of ambiguous pictures, both evaluate the subject's thinking and associational ability. The *Wechsler Intelligence Scale* is a series of six verbal subtests and five performance subtests used to evaluate the subject's intelligence. *(1:155–63; 2:228–43)*

5. **(D)** *Secondary gain* is all the sympathy, attention, and rewards that come from being ill; *primary gain* is the emotional relief, the reduction of conflict and anxiety, that is permitted by the neurotic illness.

   Secondary process thinking is logical, reality-based, and optimally produces sublimation and development.

   Sublimation is the process whereby unacceptable drives are converted into socially acceptable, growth-oriented behaviors.

   Secondary gain is produced by unconscious factors and maintained by environmental response, while the gain in *malingering* is consciously planned and sought. *(1:185; 2:1267)*

6. **(B)** *Electroconvulsive therapy* is most effective in *major depression*. This treatment is *not indicated* in *amphetamine psychosis, disorganized schizophrenia, personality disorders,* or *conversion disorders.* *(1:670–1; 2:837–8)*

7. **(D)** *Methylphenidate* is the medication most often used to treat children with the symptoms of an attention deficit hyperactivity disorder. The other medications are not indicated in this disorder. *(1:729; 2:661)*

8. **(C)** The symptoms described are those seen in an *anticholinergic psychosis.* This toxic syndrome may be caused by the tricyclic antidepressants, especially when they are used with other anticholinergic drugs. *(1:619,666; 2:798–9)*

9. **(B)** In *primary prevention*, the illness is prevented from occurring. Repainting inner-city houses after the removal of lead-containing paint is a major factor in preventing lead intoxication in children. The use of halfway houses is an example of *tertiary prevention.* Depot neuroleptics use, a crisis hotline service, and early return of a phobic child to school, are all measures to minimize the effect and severity of an existing emotional illness, all examples of *secondary prevention.* *(1:144,692; 2:680, 1155–8)*

10. **(D)** This schizophrenic patient is likely to be suffering from neuroleptic-induced dystonia, which would be relieved by *intramuscular benztropine.* Intramuscular haloperidol would worsen the symptoms, while reassurance and "talking down," and physostigmine would be ineffective. Barbiturates would merely sedate the patient. *(1:643–4; 2:779)*

11. **(C)** Whistling through the graveyard is an example of *counterphobic* behavior. These young men are scared but they deal with their fear by overreacting in the opposite emotional direction. *(1:400–1; 2:1247)*

12. **(C)** Increased intracranial pressure is about the only contraindication to the use of electroconvulsive therapy. With careful anesthesia and seizure control, this treatment can be given in the other clinical situations listed. *(1:672–3; 2:838)*

13. **(D)** *Average intelligence* is the IQ range *90 to 110.* The Intelligence Quotient (IQ) is the ratio between the Mental Age and Chronological Age, multiplied by 100. *(1:156–7; 2:238)*

$$IQ = \frac{\text{Mental Age}}{\text{Chronological Age}} \times 100$$

14. **(E)** *Neologisms*—idiosyncratic words used by a patient—are almost pathognomonic of schizophrenia. Very rarely a lesion of the superior temporal gyrus of the dominant hemisphere may produce a fluent aphasia with nonsense speech and neologisms (Wernicke's aphasia). *(1:218,330; 2:189,365)*

15. **(B)** *Agoraphobia,* from the Greek word *agora—the marketplace,* is the fear of being in places or situations from which escape would be difficult or where help would be impossible. Agoraphobia can occur with panic attacks or without panic attacks. *(1:398; 2:459–61)*

16. **(D)** *Fluoxetine,* a serotonin reuptake inhibitor antidepressant, is liable to cause nausea, stomach upset and loss of appetite early in the treatment. Headache is a common side effect. Fluoxetine would be an appropriate treatment for the symptoms of major depression experienced by this patient. *(1:650; 2:801)*

17. **(B)** When a middle-aged patient shows increasing forgetfulness, impaired self-care, and a lack of self-control, *incipient dementia* should be suspected. In early dementia, these symptoms may be apparent only when the patient is tired, stressed, or dealing with new or unexpected situations. *AIDS dementia complex—dementia due to HIV disease* can manifest with mental slowing, forgetfulness, and loss of interest in the adolescent and young adult years. *(1:245–9,274; 2:284–5,290–1)*

18. **(C)** *Paranoia* is produced by the mechanism of *projection.* The feeling that is unacceptable to the subject is projected outward and ascribed to another person. *(1:527; 2:136–7)*

19. **(C)** *Transference* is the situation in psychotherapy (and in all relationships) where the feelings the patient has from past relationships are transferred onto a new relationship object—in psychotherapy onto the psychotherapist. *(1:573; 2:171–2)*

20. **(D)** Patients with a *passive–aggressive* personality classically are stubborn, repeatedly delaying, and forgetful about things they do not wish to do or have to face. *(1:538; 2:641–3)*

The person who has an *obsessive–compulsive* personality is neat, methodical, and perfectionistic. *(1:537; 2:640–1)*

The subject with the *schizoid* personality is aloof, indifferent to others, with few friends, and does not really want friendship. *(1:528–9; 2:629–30)*

The person with a *dependent personality disorder* lacks self-confidence and passively allows others to make major life decisions for him or her. *(1:536–7; 2:639–40)*

The patient with a *borderline personality disorder* is likely to be unstable, intense, and impulsive—predictably unpredictable. *(1:533–5; 2:636–7)*

21. **(E)** A *delusion* is a false, fixed belief, not amenable to logic, and incompatible with the subject's culture and level of maturity. *(1:219; 2:190)*

22. **(C)** An *amphetamine psychosis, amphetamine psychotic disorder,* often presents with symptoms similar to paranoid schizophrenia and should be excluded in patients of all ages presenting with these symptoms. *(1:307; 2:342–3)*

23. **(B)** On a long-term maintenance basis, *mania* may be treated with *carbamazepine,* especially in patients for whom lithium is contraindicated or ineffective. *(1:382,633; 2:431,827–8)*

24. **(C)** *Testamentary capacity* is the measure of a subject's competence to make a legally valid will and should be verified by a detailed mental status examination. *(1:825–6; 2:1069–70)*

25. **(D)** In patients who are *acutely manic, electroconvulsive treatment* given daily or on alternate days, sometimes more frequently, brings symptoms under good control, usually within a few days. Although electroconvulsive therapy was used in the past to treat chronic paranoia, the treatment results were disappointing and frequently short-lived. The other syndromes listed are not treated with electroconvulsive therapy. *(1:671; 2:838)*

26. **(A)** The *rabbit syndrome,* a late-onset parkinsonian symptom in which the patient shows a parkinsonian tremor of pursed lips, is improved by *antiparkinsonian medication. (1:644; 2:780–1)*

27. **(B)** *Pigmentary retinopathy* occurs with high doses of *thioridazine.* Usually it is stated that this side effect occurs at a dose level above 800 mg daily, but it has been reported at lower dosage levels. *(1:642–3; 2:786)*

28. **(C)** *Tourette's Disorder,* manifested by recurrent motor and vocal tics, tends to start most often in the grade school years. It is more common in boys. Frequently these children are punished for disruptive behavior before the illness is diagnosed. *(1:760–3; 2:686–8)*

29. **(D)** *Sleepwalking* is not a manifestation of disturbing anxiety. It is most common in the 6 to 12 year age group and occurs during stage 3–4 sleep. If the subject is awakened during the sleepwalking, he appears to be confused and disoriented; upon awakening later, he is amnestic for the sleepwalking behavior. *(1:477; 2:749–50)*

30. **(D)** *Huntington's chorea,* an autosomal dominant, affects both sexes equally and may present initially with personality rather than neurologic changes. Suicidal risk is markedly increased in these patients and their relatives. Genetic screening can be done by amniocentesis and on family members; genetic counseling is indicated. *(1:810–1; 2:288–9)*

31. **(C)** Definite *tactile hallucinations* do *not* occur in *opiate withdrawal.* The subject undergoing opiate withdrawal will be very uncomfortable with sweating, piloerection, muscle aches and twitching, abdominal cramps, diarrhea, and vomiting but will not become psychotic or show psychotic symptoms such as delusions. *(1:220,256,300; 2:189,331)*

32. **(D)** *Monoamine oxidase inhibitors* do *not* cause the *neuroleptic malignant syndrome.* The dietary-induced side effects are rare and, in clinical practice, monoamine oxidase inhibitors produce fewer distressing side effects than tricyclic antidepressants. *(1:657–8; 2:798–801)*

33. **(C)** Hallucinations and other psychotic symptoms do not occur in a paranoid personality disorder. *Hallucinations* do occur in *mania, schizophrenia, amphetamine psychosis,* and *delirium. (1:527–8; 2:630–1)*

34. **(B)** In the course of *heroin withdrawal "cold turkey," seizures* do *not* occur. If seizures do present during a withdrawal process, it is probably because the subject was also abusing sedatives such as barbiturates or meprobamate in combination with the heroin. *(1:300; 2:331)*

35. **(E)** *Bulimia nervosa* patients are usually sexually active in contrast to anorexia nervosa patients. Some bulimics are sexually promiscuous. The bulimic subject periodically binges on high-calorie, easily eaten food. The binges are frequently terminated by vomiting or sleep, sometimes by abdominal pain, and typically are followed by much guilt and self-blame over this abnormal eating behavior. *(1:746–8; 2:760–3)*

36. **(C)** The strictly diagnosed *transvestite* does not wish to change anatomical sex: if the wish for sex change is present, the subject would be considered transsexual, *gender identity disorder in adolescents and adults.* Transvestism usually begins in childhood or adolescence. The patient dresses in the clothes of the opposite sex for sexual gratification. In DSM IV, this syndrome is named appropriately *transvestic fetshism.* In Western societies, women can cross-dress without meeting as much social disapproval and without being labeled a transvestite. *(1:446; 2:592–5)*

37. **(A)** *Coprophagia,* the eating of feces, does *not* occur in *Tourette's Disorder. Coprolalia,* the compulsive expression of obscenities, was thought to occur in the majority of patients with Tourette's Disorder, but now less severe cases are being diagnosed with less obvious symptoms. *(1:760–3; 2:686–8)*

38. **(D)** *Functional enuresis (enuresis in DSM IV)* is more common in boys, occurs in families where other family members, especially males, have a history of enuresis, and may be beneficially treated with conditioning devices. Psychotherapy may be helpful especially in helping the child and the family deal with the problems caused by the enuresis and the reactions of others. Enuresis occurs at all times of sleep and during all stages of sleep and not primarily during stage 3–4 non-REM sleep. *(1:765–7; 2:)*

39. **(D)** *Postural hypotension,* worse in the morning, is *not* a side effect of *lithium* (but is frequently seen with tricyclic antidepressants). *Polyuria* and *polydipsia,* frequent side effects disturbing to the patient, often lead to noncompliance, as does lithium-produced diarrhea, which may be worse with the slow-release lithium tablets. Lithium-induced tremor is often helped by *propranolol.* While the therapeutic adult serum lithium level is 0.8 to 1.2 mEq/L, in the elderly 0.6 to 1.0 mEq/L is an effective and safer therapeutic range. *(1:651–5; 2:820–7)*

40. **(C)** *Clomipramine* has been shown to be effective in the treatment of obsessive compulsive disorder. Improvement in the obsessive compulsive symptoms may take 6 to 12 weeks to appear, longer than it takes for an antidepressant effect to occur. Clomipramine, like the other tricyclic antidepressants, causes sedation, postural hypotension, and anticholinergic side effects. *(1:408,663; 2:478)*

41. **(D)** The patient using *disulfiram* (Antabuse) may develop toxic symptoms when exposed to any alcohol-containing compound, including aftershave, cough syrup, foods cooked in wine, and other often unsuspected day-to-day commodities.

Disulfiram therapy requires unfailing compliance so should not be used where the patient has not complied with other regimens. The patient on disulfiram treatment needs to have a good memory to keep check on the dietary requirements; patients with the memory defects seen in the Korsakoff syndrome would be most unsuitable for disulfiram therapy. Patients can be given Antabuse under very careful supervision when there is hepatic impairment, but hepatic cirrhosis would certainly not be considered to be an indication for this treatment. Pyridoxine is used to treat some of the symptoms of disulfiram toxicity. *(1:291–2; 2:326)*

42. **(C)** Patients *with psychogenic amnesia, dissociative amnesia* do not have difficulty making and retrieving new memories, unlike the patient with an organic amnesia. The patient with psychogenic amnesia can remember the way back to her room after describing to the clinical team her inability to remember major events in her past life. Recovery of memory in psychogenic amnesia is said to be typically abrupt and total (though often in clinical practice memory recovery is more gradual). An Amytal interview or hypnosis can be used to recover otherwise inaccessible memories. The patient with psychogenic amnesia is alert and in full contact with her environment. *(1:428–30; 2:560–6)*

43. **(B)** In the treatment of *alcohol withdrawal syndrome, delirium tremens,* chlordiazepoxide or other benzodiazepines are used with a high-calorie, high-carbohydrate diet with multivitamin supplement. Chlorpromazine lowers the seizure threshold, may be hepatotoxic, and is hypotensive so is contraindicated. Restraints also should not be used as the confused patient may become exhausted by struggling against them. Fluid and electrolyte replacement should be given according to the patient's needs; some of these patients are overhydrated rather than dehydrated. *(1:289; 2:324–5)*

44. **(C)** *Trazodone* may cause priapism without sexual arousal. This side effect not only can be embarrassing but can also be painful and, untreated, may lead to impotence. *(1:661; 2:800)*

45. **(D)** Symptoms similar to *panic attacks* may be caused by pheochromocytoma, hypoglycemia, hyperthyroidism, and carcinoid syndrome. Acute intermittent porphyria is more likely to produce confused or depressed states. *(1:398–9; 2:453–5)*

46. **(B)** *Paranoid personality disorder* is more common in deaf people. Subjects with this type of personality rarely seek treatment. Delusions are a symptom of psychotic thinking and do not occur in paranoid personality disorder, though the person with a paranoid personality disorder is hypersensitive, frequently litigious and often overly jealous, but not delusional. *(1:527–8; 2:630–1)*

47. **(B)** In *normal grief, bereavement,* the bereaved person shows many of the signs of depression—sadness, weeping, loss of energy, difficulty sleeping, and preoccupation with the lost loved one. There is much individual and cultural variation in the manifestations and duration of bereavement. *(1:59; 2:299–300)*

48. **(A)** The *nucleus basalis of Meynert,* a group of cholinergic cells in the forebrain, shows a marked

loss of cells in *Alzheimer's disease. (1:93,250; 2:19, 286–7)*

49. **(C)** *Diazepam* is metabolized by hepatic oxidation and has long-acting metabolites. In the elderly, metabolic breakdown tends to be slower, so diazepam has a longer half-life. The medication persists longer in obese subjects. Disulfiram, carbamazepine and isoniazid are among the medications that increase the plasma levels of diazepam. Diazepam causes anterograde amnesia for new learning—as students discover when they take diazepam to reduce pre-examination anxiety. Retrograde amnesia is a loss of past memories and is not caused by diazepam. *(1:622–6; 2:815–7)*

50. **(D)** *Abused children* are most often under age three. Their parents often describe these children as being in some way different from their siblings and rationalize the abuse as being necessary discipline. Often the child is provocative, irritating or intrusive. Usually neither parent is psychotic; the parents often come from abusive homes, show spouse abuse towards each other and are immature or have personality disorder symptoms. *(1:784–6; 2:1082–3)*

51. **(D)** *Dementia* may be caused by autoimmune deficiency syndrome, multiple sclerosis, normal pressure hydrocephalus, and Huntington's chorea. Acute intermittent porphyria is more likely to produce confusion and depression. *(1:245–6,267; 2:284–90)*

52. **(B)** Patients who attempted suicide by violent means have been shown in recent studies to have a lower level of *serotonin* metabolites in the cerebrospinal fluid. *(1:557; 2:1027)*

53. **(D)** The *autistic* child has a more favorable prognosis when the young patient is able to converse meaningfully. These autistic youngsters are prone to be interested in mechanical play and in rigid organization, to the exclusion of interpersonal relationships. Autistic children may become preoccupied with the rhythm, the beat, or even the vibration of music to the exclusion of interpersonal activities. Autistic children are often easily toilet trained; while this may make them more socially acceptable, toilet training does not have a major impact on the long-term prognosis. *(1:699–704; 2:711–7)*

54. **(A)** This is the classical picture of an *anticholinergic psychosis,* which can be produced by amitriptyline and the tricyclic antidepressants, neuroleptics, scopolamine and atropine derivatives, benztropine and the antiparkinsonian agents, especially when they are used in combination. *(1:618–9,666; 2:798–9)*

55. **(C)** *Conduct disorder* is the most frequently diagnosed disorder at child and adolescent mental health clinics. A child with a conduct disorder is showing a persistent and repetitive pattern of behavior where the basic rights of others or societal norms are violated lasting over a period of at least six months. This 10-year-old patient has initiated physical fights, been truant, and stayed away from home at night. Accordingly he meets the criteria, among many, for the diagnosis of conduct disorder. Even in DSM IV, this diagnosis lacks clear definition, is culturally biased and still describes supposedly diagnosis-defining behaviors that are shown by many non-conduct disordered children at some time in their developmental years. *(1:772–5; 2:664–70)*

56. **(A)** Increasingly, aggressive and violent behavior in children and adolescents is being treated with medications, sometimes in high doses—with limited knowledge as to the long-range side effects of these medications. Lithium carbonate has been used to decrease aggressive behaviors and to produce calming. This teenage patient is describing the common lithium side effects seen even at therapeutic doses. While none of these side effects is in itself especially disabling, these annoying side effects often lead to the patient's discontinuing the medication. *(1:487,652–5; 2:820–7)*

57. **(B)** *Lorazepam* and *oxazepam* are metabolized by glucuronide conjugation to inactive metabolites. Since they are more rapidly broken down and excreted, patients on these medications will show an acute onset of withdrawal symptoms. Hepatic oxidation, the metabolic process for diazepam, takes longer in the elderly, so patients over 60 using diazepam are more likely to experience problem side effects.

Benzodiazepine withdrawal is liable to produce rebound insomnia. The 3-hydroxy benzodiazepines, lorazepam and oxazepam, are quickly cleared and, unlike the benzodiazepines with a much longer half-life, do not accumulate and produce delayed sedation. *(1:622–6; 2:805–17)*

58. **(D)** *Delirium* and *dementia* both produce disturbances of thinking, memory deficits, and disturbances of orientation which fluctuate over the day. In dementia there is no clouding of consciousness, which is the hallmark of delirium. *(1:243–5; 2:282–5)*

59. **(D)** A *catatonic syndrome* is commonly caused by neuroleptic toxicity but may also be a manifestation of major depression or schizophrenia. Since encephalitis and other neurological disorders may cause this syndrome, careful neurological examination is essential with catatonic patients. Patients who have a borderline personality disorder may show brief stress-related paranoia or dissocia-

tive symptoms but do not show the catatonic syndrome. *(1:217,334,368–9; 2:371–2)*

60. **(D)** *Lithium* passes through the placenta and produces a higher incidence of fetal cardiac defects, most notably the Ebstein anomaly of the tricuspid valve. When pregnant women take lithium in the final weeks of pregnancy, the infant may be born with lithium toxicity. Lithium clearance is increased during pregnancy. In nursing mothers, lithium passes through the breast milk to the nursing infant. Lithium does not produce a higher incidence of Turner's syndrome. *(1:651–5; 2:820–7)*

61. **(D)** The highest incidence of *mental retardation* is in teenagers. Most mentally retarded youngsters are mildly retarded, with an I.Q. of 50 to 70; their retardation is likely not to be recognized until adolescence when they begin to have obvious academic difficulties. The encephalogram is not diagnostically helpful in most retarded children. No specific organic cause is usually found for the majority of subjects with mental retardation, especially those who are less severely retarded. Mental retardation caused by known biological causes is more likely to be severe or profound and usually is diagnosed early in life. *(1:685–942; 2:702–9)*

62. **(E)** Under stress a preschool child may show *regressed behaviors* such as enuresis, encopresis, thumb sucking, and tantrums—all manifestations of an *adjustment disorder.* Autism or autistic behaviors are not regressive behaviors and are indicative of a more serious process. *(1:494–7; 2:605–11)*

63. **(B)** *Anorexia nervosa* is 10 to 20 times more common in women than in men but the syndrome does occur in males. Anorexia nervosa is more common in certain occupations such as modeling and the ballet and in people who jog and exercise. Patients with anorexia nervosa tend to overestimate their body size.

They do not feel guilty or anxious when they do not eat and typically have reduced sexual interest. Loss of appetite occurs late in the illness; most patients with anorexia nervosa do not become anorexic until the illness has been present for some time and the symptoms and physical signs are fairly obvious. *(1:743–6; 2:755–9)*

64. **(A)** Patients with anorexia nervosa often have eating binges, *bulimia,* and are frequently deceitful about their food intake. Their laxative abuse (and vomiting) may precipitate electrolyte imbalance. Anorexia nervosa patients tend to be compulsive and perfectionistic. Anorexia nervosa patients with an early age of onset tend to have a better prognosis than those who develop the syndrome later in life. It has been suggested that diet-

ing and preoccupation with being slim is more age-appropriate in adolescents and young adult women; in older women this preoccupation is less age-appropriate and may indicate more serious psychopathology. *(1:743–6; 2:755–9)*

65. **(B)** *Suicidal risk* is increased when the patient is elderly, male, unmarried or divorced, or has a history of prior suicide attempts. Suicide is more common in patients who are alcohol or drug abusers.

Females attempt suicide more frequently, but males are more at risk for successful suicide. *(1:551–9; 2:1023–5)*

66. **(A)** *Rett's disorder* occurs primarily in females. It is a rare type of *pervasive developmental disorder* manifested by loss of development after a seemingly normal early infancy, by delay or loss of language development and motor skills and by the development of autistic-like behaviors and mannerisms. Head growth slows often with onset of seizures. *(1:688)*

67. **(D)** *Physostigmine* can be used to reverse or to treat the most serious symptoms of anticholinergic toxicity. Physostigmine can also produce life-threatening side effects so must be used with caution. *(1:619,666; 785,798–9)*

68. **(A)** In the management of *separation anxiety disorder,* school phobia, early return to school is imperative, even if the child merely sits or studies in the principal's or the counselor's office. Assignment of a homebound teacher tends to perpetuate the school absence and may delay or make more difficult an eventual return to school. There should always be a careful evaluation of the school environment, the classroom situation, the family, and the child to ascertain factors that might produce or maintain separation anxiety and phobic fear. Methylphenidate is used in treating attention deficit disorder but is not indicated just in school refusal. Pimozide, an antipsychotic, is used in the treatment of Tourette's Disorder and also would not be indicated for separation anxiety disorder. *(1:733–6; 2:673–7)*

69. **(C)** In patients with *obsessive–compulsive disorder*, isolation, undoing and reaction are primary emotional defenses. These patients are likely to show more than the usual magical thinking and ambivalence. Somatization is not specifically associated with obsessive–compulsive subjects. *(1:404–9; 2:472–9)*

70. **(D)** In the elderly, *depression* may coexist with dementia. Depression can also cause a "pseudodementia" syndrome. The incidence of suicide is highest in the elderly, especially in males. Depression in the elderly does respond to antidepres-

sants, typically in lower than the usual adult dose and usually responds well to electroconvulsive therapy. *(1:812; 2:1128–33)*

71. **(E)** This is the symptomatic picture seen in evolving *neuroleptic malignant syndrome.* In drug-induced catatonia or dystonia, significant fever would not be present. A hypertensive crisis does not occur with haloperidol use and does not present with these symptoms. Acute dystonia or tardive dyskinesia have different symptoms. *(1:646; 2:783–4)*

72. **(B)** Your diagnosis is best confirmed by demonstrating *elevated serum creatine phosphokinase.* When a neuroleptic malignant syndrome is fully developed, there is likely to be complete breakdown of body homeostasis and most tests will then be abnormal. *(1:646; 2:783–4)*

73. **(D)** *Bromocriptine,* a dopamine antagonist, is most commonly used to treat neuroleptic malignant syndrome.
    Dantrolene, a muscle relaxant, is also used. Neuroleptics must be discontinued and intensive supportive treatment instituted. *(1:646; 2:783–4)*

74. **(B)** This is the classical history of the development of withdrawal symptoms in a *chronic* (unsuspected) *alcoholic. (1:288–9; 2:323)*

75. **(B)** *Chlorpromazine* is not used in treating delirium tremens or alcohol withdrawal symptoms because it lowers the seizure threshold and makes seizures more likely, causes hypotension, and is potentially hepatotoxic in a patient whose liver is compromised already by the chronic alcoholism.
    Benzodiazepines, high-calorie, high-carbohydrate diet with vitamin supplement and fluid and electrolyte replacement as needed is the usual treatment. Supportive psychotherapy is helpful for the patient and family. *(1:289; 2:324–5)*

76. **(A)** This patient is presenting with the type of short-term memory deficit seen in *Korsakoff's syndrome.* Signs of cerebellar dysfunction, peripheral neuropathy, and cirrhosis may be present due to chronic alcohol abuse. *(1:290–1; 2:323)*
    The *Ganser syndrome,* the syndrome of the approximate answer—"Two and two is five"—was first described as a response of prisoners to interrogation. *(1:435–6; 2:582)*
    The *Capgras' syndrome,* the syndrome of twins or impostors, is most often seen in paranoid patients who claim that someone they know well is not really the person they are talking to or seeing but rather someone else, looking exactly like the known person, a twin or someone impersonating that other person. *(1:361; 2:394)*

In the *Munchausen syndrome,* the patient deliberately feigns symptoms in order to get medical attention or treatment. *(1:480–1; 2:549–52)*
    Klinefelter's syndrome, an XXY chromosome disorder, produces a male with testicular atrophy, small penis, and, sometimes, adolescent gynecomastia. Many of these patients have emotional disorders and often mental retardation. *(1:754; 2:58)*

77. **(B)** This patient is *confabulating.* Automatically he is producing false memories to compensate for his memory deficit. *(1:203,290; 2:323,1273)*

78. **(E)** Most brain-damaged children are not hyperactive; reduced activity is more likely to be a problem with brain-damaged youngsters. Children with *attention deficit hyperactivity disorder* are much more commonly male. Impulsivity is a major symptom in this syndrome, as is difficulty maintaining attention at different tasks. Typically these symptoms are noted in the preschool years, though often these youngsters are not brought for evaluation until their disruptive classroom behavior causes a problem. *(1:725–30; 2:651–64).*

79. **(A)** Tolerance does not develop to *methylphenidate* in the treatment of attention deficit hyperactivity disorder. Methylphenidate may cause weight retardation and possibly height retardation. With this in mind, drug holidays during vacations and holidays are recommended unless the child becomes intolerably hyperactive when off the medication. Increasingly it is noted that a significant number of these patients continue to show symptoms and are benefitted by methylphenidate in the adolescent and adult years. Methylphenidate and the stimulant medications may induce symptoms of Tourette's Disorder. *(1:729; 2:660–3)*

80. **(A)** *Suicide risk* is not increased when the possibility is raised with the patient. The risk of suicide is greater where there have been prior suicide attempts. When a patient is deeply, overwhelmingly depressed, he is likely to be too immobilized by the depression to act suicidally. As the patient begins to improve, he may be less overwhelmed, less immobilized, but still deeply suicidal—and now more able to act on the suicidal feelings. Suicidal risk is higher in elderly patients, especially those who are divorced or widowers. *(1:551–9; 2:1021–35)*

81. **(E)** *Tricyclic antidepressants* will cause anticholinergic side effects (dry mouth, constipation, and urinary problems) within the first week of treatment and, even at therapeutic levels, have quinidine-like effects on the heart. It is likely to take two to three weeks before there is significant mood elevation; the patient often notices an improve-

ment in appetite and sleeping before improvement in mood. Food-induced hypertensive crises do not occur with tricyclic antidepressants but do occur with monoamine oxidase inhibitor antidepressants. *(1:664–6; 2:789–801)*

82. **(D)** *Electroconvulsive therapy* would be a safe and efficient treatment. With careful management, age and hypertension do not contraindicate the use of electroconvulsive therapy. Dementia is not worsened by electroconvulsive therapy. *(1:669–673; 2:836–41)*

83. **(D)** *Goiter* is a well-recognized side effect of *lithium* use. In some patients receiving lithium, hypothyroidism may develop, requiring either discontinuation of the lithium or supplemental thyroid intake. *(1:653; 2:824–5)*

84. **(F)** *Withdrawal convulsions* may occur after chronic *meprobamate* use (and on withdrawal from other sedatives such as alcohol, barbiturates, and benzodiazepines). *(1:621–2; 2:818)*

85. **(C)** *Pigmentary retinopathy* is liable to occur in patients given *thioridazine* in doses over 800 mg/day. Permanent retinal changes can develop within several weeks and have been reported in patients at even lower dose levels. *(1:642–3; 2:786)*

86. **(A)** *Hypomania* and manic states may be precipitated by *L-dopa*, bromocriptine, and amantadine, all dopamine antagonists. Confusion, disorientation, and depression may also be seen in patients receiving L-dopa. *(1:72–3,377–8)*

Answers 87 through 89 deal with neuroleptic side effects. (1:641–6; 2:779–87)

87. **(D)** *Tardive dyskinesia*, most easily recognized by visual inspection, often presents with orofacial-lingual dyskinesias such as tics and grimaces, lip smacking, chewing movements, and tongue protrusion with choreiform or athetoid movements of the limbs and trunk. *(1:644–6; 2:781–3)*

88. **(C)** In the *rabbit syndrome*, the subject shows neuroleptic-induced lip pursing with a slow, steady parkinsonian-rate perioral lip tremor—like the lip movements of a rabbit. This syndrome is responsive to the antiparkinsonian drugs. *(1:644; 2:780–1)*

89. **(A)** *Akathisia* is manifested by restlessness and the inability to keep still. The subject may feel this constant need to move to be irritating and distressing. These symptoms may be misdiagnosed as manifestations of anxiety. *(1:644; 2:779–80)*

Answers 90 through 93 deal with defense mechanisms. (1:183–4; 2:136–8)

90. **(B)** In *displacement*, feelings are transferred or redirected onto a more acceptable object. In this way, otherwise unacceptable or dangerous feelings are allowed open expression. *(1:184; 2:1249)*

91. **(G)** In *sublimation*, unacceptable feelings or drives are repressed but the energy behind these emotions is redirected into socially useful and growth-promoting goals. *(1:184; 2:138)*

92. **(C)** When a person is struggling emotionally with unacceptable or conflictual feelings, these emotions may be dealt with by *reaction formation*, whereby the subject responds to the situation outwardly with feelings and behaviors opposite to the underlying emotions, frequently in an exaggerated fashion. *(1:184; 2:136)*

93. **(F)** The term *conversion disorder* is one of the few psychiatric diagnoses that suggest a psychological process or mechanism. In conversion, psychological feelings are thought in some way to be converted into a physical symptom, a loss or alteration of function, that relieves the emotional conflict. In this situation described, the man's right-arm paralysis successfully prevents him from acting out his unacceptable urges to hit his wife for whom he cares—the primary gain of the conversion symptom is the resolution of his emotional conflict. *(1:419; 2:537)*

Answers 94 through 97 deal with neuropathology.

94. **(F)** In *Wernicke's syndrome*, most often due to chronic alcoholism, necrosis and hemorrhage in the mammillary bodies and adjacent to the aqueduct and the ventricular system may be found. *(1:71–2,290; 2:323)*

95. **(A)** *Wilson's disease, hepatolenticular degeneration*, is an autosomal recessive disorder of copper metabolism, leading to degeneration and cell loss in the putamen and caudate (the lenticular nuclei of the brain). *(1:73; 2:290)*

96. **(E)** In *Tourette's Disorder* there is no gross neuropathology, though recent studies indicate a possible neurotransmitter defect. *(1:761; 2:687)*

97. **(D)** Autopsy of the patient with *Alzheimer's disease* will show general brain atrophy, which is likely to be most prominent in the frontal and temporal lobes. *(1:250; 2:285–8)*

Answers 98 through 101 deal with the paraphilias, sexual deviations. (1:443–8; 2:592–5)

98. **(F)** The *exhibitionist,* usually a male, gains sexual gratification through genital exposure to strangers, usually of the opposite sex. Typically exhibitionists pose no physical danger to others unless they are prevented from escaping. *(1:445; 2:592–5)*

99. **(C)** The *transvestite fetishist* gains sexual pleasure through dressing in the clothes of the opposite sex. These patients are almost exclusively males. *(1:446; 2:592–5)*

100. **(B)** The *transsexual,* the patient with *gender identity disorder,* is dissatisfied with his or her anatomical sex, believes that he or she is really a member of the opposite sex, and seeks surgical and hormonal sex change to make the physical appearance coincide with the sexual self-image. *(1:752–3; 2:588–92)*

101. **(E)** The *pedophile* achieves sexual excitement and gratification by engaging in sexual activities, homosexual or heterosexual, with prepubertal children. *(1:444–5; 2:592–5)*

Answers 102 through 104 deal with the less frequently used medications.

102. **(B)** Especially when lithium is ineffective or contraindicated in the treatment of a *manic patient, carbamazepine* may be used. *(1:382,632–5; 2:431, 827–9)*

103. **(D)** In treating *attention deficit hyperactivity disorder,* methylphenidate is the usual initial medication. Where this drug treatment is ineffective or causes unacceptable side effects, *pemoline* is often prescribed. *(1:729; 2:661)*

104. **(A)** *Akathisia,* neuroleptic-induced motor restlessness, often does not respond to antiparkinsonian medication. *Amantadine* may be more effective in producing symptom relief. *(1:617–8; 2:779–80)*

Answers 105 through 107 deal with schizophrenic syndromes. (1:332–6; 2:371–4)

105. **(A)** Waxy flexibility, negativism, and mutism are characteristic of *catatonic schizophrenia* (but are now more frequently seen in drug- or neuroleptic-induced catatonic states). *(1:334; 2:371–2)*

106. **(D)** The *disorganized schizophrenic* typically shows the layman's idea of psychosis—silly, giggling, bizarre, responding to inner stimuli and socially very disabled. *(1:332–4; 2:371)*

107. **(E)** *Paranoid schizophrenics* are often hypersensitive and suspicious, jealous, resentful and sometimes litigious. Occasionally they may be hostile and violent in response to their paranoid beliefs. Frequently paranoid delusions seen in these patients are grandiose in nature—these patients believe that they are victimized or persecuted because they are in some way special. *(1:334–5; 2:371)*

Answers 108 through 110 deal with medication side effects.

108. **(B)** *Reserpine* causes dose-related agitation, depression, suicidal feelings and suicidal behavior. *(1:89,259)*

109. **(A)** *Lithium carbonate* at therapeutic levels is likely to cause finger tremor (which may be treated with propanolol), slowing of cognition—a dulling effect, and a worsening of psoriasis and acne. *(1:652–5; 2:821–6)*

110. **(C)** *Nortriptyline* and other tricyclic antidepressants are prone to cause sedation and urinary retention (which can pose major problems for males who are developing bladder obstruction due to prostatic hypertrophy). Glaucoma can be precipitated or markedly worsened due to the anticholinergic effect of the medication. *(1:665–7; 2:798–801)*

111. **(E)** *Conduct disorder* is more commonly diagnosed in boys than in girls. This boy is repeatedly truant, he is getting into fights, and he has been stealing. If these violations of age appropriate rules and norms of society have been recurring for more than six months, this young patient would be diagnosed as having a conduct disorder. If these conduct problems started before age 10, his conduct disorder would be designated *childhood onset type.* If the symptoms started after age 10, his disorder would be specified as *adolescent onset type.* (1:722–5; 2:664–70)

112. **(C)** *Trichotillomania,* a disorder that usually starts in childhood and is more common in females, is manifested by the recurrent compulsive pulling out of one's own hair. Often these patients chew or swallow the hair, sometimes in a ritualistic fashion. Usually the hair is pulled from the scalp but hair pulling can be done in any area of body hair, including rectal or pubic hair by patients who are more disturbed emotionally. (1:491–3; 2:617–9)

113. **(G)** Children, and patients of any age, who have *separation anxiety disorder* often develop physical symptoms when separation is approaching or has occurred. Thus, children with separation anxiety disorder, school phobia, are likely to develop symptoms on Sunday (in anticipation of separation). As the school week draws to a close on Thursdays and Fridays, the symptoms are likely to subside. Stressful situations at school are liable to magnify or reinforce the separation anxiety. *(1:733–6; 2:673–7)*

114. **(D)** Children with *autistic disorder* are usually slow in developing communicative language and may be considered as possibly being deaf. Autistic disorder children may look physically very healthy. A four-year-old child who is relating meaningfully to caring adults is unlikely to go off with an absolute stranger without anxiety or fuss. The lack of age-appropriate healthy separation anxiety should raise questions about the child's relationship ability. Autistic children are often fascinated by moving objects and may continue occupied for hours with a repetitiously moving toy; at the same time autistic children are often bothered by anything that changes their environment. *(1:699–704; 2:711–7)*

115. **(C)** Because the 7-hydroxy metabolite of *amoxapine* is an active dopamine blocker, amoxapine has many of the side effects seen with the dopamine blocking neuroleptics, including akinesia, akathisia, parkinsonism and tardive dyskinesia. Amoxapine can also cause galactorrhea. *(1:665–6; 2:801)*

116. **(A)** *Phentolamine* is effective emergency treatment for the tyramine induced hypertensive crisis in patients taking monoamine oxidase inhibiter antidepressants. Phentolamine can cause cardiac arrhythmias and marked hypotension. *(1:657–8; 2:802–3)*

117. **(E)** Maprotiline may induce seizures at high therapeutic dose levels or when the dose levels are raised quickly. Because of this side effect, it may be more difficult to maintain patients on maprotiline at the needed dose levels for adequate time to produce therapeutic effect. *(1:666; 2:801)*

118. **(A)** The patient is showing a *major depression with mood congruent psychotic features*. She is severely depressed. She shows markedly diminished interest in activities. She has lost weight, is not eating and is refusing fluids. She expresses bizarre somatic delusions where the delusional symptoms are congruent with her depressed mood state. *(1:366–75; 2:403–11)*

119. **(D)** The *sleep apnea syndrome, breathing-related sleep disorder* can often be diagnosed from the history given by the subject—typically an obese, middle-aged male—of feeling sleepy, tired, and irritable during the day—and from the bed partner that this man snores heavily and grunts or gasps during his sleep. *(1:474; 2:746–7)*

120. **(F)** This teenage girl was faced with conflictual feelings about loving and respecting her father but at the same time being violently angry with his intrusive but possibly correct comments about her private sexual feelings. Rather than scream back at him, she develops a *conversion disorder*. She loses her voice. The conflict between loving and enraged feelings is relieved—and this is the *primary gain* from the symptom. All the attention she will now receive from the family and from the possibly contrite father will be the *secondary gain* of the disorder. *(1:418–20; 2:535–40)*

Practice Test Subspecialty List

DEFINITIONS

2,3,5,9,11,14,18,19,21,69,77,87,88,89,90,91,92,93

PSYCHOLOGICAL TESTING

4,13,61

CHILD AND ADOLESCENT PSYCHIATRY

7,28,29,36,37,38,50,53,55,56,61,62,66,68,78,79,96,103,
111,112,113,114,120

ADULT PSYCHOPATHOLOGY

1,14,15,17,20,22,30,31,33,34,35,36,42,45,46,47,48,51,52,
58,59,63,64,65,70,71,72,73,74,75,76,79,80,81,82,94,95,97,
98,99,100,101,102,104,105,106,107

SOMATIC TREATMENTS

1,6,8,10,12,16,22,23,25,26,27,32,39,40,41,43,44,49,54,56,
57,60,67,73,75,77,79,81,82,83,84,85,86,87,88,89,102,103,
104,108,109,110,115,116,117,118,119

**SOCIAL PSYCHIATRY AND FORENSIC
PSYCHIATRY**

9,24

NAME _____
       Last   First   Middle

ADDRESS _____
                    Street

_____
City   State   Zip Code

DIRECTIONS

MAKE ERASURES COMPLETE

Mark your social security number from top to bottom in the appropriate boxes on the right. Refer to the section "HOW TO TAKE THE PRACTICE TEST" in the Introduction to the book for more information. PLEASE USE A NO. 2 PENCIL ONLY.

SOC SEC NUMBER

| 0 1 2 3 4 5 6 7 8 9 |
| 0 1 2 3 4 5 6 7 8 9 |
| 0 1 2 3 4 5 6 7 8 9 |
| 0 1 2 3 4 5 6 7 8 9 |
| 0 1 2 3 4 5 6 7 8 9 |
| 0 1 2 3 4 5 6 7 8 9 |
| 0 1 2 3 4 5 6 7 8 9 |
| 0 1 2 3 4 5 6 7 8 9 |
| 0 1 2 3 4 5 6 7 8 9 |

1. Ⓐ Ⓑ Ⓒ Ⓓ Ⓔ
2. Ⓐ Ⓑ Ⓒ Ⓓ Ⓔ
3. Ⓐ Ⓑ Ⓒ Ⓓ Ⓔ
4. Ⓐ Ⓑ Ⓒ Ⓓ Ⓔ
5. Ⓐ Ⓑ Ⓒ Ⓓ Ⓔ
6. Ⓐ Ⓑ Ⓒ Ⓓ Ⓔ
7. Ⓐ Ⓑ Ⓒ Ⓓ Ⓔ
8. Ⓐ Ⓑ Ⓒ Ⓓ Ⓔ
9. Ⓐ Ⓑ Ⓒ Ⓓ Ⓔ
10. Ⓐ Ⓑ Ⓒ Ⓓ Ⓔ
11. Ⓐ Ⓑ Ⓒ Ⓓ Ⓔ
12. Ⓐ Ⓑ Ⓒ Ⓓ Ⓔ
13. Ⓐ Ⓑ Ⓒ Ⓓ Ⓔ
14. Ⓐ Ⓑ Ⓒ Ⓓ Ⓔ
15. Ⓐ Ⓑ Ⓒ Ⓓ Ⓔ
16. Ⓐ Ⓑ Ⓒ Ⓓ Ⓔ
17. Ⓐ Ⓑ Ⓒ Ⓓ Ⓔ
18. Ⓐ Ⓑ Ⓒ Ⓓ Ⓔ
19. Ⓐ Ⓑ Ⓒ Ⓓ Ⓔ
20. Ⓐ Ⓑ Ⓒ Ⓓ Ⓔ
21. Ⓐ Ⓑ Ⓒ Ⓓ Ⓔ
22. Ⓐ Ⓑ Ⓒ Ⓓ Ⓔ
23. Ⓐ Ⓑ Ⓒ Ⓓ Ⓔ

24. Ⓐ Ⓑ Ⓒ Ⓓ Ⓔ
25. Ⓐ Ⓑ Ⓒ Ⓓ Ⓔ
26. Ⓐ Ⓑ Ⓒ Ⓓ Ⓔ
27. Ⓐ Ⓑ Ⓒ Ⓓ Ⓔ
28. Ⓐ Ⓑ Ⓒ Ⓓ Ⓔ
29. Ⓐ Ⓑ Ⓒ Ⓓ Ⓔ
30. Ⓐ Ⓑ Ⓒ Ⓓ Ⓔ
31. Ⓐ Ⓑ Ⓒ Ⓓ Ⓔ
32. Ⓐ Ⓑ Ⓒ Ⓓ Ⓔ
33. Ⓐ Ⓑ Ⓒ Ⓓ Ⓔ
34. Ⓐ Ⓑ Ⓒ Ⓓ Ⓔ
35. Ⓐ Ⓑ Ⓒ Ⓓ Ⓔ
36. Ⓐ Ⓑ Ⓒ Ⓓ Ⓔ
37. Ⓐ Ⓑ Ⓒ Ⓓ Ⓔ
38. Ⓐ Ⓑ Ⓒ Ⓓ Ⓔ
39. Ⓐ Ⓑ Ⓒ Ⓓ Ⓔ
40. Ⓐ Ⓑ Ⓒ Ⓓ Ⓔ
41. Ⓐ Ⓑ Ⓒ Ⓓ Ⓔ
42. Ⓐ Ⓑ Ⓒ Ⓓ Ⓔ
43. Ⓐ Ⓑ Ⓒ Ⓓ Ⓔ
44. Ⓐ Ⓑ Ⓒ Ⓓ Ⓔ
45. Ⓐ Ⓑ Ⓒ Ⓓ Ⓔ
46. Ⓐ Ⓑ Ⓒ Ⓓ Ⓔ

47. Ⓐ Ⓑ Ⓒ Ⓓ Ⓔ
48. Ⓐ Ⓑ Ⓒ Ⓓ Ⓔ
49. Ⓐ Ⓑ Ⓒ Ⓓ Ⓔ
50. Ⓐ Ⓑ Ⓒ Ⓓ Ⓔ
51. Ⓐ Ⓑ Ⓒ Ⓓ Ⓔ
52. Ⓐ Ⓑ Ⓒ Ⓓ Ⓔ
53. Ⓐ Ⓑ Ⓒ Ⓓ Ⓔ
54. Ⓐ Ⓑ Ⓒ Ⓓ Ⓔ
55. Ⓐ Ⓑ Ⓒ Ⓓ Ⓔ
56. Ⓐ Ⓑ Ⓒ Ⓓ Ⓔ
57. Ⓐ Ⓑ Ⓒ Ⓓ Ⓔ
58. Ⓐ Ⓑ Ⓒ Ⓓ Ⓔ
59. Ⓐ Ⓑ Ⓒ Ⓓ Ⓔ
60. Ⓐ Ⓑ Ⓒ Ⓓ Ⓔ
61. Ⓐ Ⓑ Ⓒ Ⓓ Ⓔ
62. Ⓐ Ⓑ Ⓒ Ⓓ Ⓔ
63. Ⓐ Ⓑ Ⓒ Ⓓ Ⓔ
64. Ⓐ Ⓑ Ⓒ Ⓓ Ⓔ
65. Ⓐ Ⓑ Ⓒ Ⓓ Ⓔ
66. Ⓐ Ⓑ Ⓒ Ⓓ Ⓔ
67. Ⓐ Ⓑ Ⓒ Ⓓ Ⓔ
68. Ⓐ Ⓑ Ⓒ Ⓓ Ⓔ
69. Ⓐ Ⓑ Ⓒ Ⓓ Ⓔ

70. Ⓐ Ⓑ Ⓒ Ⓓ Ⓔ
71. Ⓐ Ⓑ Ⓒ Ⓓ Ⓔ
72. Ⓐ Ⓑ Ⓒ Ⓓ Ⓔ
73. Ⓐ Ⓑ Ⓒ Ⓓ Ⓔ
74. Ⓐ Ⓑ Ⓒ Ⓓ Ⓔ
75. Ⓐ Ⓑ Ⓒ Ⓓ Ⓔ
76. Ⓐ Ⓑ Ⓒ Ⓓ Ⓔ
77. Ⓐ Ⓑ Ⓒ Ⓓ Ⓔ
78. Ⓐ Ⓑ Ⓒ Ⓓ Ⓔ
79. Ⓐ Ⓑ Ⓒ Ⓓ Ⓔ
80. Ⓐ Ⓑ Ⓒ Ⓓ Ⓔ
81. Ⓐ Ⓑ Ⓒ Ⓓ Ⓔ
82. Ⓐ Ⓑ Ⓒ Ⓓ Ⓔ
83. Ⓐ Ⓑ Ⓒ Ⓓ Ⓔ
84. Ⓐ Ⓑ Ⓒ Ⓓ Ⓔ
    Ⓕ Ⓖ
85. Ⓐ Ⓑ Ⓒ Ⓓ Ⓔ
    Ⓕ Ⓖ
86. Ⓐ Ⓑ Ⓒ Ⓓ Ⓔ
    Ⓕ Ⓖ
87. Ⓐ Ⓑ Ⓒ Ⓓ Ⓔ
88. Ⓐ Ⓑ Ⓒ Ⓓ Ⓔ
89. Ⓐ Ⓑ Ⓒ Ⓓ Ⓔ

90. (A) (B) (C) (D) (E) (F) (G)

91. (A) (B) (C) (D) (E) (F) (G)

92. (A) (B) (C) (D) (E) (F) (G)

93. (A) (B) (C) (D) (E) (F) (G)

94. (A) (B) (C) (D) (E) (F)

95. (A) (B) (C) (D) (E) (F)

96. (A) (B) (C) (D) (E) (F)

97. (A) (B) (C) (D) (E) (F)

98. (A) (B) (C) (D) (E) (F)

99. (A) (B) (C) (D) (E) (F)

100. (A) (B) (C) (D) (E) (F)

101. (A) (B) (C) (D) (E) (F)

102. (A) (B) (C) (D) (E)

103. (A) (B) (C) (D) (E)

104. (A) (B) (C) (D) (E)

105. (A) (B) (C) (D) (E)

106. (A) (B) (C) (D) (E)

107. (A) (B) (C) (D) (E)

108. (A) (B) (C) (D) (E)

109. (A) (B) (C) (D) (E)

110. (A) (B) (C) (D) (E)

111. (A) (B) (C) (D) (E) (F) (G) (H)

112. (A) (B) (C) (D) (E) (F) (G) (H)

113. (A) (B) (C) (D) (E) (F) (G) (H)

114. (A) (B) (C) (D) (E) (F) (G) (H)

115. (A) (B) (C) (D) (E)

116. (A) (B) (C) (D) (E)

117. (A) (B) (C) (D) (E)

118. (A) (B) (C) (D) (E) (F)

119. (A) (B) (C) (D) (E) (F)

120. (A) (B) (C) (D) (E) (F)